Managing and Leading
Innovation in Health Care

For Baillière Tindall

Commissioning Editor: Jacqueline Curthoys/Susan Young
Project Development Manager: Karen Gilmour
Project Manager: Jane Dingwall
Design Direction: Judith Wright

Managing and Leading Innovation in Health Care

3|0|0|

Edited by

Elizabeth Howkins BA MSc RGN RHV CPT PGCEA

Senior Lecturer in Primary Care, Department of Health and
Social Care, University of Reading, Reading

Cynthia Thornton MSc RGN DN PWT PGCEA DNT

Director of Postgraduate Studies, Department of Health and
Social Care, University of Reading, Reading

Foreword by
Sarah Mullally

Chief Nursing Officer for England, Department of Health, London, UK

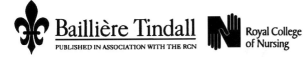

Baillière Tindall
PUBLISHED IN ASSOCIATION WITH THE RCN

Royal College
of Nursing

Baillière Tindall
An imprint of Elsevier Science Limited. All rights reserved

© Harcourt Publishers Limited 2002

is a registered trademark of Elsevier Science Limited

First published 2002

ISBN 0 7020 2552 6

British Library Cataloguing in Publication Data
A catalogue record for this book is available from the British Library

Library of Congress Cataloging in Publication Data
A catalog record for this book is available from the Library of Congress

Note
Medical knowledge is constantly changing. As new information becomes available, changes in treatment, procedures, equipment and the use of drugs become necessary. The editors, contributors and publishers have taken care to ensure that the information given in this text is accurate and up to date. However, readers are strongly advised to confirm that the information, especially with regard to drug usage, complies with the latest legislation and standards of practice.

 your source for books,
journals and multimedia
in the health sciences
www.elsevierhealth.com

The
publisher's
policy is to use
**paper manufactured
from sustainable forests**

Printed in China

Six Steps to Effective Management series

Series editor: *Ann Young*

Managing the Business of Health Care
Edited by Julie Hyde and Frances Cooper

Managing Diversity and Inequality in Health Care
Edited by Carol Baxter

Managing and Implementing Decisions in Health Care
Edited by Ann Young and Mary Cooke

Managing Communication in Health Care
Edited by Mark Darley

Managing and Leading Innovation in Health Care
Edited by Elizabeth Howkins and Cynthia Thornton

Managing and Supporting People in Health Care
Edited by Margaret Buttigieg and Surrinder Kaur

About the series

The Six Steps to Effective Management series comes at a time when the speed and extent of change within health care have rarely been greater, and the challenges facing nurses and everyone working within the health care sector are extensive. The series identifies and discusses those challenges and suggests ways of managing them. It aims to be unique in that it links theory with practice through the application of evidence where available and includes case studies which build on sound and relevant theoretical material.

All nurses are required by the clinical governance agenda to have a grasp of management principles. The *Six Steps to Effective Management* series is both practical enough to appeal to the practitioner and theoretical enough to be useful to those undertaking courses at undergraduate or diploma level. The books are relevant to all nurses.

The series comprises six volumes that are carefully constructed to contain a mix of theoretical and practical approaches, research and case studies, including a variety of perspectives from different sectors of health care. Each volume is relevant, realistic and practical to encourage reflection and critical thinking to prepare readers for flexible and adaptable styles of management.

For more information on this series please contact: Harcourt Health Sciences Health Professions Marketing Department on +44 20 7424 4200.

Contents

Section Three   DEVELOPING SKILLS IN INNOVATION   161

Section Four   MANAGING KNOWLEDGE IN HEALTH CARE   247

Contents

Six Steps to **Effective Management**

**Section Five OLD PROBLEMS,
NEW SOLUTIONS** 337

Contents

Contributors

Colin Beacock RGN RNLD CertEd DipN(Lond) MA
Policy Analyst, RCN Policy Unit

Colin Dale MA RN DipN(Lond) CertEd RNT DMS CertCoun
Freelance Nurse Consultant

Ann Ewens PhD MA(Ed) BSc(Hons)Nursing RGN DipN
Lecturer in Primary Care, Department of Health and Social Care,
University of Reading, Reading

Chris Flood BSc RGN RN(MH) DipNursing
Research Associate in Health Economics, Health Economics Group,
University of East Anglia

James Gardner RMN CertHMS MBA
General Manager, North Yorkshire Centre for Forensic Psychiatry,
Wakefield

Barbara Goodfellow RGN DND RNT BA(Hons) MSc
Senior Lecturer, Department of Health Sciences, University of East
London, London

Elizabeth Howkins BA MSc RGN RHV CPT PGCEA
Senior Lecturer in Primary Care, Department of Health and
Social Care, University of Reading, Reading

Julie Hughes RGN RSCN CPT PGCEA BSc(Hons)
Community Practice Lecturer, Department of Health and Social Care,
University of Reading, Reading

Sue Merrylees RNMH CertEd MA
Subject Leader (Nursing), Department of Nursing and Applied Health
Studies, University of Hull, Hull

Shirla Philogene OBE MSc RN RM QN RHV
Principal, Montrose Associates, London

Sharon Pickering BA(Hons) RGN BSc(Hons) MSc DipN(Lond) PGDip(HSSM)
Project Manager, Workforce Taskforce, NHSE Trent, Sheffield

Thoreya Swage MBBS MA
Independent Consultant in Health Care Management, Farnham
Honorary Fellow, Department of Health and Social Care,
University of Reading, Reading

Six Steps to **Effective Management**

Ben Thomas BSc MSc RMN RGN RNT DipN FRCN
Director of Nursing, Somerset Partnership NHS and Social Care Trust
Principal Lecturer, University of Plymouth

Jeanette Thompson MA BSc(Hons) RNMH PGDip(HSSM) PGDip Manchester
CertEd DipN(Lond) ITEC
Lecturer, Learning Disabilities, Department of Health Sciences,
University of York, York

Cynthia Thornton MSc RGN DN PWT PGCEA DNT
Director of Postgraduate Studies, Department of Health and Social
Care, University of Reading, Reading

John Turnbull MSc BA RNMH
Director of Nursing and Performance, Oxfordshire Learning Disability
NHS Trust, Headington, Oxford
Lecturer, Department of Health and Social Care, University of
Reading, Reading

Application contributors

Linda Chapman RGN DPNS BSc(Hons) PGCEA
Community Practice Lecturer, Department of Health and Social Care,
University of Reading, Reading

Ginny Collings MSc RGN RM RHV DipPrimCare DipProfNursStud HealthEdCert
Project Co-ordinator, Health Visitor, Bournemouth Primary Care Trust,
Bournemouth

Pamela Denicolo PhD BA(Hons) MILT HonMRPSGB
Faculty Director of Postgraduate Research, Faculty of Education and
Community Studies, University of Reading, Reading

Brendan Docherty MSc BSc(Hons) RN FETC PGCE
Critical Care Manager, Queen Elizabeth Hospital, London NHS Trust,
Honorary Lecturer, City University

Ann Ewens PhD MA(Ed) BSc(Hons)Nursing RGN DipN
Lecturer in Primary Care, Department of Health and Social Care,
University of Reading, Reading

Mary Hollins RGN SNCert CPT
School Nurse Coordinator, South Ockenden Health Care, South Ockenden

Elizabeth Howkins BA MSc RGN RHV CPT PGCEA
Senior Lecturer in Primary Care, Department of Health and Social Care, University of Reading, Reading

Judith James MA BMBCh DCH DRCOG MRCGP
General Practitioner, Parkside Family Practice, Reading

Prabha Lacey BSc PGC(Evidence-based Health)
Project Manager, Primary Care Collaborative, Bracknell Forest PCT

Linda Lilley BEd(Hons) RGN RNT
Assistant Director of Nursing and Practice Development, Kettering General Hospital, Kettering

Anne Owen MA DMS RGN RM RHV
Director of Clinical Services, Wokingham Primary Care Trust, Wokingham

Sally Patrick BSc(Hons) RGN RM DipNP
Lead Nurse of the Slough NHS Walk-in Centre

Joanna Richards BA(Hons) PGDip RGN RM RHV
Research Student, Department of Health and Social Care, University of Reading, Reading

Thoreya Swage MBBS MA
Independent Consultant in Health Care Management, Farnham
Honorary Fellow, Department of Health and Social Care, University of Reading, Reading

John Turnbull BA MSc RNMH
Director of Nursing and Performance, Oxfordshire Learning Disability NHS Trust, Headington, Oxford
Lecturer, Department of Health and Social Care, University of Reading, Reading

Application contributors

Foreword

The importance of effective leadership, innovation and change management cannot be underestimated. These are crucial factors that ensure the central tenet of the NHS Plan – that care and treatment must be dictated by the needs of the patient – will be realised. The NHS is being repositioned around the patient – making the NHS patient-centred. This calls for a major transformation across the NHS with changes in traditional structures, systems, roles and ways of working. Transformation does not just happen. It requires effective leadership. All nurses have a part to play in improving patient care and the experience of service users and carers. This book addresses how nurses can take on new roles and develop their leadership potential to innovate and provide effective leadership at all levels.

In order to do this leadership needs to be clearly supported and valued within the culture of healthcare organisations. Leadership involves a willingness to take risks and an ability to stay open to new experiences. Managing change involves learning from failure as well as from success. Effective leadership thrives in learning organisations – organisations that provide space for individuals and teams to reflect, to learn from and build on experience, drawing on best practice to improve the patient's experience of health care. In order to develop effective leadership skills nurses need the freedom to learn and the support systems that allow them to confront challenges – they need room to think, and to be creative in finding new ways to improve care.

A shared understanding of the qualities necessary for effective leadership is required. Effective leaders also need to understand the reasons for their own effectiveness. From the wide range of leadership models and approaches to change and innovation reviewed in this volume it is neither appropriate nor desirable to identify a single approach or style to apply as a blueprint across the NHS. Indeed, the most effective leaders are probably able to use a range of styles in dealing with different situations. However, for effective nurse leadership, several common factors can be acknowledged. Leadership, is not an isolated activity but depends on the relationships and interactions among individuals working on a task in a team. Leadership is a team function although it is clear individual characteristics play an important part. Effective leadership depends on maintaining a dynamic balance between these elements – it is the interplay between the individual's attributes, the team and the task that are central to an understanding of effective leadership in a modern, patient-centred NHS.

In its broadest sense the task is to improve the patient's experience of health care. Leadership involves understanding the task so individuals can be supported in their progress and achievement. Exactly how we approach the task will vary from setting to setting. We cannot rely on simply recreating old systems and fall back on familiar routines. This means developing new roles, finding new solutions without the certainty and support that comes with familiarity. It will require new ways of working, new roles and working in different ways.

Rethinking the way we work – working outside the familiar boundaries – will mean making difficult decisions and, at times, unpopular choices. Effective leadership in the NHS will involve moving away from approaches that merely prevent services from failing to those that encourage development, innovation and excellence in achieving our task.

The NHS of the future is based on partnership working and collaboration, and the relationship between effective leadership and teamwork will become increasingly important. As part of a clinical team, whether it is in the community, on a hospital ward, or a top management team where the nurse is working at executive level, effective leaders will be team players. We need leadership that understands the relationship between individuals and the way people work together, leadership that empowers others to reach their potential within the team context.

Leadership involves making sense of the challenges that an organisation faces and communicating this to patients and the public, to colleagues and managers. There is a need for leaders who are able to see the whole picture, and create a common vision with others. They will be able to articulate how the team relates to the organisational structures, systems and functions. Increasingly, this means a greater emphasis on partnerships working with agencies that complement NHS organisations including social care, the voluntary and independent sectors. Qualities that facilitate understanding and cohesiveness are particularly important in complex areas of health care requiring

Foreword

interagency cooperation where problems may not be susceptible to solution by a single agency and where new teams are created to find solutions.

Much has been written on the personal attributes and characteristics of the effective leader. They include skills that recognise the complexity of modern organisations; that focus on defining and communicating mission and strategy through teams and networks. Other attributes include the ability to bring together people from diverse backgrounds to work together on a common concern, to define and achieve common goals; to inspire others to follow their vision. These are not based solely around magnetism or charisma but on the ability to motivate, to empower and to bring out the best in others so the next steps they take are based on the confidence of their own experience.

Achieving a shared understanding of effective leadership is a challenge in itself. But there are barriers to the full development of leadership potential in the NHS and this presents a challenging agenda. Attitudes to risk, to failure and fears of their consequences may inhibit key leadership behaviours. Working in different ways and developing new roles often calls for radical goals and unconventional approaches. These may have inherent risks and be discouraged because of this. Intolerance of failure in a culture of blame is likely to inhibit innovation, leadership potential and the wider development of learning organisations. These barriers must be removed or reduced as much as possible. Today, effective leadership is unlikely to come about through the hierarchical structures of traditional methods. It will involve more collaboration, managing change through others while retaining a clear focus on the patient's experience of care. It is about playing to strengths but realising limitations and identifying areas for improvement. We already have some excellent examples of strong leadership within the NHS but we need to ensure that the health service attracts and keeps the best leaders. Leaders need sufficient freedom to lead and to be supported and challenged by others within and beyond their organisations. So we need to develop an environment that nurtures and rewards leadership and that recognises the benefit of talent and energy – so that leadership in nursing is confident, creative and celebrated at all levels of the NHS. This book is an essential resource for all nurses who are prepared to face this challenge and engage with the process ahead.

Sarah Mullally

Preface

The advent of the new millennium has been prefaced by a period of previously unknown expressed dissatisfaction with the National Health Service (NHS). Consumers have become increasingly empowered and articulate in questioning standards in relation to both professional expertise and inadequate and poor quality service provision. This, coupled with the constantly rising cost of the delivery of health care within the NHS, has forced the provision of health care to be viewed as a priority within the current political agenda, resulting in the introduction of a plethora of health policy initiatives.

Two White Papers, *The New NHS: Modern, Dependable* (1997) followed by *The NHS Plan* (2000) have tried to introduce a change in the ideological stance in an attempt to place the consumer at the centre of the health care system. More overt systems of accountability for professional practice and the use of resources have been introduced. Cost-effectiveness, although remaining as a strong driver, is coupled with an emphasis on the need for innovation and creativity in the delivery of health care.

The opportunities for nurses are immense but in order to facilitate an effective response the government foresaw the need for a modernisation programme. A framework is provided in the White Paper, *Making a Difference* (1999). The contribution of nursing is indisputably valued but there are important conditions that demand changes in both nursing practice and the education and professional development of nurses. New senior nursing posts provide incentives for experienced nurses to remain in the clinical setting. Extended roles, the nurse-led 'walk-in centres' and the introduction of nurse prescribing have all enlarged the facility for increased autonomy. Collaboration and interdisciplinary working is viewed as an essential element of health care that is focused primarily upon the needs of the patient.

Innovation and change are set to be integral components in the development and delivery of health care. Frameworks are in place to safeguard standards, to provide an evidence base for health care practice and to promote effective use of health care resources. Nurses working at every level of the organisation will need leadership skills in order to take up opportunities to make a vital contribution to the delivery of health care. The application chapters are an essential part of this book and provide real evidence that many nurses have leadership skills, are engaging in the business of innovation and change and are making a difference in the provision of health care.

The book explores factors that are central to managing and leading innovation in health care. The cultural shift that is needed to drive the modernisation agenda raises the importance of leadership within nursing so that the profession can grasp the opportunities and 'make a difference' to health care. Throughout the book reference will be made to the concept of creativity. Creativity can be a mechanism for freeing up staff who for so long have been constrained by hierarchical organisations and have not been allowed to be creative. Or it can be viewed as a possible solution to solve some of those intractable problems that characterise health care. The concept of creativity is explored both from a theoretical and a practice perspective. Many authors present a variety of approaches, which we hope will challenge, inform and inspire readers.

How the book is arranged

In designing the outline of the book a logical approach for the reader was envisaged, but structured in a way that moves the thinking forward. There are 14 chapters, called theory chapters, which provide a critical evaluation of the underlying knowledge and theories in relation to nurses and nursing practice. Immediately following each theory chapter is an application chapter, which is an account of practice. Exceptions are Chapter One, which deals with policy, and Chapter Nine where the application is integral to the chapter. The people approached to write the application chapters were not constrained by any format, only encouraged to share their exciting changes in practice and to celebrate their innovations by making them part of this book. The book is not intended to be a 'how to do it', but readers should discover possibilities that encourage creative developments within their own practice as they dip in and out of the wealth of material presented here.

The book is structured into five sections and a concise introduction will preface each part. Section One, The Creative Challenge, sets the context for the book and addresses some of the issues in managing change and innovation in health care. In Section One there are three theory chapters which address policy aspects, the concept of caring and then the changing professional role of the nurse. Section Two picks up some of the issues about changing relationships in health care. There are three theory chapters that discuss the nature and purpose of leadership, the place of negotiation in organisational change and the challenges that face nurses in relation to collaboration and working together. Section Three is about developing skills for innovation, how changes can be sustained and embedded in practice. There are three theory chapters: one on educational issues, one on managing change and a chapter that addresses some of the barriers to change by the use of a case study. Section Four, Managing Knowledge in Health Care, links the importance of the infrastructure with managing the knowledge of change. The three theory chapters address evidence-based practice, the potential for the use of information technology for nurses in primary care and how research and development can be used in practice to facilitate change. Section Five is about the future, acknowledging that many of the problems will be familiar but that there are new solutions to these old problems. There are two theory chapters in this section, one on creative solutions to quality improvement and the other on releasing the creative potential of people in health care organisations.

References

Department of Health 1997 The new NHS: modern, dependable. Department of Health, London
Department of Health 1999 Making a difference: strengthening the nursing, midwifery and health visiting contribution to health and healthcare. Department of Health, London
Department of Health 2000 The new NHS plan. Department of Health, London

Elizabeth Howkins and Cynthia Thornton

Section **One**

THE CREATIVE CHALLENGE

OVERVIEW

This section will form the foundation for the book, from which the following sections will evolve. Innovation and change are integral components of the National Health Service (NHS) and important elements of current nursing practice. Creativity is the generating force that energises the change process. It is powerful and has the ability to facilitate positive development and growth. Alternatively if thwarted then the negative reaction may be destructive to the person and detrimental to the health care environment.

There are a plethora of influences that affect the NHS and the delivery of health care within the United Kingdom (UK). These include: the philosophy which underpins political policies; the financial state of the national economy; the voice of professional bodies; and the demands of stakeholders, including patients and carers. Together they form the context in which health care is delivered. Chapter One provides a foundation for the book and raises the issues that are pertinent to the political context of managing innovation and change in health care. It will provide the reader with insight into the challenge that faces nurses at all levels of professional practice. Issues will be introduced that will form the focus for in-depth evaluation in later chapters. An argument will be developed that supports the value of nursing both as an autonomous profession and as part of the collaborative health care practice required to meet the complex needs of many of the current consumers of health care.

Caring as a concept is central to the theory and practice of nursing. Chapter Two provides a critical exploration of this concept. Definitions of caring are addressed and questions are raised in relation to some of the anomalies that may arise when considering the art and science of nursing. Information technology is viewed as a positive attribute in relation to communication but is it detrimental to the compassionate aspects of care? Is there a place in the modern NHS for creative nursing care and does the professional's perception of what is of greatest value align with the perception of the patient or carer who is the recipient of that care?

The application chapter is a personal experience of care. It highlights some interesting aspects that might well challenge the professional view of priorities. This cameo from real-life experience supports the notion of reflexivity and of partnerships in care.

The final chapter in this section considers the professional status of nursing today. Some conflicting issues will be addressed: has the movement towards evidence-based practice, the introduction of nurse prescribing, and the extension of nursing roles to relieve doctors enhanced the professional status of nursing or is it being drawn steadily back to sit under the wing of the medical model? Has increased autonomy and accountability provided the nurse with the vehicle to create effective innovations that will promote both the quality of care and the status of the professional nurse?

The two applications demonstrate how nurses are working in different, autonomous, nurse-led situations. In Application 3.1 Ginny Collings describes a health improvement initiative which evolved from consumer consultation. In Application 3.2 Sally Patrick outlines the development of the Slough Walk-in Centre. In each case the patient is central to the service that is provided. Innovation and change are essential features in response to identified community needs.

The creative challenge

Chapter **One**

Creativity in health care

Elizabeth Howkins and Cynthia Thornton

- Creativity in health care
- Modernisation agenda
- Cultural shift

- User participation
- Working in partnership
- Leadership

O V E R V I E W

This chapter sets the scene for the whole book by exploring the context of the culture change and innovation in health care. It addresses aspects of partnership working and modernisation for nurses as they embrace a new culture and come of age as a profession. The importance of leadership in facilitating a change in the culture of nursing is addressed and linked to the creative challenge that is a theme throughout the book. Reference is made throughout the chapter to many of the written contributions that provide the depth and insight that go to make this book special and important in the field of health care. In the final section the strands of the chapter will be brought together in a discussion on leadership and creative challenge.

INTRODUCTION

Creativity in health care means adopting and implementing new ways of thinking in order to change the way nurses work. This calls for a need to rethink and perhaps reject routine ways of working, to question traditional approaches to problem solving and to adopt a willingness to work outside the conventional boundaries. Health care leadership is vital to the NHS modernisation agenda as it depends on a cultural shift to change attitudes within the organisation, to facilitate creativity, and to support people in making difficult decisions. The opportunities for nurse leaders are both exciting and challenging.

Innovation and change are set to be integral components in the government's modernisation programme. *Making a Difference* (DoH 1999a) was a precursor to *The NHS Plan* (DoH 2000) and laid out an agenda for the modernisation of nursing; this gives nurses a real opportunity to throw off the 'cloak' of tradition and outdated ideals and embrace a new culture and new professionalism.

THE CONTEXT OF THE CHANGING CULTURE

The NHS is a huge organisation and has been subjected to endless reorganisation over the years with the intention of improving patient services. All the various changes have still not produced a health service fit for the 21st century. The organisation of the NHS has been based on a hierarchical style of management where tradition, vested interests and inefficiency seemed to thrive. The recognition of the necessity of a cultural shift by all factions of the NHS must be achieved if the modernisation plan is to succeed. Because the modernisation agenda means a change of attitude to focus on the patient rather than on the professional, to partnership based on respect and trust and to becoming a learning organisation, the task appears formidable. Getting people to embrace change is known to be difficult, as it poses a level of threat, whereas retaining the status quo always feels safer.

The prime minister, in his speech to the 2001 Labour party conference, said of the public sector that 'It is not the reform that is the enemy of public services; it is the status quo' (Blair 2001, p. 5). The rhetoric, the policies and ideas will not change anything unless everyone acknowledges that change must occur and then become committed to the change. It is at grassroots that this must happen, through innovative leadership but supported by a changing organisation. The present system and structures work against the goals of reform – they inhibit innovation and creativity. This point was enlarged upon in the Blair speech:

> There are too many old demarcations, especially between nurses, doctors and consultants; too little use of new technology; too much bureaucracy; too many outdated practices; too great an adherence to the way we've always done it rather than the way public servants

would like to do it if they got the time to think and the freedom to act. (Blair 2001, p. 5)

It is the ideals expressed in the last phrase 'time to think and the freedom to act' that most positively facilitate change, but the recognition that they are essential components has to be acknowledged by the organisation. The significance of creating a thinking organisation is discussed and analysed in Application 14.1.

The challenge is to change the culture of a bureaucratic organisation such as the NHS – which is characterised by being 'centralised, hierarchical, authoritarian, closed, formal, tightly controlled, top down and reactive' (Truman 2001, p. 12) and therefore likely to block any creativity – to one which should encourage creativity. People are no longer prepared to work in a mechanistic organisation where they are given orders, work only for monetary rewards and remain in the same job for life. Organisations today can be described as moving towards a 'systemic management' (Mullins 1989) characterised by growth, development and change. Such organisations have a central vision, mission or strategic plan, the organisation forms networks, people work across professional barriers and decision making is diffused throughout the organisation, i.e. an organisation that is more amenable to change. Some NHS organisations have moved towards systemic management, but many have far to go.

Two useful concepts in understanding how social life is changing are modernity and post-modernity. The guiding principles of modernity are 'a belief in progress, technical expertise, order and values that are universal' (Biggs 2000, p. 366). The idea of modernity is one where boundaries are fairly impermeable and identities fixed by the groups that one belongs to (such as race, gender and class) and the expected group behaviour. In health care this means professional roles remain distinct and separate: there is doctor's work which is male and prestigious whereas nurses (who are mainly female) have a subservient role. 'Post-modernity, on the other hand, marks a shift towards a much more fluid state of affairs' (Biggs 2000, p. 366), where relationships can form when needed and be discarded when other situations arise. The boundaries between groups become more permeable, allowing different professions, agencies and users to communicate with one another and thus increase awareness of each other's perspective. It is a position that moves towards user participation and encourages interprofessionalism. Biggs does, however, raise the point that although postmodernity gives birth to a new openness as boundaries are redrawn he does wonder whether there will still be an existence of

Creativity in health care

'in groups' and 'out groups'. But post-modernity does offer a framework to examine what is happening in health care and the potential for a new openness, user participation and working in partnership.

The context of the changing culture is certainly ambitious in that it addresses relationships and expects an attitude change which, if achievable, will be slow. But for nurses it really does offer a golden opportunity to change, to break down their professional barriers and work with others, to throw off the medical dominance and celebrate a new professionalism.

WORKING IN PARTNERSHIP

'Ideological boundaries or institutional barriers should not be allowed to stand in the way of better care' (DoH 2000, NHS plan 11.2). This statement builds on the principle of post-modernity that sees boundaries as permeable and the need for other identities to develop to meet health and social care needs. Working in partnership logically follows the more fluid arrangement of new and changing relationships required by the NHS plan (DoH 2000). But the notion is not new, it was established as a 'duty of care' in 1997 as part of the White Paper *The New NHS* (DoH 1997) and outlined such activities as joint working, interagency work and collaborative work between health and social care. Its relevance is not questioned but partnership has now moved to central stage of the NHS plan.

Partnerships are 'characterised by joined-up government and integrated and accessible services' (Ashcroft 2001, p. 50). The potential for change is far-reaching for staff, patients and agencies. There are issues of blurring of roles, taking up new roles and discarding old roles, which can be both positive and negative for the health and social care professions. As new services are set up there will be concerns about accountability and the relationship between professions, the public and the government. Ashcroft effectively uses a reference to the holy trinity to sum up the potential complexity of this change. He writes:

> Health care partnerships may come to resemble the theology of the trinity which oscillates between trying to distinguish distinct persons out of a fundamental unity, or trying to establish unity from distinct persons. (Ashcroft 2001, p. 50)

Partnership is about relationships between agencies, professionals and patients. In practical terms this involves a whole array

The creative challenge

of arrangements, strategic organisations, community networks, legal partnerships, and service delivery organisations. An example of a strategic organisation is a health action zone that would have been set up to target health and social care in disadvantaged areas and to meet specific complex need. Partnerships may grow out of a local community, such as those described in Applications 3.1 and 5.1. The strength of both these initiatives is the patient/client involvement, which provides the focus for the partnership.

A larger and more complex partnership is the creation of primary care trusts (PCTs). This development offers primary care a golden opportunity to build something new in terms of organisational design, unhampered by traditional NHS structures. At the present time the new PCTs are emerging in different ways: some have developmental and expansionist plans while others will have direct survival needs, for example financial and clinical support. However Beenstock & Jones (2000) argue that whatever form the PCT takes it should aim to create itself into a 'learning organisation that develops, transforms through the development of its members . . . which means that staff through their work, make contributions, not just to their organisations, but through them to the wider society' (Beenstock & Jones 2000, p. 29). The significance of ensuring the new organisation is a learning organisation should mean that staff feel valued, empowered and can realise their own leadership potential. Staff will also learn that working in partnership with patients is normal practice and that networking with wider society adds value to their organisation and thus to patient care. The issues of developing a learning organisation are addressed in detail in Chapters 8 and 9.

Although the examples of developing partnership show a certain positive 'spin' there are reservations. The government wants to 'reject the command-and-control approach to policy making as decidedly "Old Labour" ' (Hudson 2000, p. 20) and avoid the growing resentment of centralisation. Public discontent at the state of the NHS and allowing organisations the freedom to develop in their own ways, with great variations in local arrangements, could mean an election loss for the Labour party. A system of traffic lights has been introduced 'in which organisations (or partnerships) on green can expect "earned autonomy", while those on red can look forward to escalating interventions' (Hudson 2000, p. 20). But the tightening of political control has to be balanced by the need to let new organisations flourish in the network environment so that different modes of partnership can grow.

Working in partnership is exciting and does offer real opportunity for the professionals and the public to create organisations that really are receptive to patient care, are able to adapt their ways of working to meet patient need and can respond positively to patients' demands. But how does the working in partnership and the changing culture relate to nursing innovation and change?

MODERNISING NURSING: A NEW CULTURE AND A NEW PROFESSION?

The modernisation process depends upon a culture shift and attitude change by the professionals delivering health care. The need for change is certainly recognised by the health policy makers, managers, nurse leaders and academics, but this is not necessarily a view that is embraced by nurses at grassroots. The day-to-day pressures of the workplace are felt in staff shortages which means heavy workloads and lack of time to provide the ideal level of nursing care for patients. At the same time changes in society mean patients now expect a higher level of care, more informed care and to be part of the decision-making process for their care – in many ways a far healthier relationship than the one where the professional was always right and the agenda was from a professional perspective, thus often ignoring the patient's needs.

In developing the NHS plan it was important to make sure that the pressures on staff were recognised, patient expectations made clear and resource issues became transparent. The resulting policy document would then have some chance of being owned by all. The preparation of the NHS plan incorporated a high level of consultation with the public, NHS staff and other expert stakeholders, producing an inclusive process where everyone had a 'chance to express their views and to highlight their concerns and aspirations' (Mullally 2001, p. 23). The resulting White Paper goes a long way in addressing the shift from a professional to a patient-centred focus and raising the issues of recruitment and retention of nursing staff. But the key to any policy document is neither the rhetoric, nor the words, but its implementation.

Pippa Gough (2001), in her speech to English Chief Nursing Officers, identified three dimensions in the modernisation process (Box 1.1), each of which will be discussed here in relation to nursing.

Box 1.1 Dimensions in the modernisation process

- Creating a health service which places the patient at the heart
- To stop the scandals and horror around professional neglect, incompetence and misconduct
- Workforce shortfalls by reconfiguration of the health care workforce

---

The creative challenge

Creating a health service which places the patient at the heart

Shaping services around the needs of the patient to ensure that the 'right care is provided in the right place, by the right person and with the best possible outcomes for the patient' is sensible and begs the question that if it is so obvious why hasn't it happened before? The answer lies in the vested interests of each profession to protect what they see as special to them, to build up barriers and create systems that sustain their distinctiveness. But in the world of health care today the level of complexity needs a team approach so that knowledge is shared, duplication of care is avoided and a whole-system approach can be implemented.

The changes in social life, in health care and the recognition that carers and patients have a responsibility for their own health have had a tremendous impact on the sense of professionalism. Health professionals can no longer remain isolated (Fish & Coles 1998) but have to work as part of a team and with a range of other professions. In reality nurses have been more ready to embrace teamwork than their medical colleagues but slower to develop leadership roles in multidisciplinary teams.

Another educational development that has helped nurses to shift their focus to patient-centred care has been the endorsement of reflective learning as part of all educational programmes. Reflective practice 'involves a careful consideration of one's own practice by systematic critical enquiry' (Fish & Coles 1998, p. 68). Fish & Coles argue that most professionals have not been helped to understand their professionalism but they all have a 'deep-seated need to understand (and account for) their professionalism' (Fish & Coles 1998, p. 10) (the essential place of educational preparation for nurses is addressed in Ch. 7). In 1995 Celia Davies acknowledged that nurses could be the first to take on the new model of reflective practitioner, describing this as someone who is 'engaged, embodied and creating an active problem-solving environment' (Davies 1995, p. 185). Many nurses in leadership roles are using this model but it still needs to become part of all nursing practice.

To stop the scandals and horror around professional neglect, incompetence and misconduct

The second dimension of professional dominance has become a reality through a catalogue of high-publicity cases such as the Shipman murders, the Bristol Hospital Inquiry and the Allit murders. The murder trials of Shipman and Allit seemed at the time both horrific and unbelievable in that highly qualified health professionals could murder their own patients. The rights and wrongs of the cases are beyond description but the message that the public received was that you cannot trust the professional. The Bristol Hospital situation differed in that murder was not intended but nevertheless babies died or were left brain damaged as a result of gross professional incompetence. But the messages to the public were the same and became more worrying as the incompetent care continued, even when colleagues became aware of the seriousness of the situation (Kennedy 2001). The resulting inquiry was far-reaching and affects almost every aspect of the NHS. The rebuilding of 'trust between the public, health care professionals and the NHS will take time and major changes in attitude' (Burr 2001, p. 10). The inquiry identified inappropriate attitudes as a key problem but acknowledged that changing attitudes is not easy. Structures are being put in place to help change the culture from one of blame to a culture where it is accepted that everyone makes mistakes at times and it is what we learn from the mistake that is important.

The introduction of clinical governance through the White Paper *A First Class Service* (DoH 1998) should have a significant impact on making organisations 'accountable for continuously improving the quality of their services and safeguarding high standards of care' (DoH 1998, p. 33). The broader issues of evidence-based practice are addressed in Chapters 10 and 12.

Nurses have a system of self-regulation that allows the profession to regulate its own members in order to protect the public from poor or unsafe professional practice. Clinical governance is a framework which helps nurses to maintain and improve standards of care by bringing together existing quality assurance and audit processes. This framework is supported by self-regulation. The principles underpinning professional self-regulation are inextricably linked to those underpinning clinical governance (UKCC 2001). To maintain registration nurses have to keep a professional profile of their achievements, their learning and how they can demonstrate that they are 'fit for practice'. This profile has to be available for submission to the nurse-regulating body, the Nursing and Midwifery Council (formerly UKCC).

The issues of quality in health care are complex but fundamental. Although systems can be put in place to address quality issues there needs to be a move away from approaches that merely prevent services from failing, to one that encourages development, innovation and excellence. Chapter 13 emphasises the importance of ownership at grassroots, interpretation to meet local needs and a form of implementation that will really engage staff to ensure success in raising the quality of patient care in the NHS.

Workforce shortfalls by reconfiguration of the health care workforce

The lack of doctors, nurses and professions allied to health is a reality and the strategy to increase the numbers is laid out in the NHS plan. But the issue of addressing shortfalls by reconfiguration of the health care workforce is different. All health care professionals are being urged to 'break down professional boundaries, to work more flexibly, to be less tribal, to develop new roles' (Gough 2001, p. 9). This does not call for dissolution of professions but to find a more flexible and collaborative approach (role change, blurring of professional boundaries and the threat to the professional identity are discussed in Ch. 6).

Roles have begun to change over the last few years, particularly in nursing. The drive to keep the expertise in the clinical role has been addressed by the creation of nurse consultant posts. There are nurse practitioners who run their own practice and employ doctors, occupational therapists, counsellors and other health professionals. The creation of nurse-led walk-in centres (Application 3.2) is an example of nurse autonomy but more importantly running a service to meet local patient need and to increase access to health care. The introduction of nurse-prescribing rights offers further scope in developing the autonomy of the nurse. The initial implementation programme was restricted to district nurses and health visitors who are able to prescribe from a limited nurse prescribing formulary (NPF). However, in response to the recommendations made by the Second Crown Report (DOH 1999b) government legislation has supported a considerable expansion of the NPF to include all general sales lists (GSL) and pharmacy medicines (P) and prescription only medicines (POMs) that are linked to specified medical conditions in four areas:

- minor illness
- minor injuries
- health promotion and maintenance
- palliative care.

In addition the government has announced its intention of taking steps to allow 'supplementary prescribing' by nurses to allow them to treat more complex conditions, such as in mental health care and

Creativity in health care

the management of chronic disease, following an initial assessment of the patient by a doctor.

The new phase in prescribing will enable nurses who practise in the above areas and who need to prescribe in order to complete an episode of care to be fully autonomous in their practice. As well as including a wide range of nurses from both the acute sector and primary care, legislation suggests that other professional groups allied to medicine, for example physiotherapists will, in future, also be able to apply for prescribing rights. The tradition of prescribing rights being restricted to doctors and dentists will no longer exist and the cultural shift that will occur exemplifies not only a greater autonomy for nurses but also a blurring of professional roles.

All these developments offer career opportunities to nurses which should in turn encourage them to remain in clinical practice or to know that they will be supported in developing new roles which can meet patient need and health care innovation in imaginative ways. As health care professionals work together to find new roles they should strengthen their professions, not weaken them.

Recruitment and retention of nurses and all health professions is vital. The main reason nurses leave is more to do with working environment than pay (Meadows et al 2000). In order to attract staff and make sure they stay and make their career in the NHS, their individual needs must be addressed, strategies put in place to identify and prevent bullying at work, a culture created where everyone has an opportunity to have their opinion heard, to know that they work in a learning organisation and that everyone can be part of a decision-making process, such as shared governance. An example of this is described in Application 8.1.

Health professionals have begun to work in other ways to address health care workforce issues but they must be supported in any change. The modernisation agenda incorporates partnership, lifelong learning, flexibility and collegiateness, all concepts that rely on a nurturing culture.

NURSING: COMING OF AGE IN A NEW CULTURE

Posing the heading of the previous section (Modernising nursing: a new culture and a new profession?) as a question was intentional. We endorse the need for a new culture but see the profession coming of age rather than being a new profession. People will always need nursing and nursing care but the challenge now for the profession is to modernise nursing to ensure that people receive compassionate care in a 'humane, well-informed and competent way' (Gough 2001, p. 9). Chapter 2 explores the challenges to creative caring posed by increasing technology and the pressure to produce measurable outcomes while the concept of leadership in developing and supporting the changing professional role of the nurse is explored in Chapter 3.

Encouraging criticality and lateral thinking is now part of the educational preparation for nurses and should facilitate all nurses to become lifelong learners and help sustain a learning culture to foster creativity. But in order to have creativity and vision, the level of thinking must be improved and time routinely given for reflection – a view endorsed by the chief nurse, Sarah Mullally, who wrote: 'Visioning requires headroom, space for creativity, time for reflection' (Mullally 2001, p. 26).

LEADERSHIP AND THE CREATIVE CHALLENGE

The NHS of the future will be based upon partnership working, collaboration and joint working. All of these depend on developing a more facultative working environment than the hierarchical, authoritarian and controlled model of the past. The concept of leadership is at the heart of managing a culture change and developing people. The NHS chief executive, Nigel Crisp, stated that leadership:

> . . . is about setting direction, opening up possibilities, helping people to achieve, communicating and delivering. It is also about behaviour. What we do as leaders is even more important than what we say. (Hayes 2001, p. 1)

In order to show that they are serious about the leadership issue the government, through the Department of Health, is rolling out a 3-day programme called Leading Empowered Organisations (LEO). The focus of the course is on accountability, authority and responsibility and how the three link together in the leadership role. There are critics of the programme, saying it is 'too woolly' (Duffin 2001, p. 12) and not easily applied to practice; some managers just cannot support the programme because of staff shortages. But for many the experience of doing the course is that they return to work feeling 'awakened'. However, they are not always able to put what they have learnt into practice which inevitably leads to frustration. It also indicates that the organisations are not

Creativity in health care

13

yet ready to really embrace leadership at all levels. It is therefore debatable whether a 'taster' really works when issues and theories of leadership need time and application to practice. An example of matching education with the reality of the workplace is presented in Application 4.1.

Chapter 4 discusses approaches to leadership and explores four styles: transactional, transformational, renaissance and connective. The move from a transactional style, which involves maintaining the status quo of the organisation, to a transformational style is addressed, proposing that the latter is particularly suited to present changes in health care as it incorporates management of change and leaders who inspire people to follow their clear vision. Leadership theory must, however, be developed and expanded to include power differentials, to acknowledge that transformational style can be viewed as liberating the oppressed nurse and service user but ignoring the important role of influencing policy and creating social networks across professions and agencies.

The essential link to influencing policy and creating social networks is further developed in Chapter 5 where the importance of negotiation in managing change and developing leadership in the workforce is explored in-depth. In order to enhance leadership qualities the process of negotiation has to become a regular feature of modern nursing practice. Negotiation is a mechanism by which leadership skills are developed to enhance accountability and autonomy in health and social care services. It is an essential component of organisational development through which shared learning, common understanding and communications become established features of the organisational culture.

Creativity is the generating force that energises the change process. It is powerful and has the ability to facilitate positive growth and development. It is also a symbol of freedom for those working in the NHS. Chapter 14 analyses the symbolic and literal use of the word 'creativity' and explores how to help people working in health care organisations to release their creative potential. Creating the conditions in which staff feel free to think for themselves and encourage others to do so will inevitably improve their motivation and commitment.

In order for new cultures to flourish there has to be new thinking. Organisations will need to think outside and work across organisational boundaries, to think and work in completely new ways. People are 'constrained by conventional organisations, labels and assumptions' (Clarke & Stewart 2000, p. 379); they need to think the unthinkable or 'to entertain the unconventional and pursue the radical'. The difficulty in moving with this radical agenda

The creative challenge

is that the endpoint is unknown. But the process does need to happen to address intractable problems in health care. The task for leaders will be managing uncertainty.

The notion of working in an organisation that will support creativity becomes both exciting and daunting. Encouraging creativity – supporting visionary ideas, allowing staff to think the unthinkable, removing barriers, overcoming blocks, breaking rules and celebrating imaginative ideas – all sounds very unfamiliar in the NHS. But to bring about change and innovation in health care this is exactly what needs to happen.

CONCLUSION

This chapter explored some of the issues that are impinging on nurses as they embrace the modernisation agenda. By setting the issues in the context of organisational change and changes in social life it was possible to appreciate that the time is now right to support a change in attitudes and culture shift, but the degree of resistance to change and the time needed to change attitudes was acknowledged as problematic. Partnership working is now firmly centre stage in the NHS plan and involves building relationships between agencies, professionals and patients. Although much of the rhetoric about partnership working indicates sharing, flexibility and innovation there remains a real concern for quality patient care. It is therefore a fine balancing act by the health economy in encouraging new organisations to flourish but at the same time keeping control at the centre so that any 'failing' organisation is monitored and quickly turned around.

Modernising nursing means that nurses have to acknowledge the shift in culture, the need to work in partnership, to be patient centred, to adopt clinical governance and self-regulation as part of practice and to change and develop nursing roles to meet the health needs of the community. All this is well within the scope and ability of nurses as the profession comes of age. Leadership at every level of the profession will help to facilitate the change but also give nurses the confidence to know that they really can make a difference to health care. Creativity is the generating force that can energise the change process and encourage new ways of thinking to bring about improved patient care.

References

Ashcroft J 2001 Releasing the dividend of 'new' partnerships. In: Meads G, Meads T (eds) Trust in experience. Radcliffe Medical Press, Abingdon

15

Beenstock J, Jones S 2000 Time to shape up. Health Service Journal August 24: 28–29

Biggs S 2000 User voice, interprofessionalism and postmodernity. In: Davies C, Finlay L, Bullman A (eds) Changing practice in health and social care. Open University Press and Sage, London

Blair T 2001 Prime minister's speech to Labour party. Guardian Newspaper October 3: 4–5

Burr S 2001 Making a difference: Bristol Royal Infirmary. Nursing Management 8(7): 8–10

Clarke M, Stewart J 2000 Handling wicked issues. In: Changing practice in health and social care. Open University Press and Sage, London

Davies C 1995 Gender and the professional predicament in nursing. Open University Press, Buckingham

Department of Health 1997 The new NHS: modern, dependable. Department of Health, London

Department of Health 1998 A first class service: quality in the NHS. Department of Health, London

Department of Health 1999a Making a difference: strengthening the nursing, midwifery and health visiting contribution to health and health care. Department of Health, London

Department of Health 1999b Review of the prescribing, supply and administration of medicines (2nd Crown Report). Department of Health, London

Department of Health 2000 The NHS plan. Department of Health, London

Duffin C 2001 Hear LEO's roar. Nursing Standard 15(21): 12–13

Fish D, Coles C 1998 Developing professional judgement in health care. Butterworth-Heinemann, Oxford

Gough P 2001 Changing culture and deprofessionalisation. Nursing Management 7(9): 8–9

Hayes L 2001 Leadership in nursing. The Queen's Nursing Institute Newsletter 11(3): 1

Hudson B 2000 Wicked steps to partnership. Health Service Journal August 3: 20

Kennedy I 2001 Learning from Bristol. The report of the Public Inquiry into children's heart surgery at the Bristol Royal Infirmary 1984–1995. The Stationery Office, London

Meadows S, Levenson R, Baeza J 2000 The last straw, explaining the NHS nursing shortage. King's Fund Publishing, London

Mullally S 2001 Leadership and politics. Nursing Management 8(4): 21–27

Mullins L 1989 Management and organisational behaviour, 2nd edn. Pitman, London

Truman P 2001 A question of style. Nursing Management 7(8): 10–12

United Kingdom Central Council for Nursing, Midwifery and Health Visiting (UKCC) 2001 Professional self-regulation and clinical governance. UKCC, London

The creative challenge

Chapter **Two**

Creativity and caring

Barbara Goodfellow

- Caring as a distinctive aspect of professional nursing
- The contested definitions of caring
- The relative role of cognition and intuition in creative caring

- The importance of reflection
- How can the current challenges to creativity in caring be taken and used to support good nursing?

OVERVIEW

This chapter, first, briefly considers the historical roots of caring within the western tradition, then goes on to explore meanings and paradigms of caring currently debated within the nursing literature. Creative caring in relation to the science and the art of nursing is discussed as is the importance of cognition, intuition and reflection within this process. Finally, the possible challenges to creative caring such as the innovations in technology and pressure to produce measurable outcomes are noted, as is the way in which these might be taken and used creatively to support caring, compassionate nursing.

INTRODUCTION

The aim of this chapter is to provide a critical discussion of caring as a creative human enterprise. There is general agreement that nurses are caring people; many are drawn to the profession for that reason. Caring as a concept is central to the theory and practice of nursing and in recent years a debate has centred around caring as a theoretical construct (Leininger 1988, Morse et al 1990, Watson 1985). Emerging from the literature is the conviction that caring is a distinctive aspect of professional nursing. At the same time the imperatives of facilitated self-care and partnership as well as innovations in technology have arrived, necessitating a reconceptionalisation and reformulation of the discipline of caring within nursing and with it the need for the profession to be more creative in its approach to care.

Historically western traditions of caring prior to the 18th century were founded primarily on Christian paradigms. The patient, whether sick mentally or physically, was taken to a 'safe' place or sanctuary that provided respite and care. The sick were nurtured, both physically and spiritually, by carers. They had a remit to provide non-judgemental companionship. The relationship between carer and cared for was an ethical or 'loving' relationship (Peacock & Nolan 2000). It has been argued that the devaluing of caring in health care is evident from the middle of the 19th century with the rise of scientific positivism. From that time traditional ways of caring for sick people, not susceptible to scientific investigation and intervention, were either abandoned or discouraged. Jewson (1976) charts the development of modern curative medicine from a time of 'bedside medicine' at the end of the 18th century when only a wealthy few could retain the services of a doctor, through to the early years of the 19th century when the reductionist, mechanistic approach was beginning to be applied in medical schools. The emergence of what Jewson called 'hospital medicine' based on these Cartesian principles can be seen as the root of the dominance of biomedicine in modern health care systems and the establishment of doctors as the most powerful group of health professionals. Along with this transformation of medicine, where the focus was on the specialism of the doctor in relation to particular organs rather than on the patient, came the effect of depersonalising health care and stressing a concern for cure at the expense of care. In Jewson's third category – 'laboratory medicine' – the focus moved from organs to component cells and tissues with clinical diagnosis increasingly structured around the requirements of the laboratory and the application of technical procedures. The question is, where is nursing and care located in these developments?

DEFINITIONS OF CARING

Traditionally for many theorists, care, as opposed to cure, has been the critical factor in differentiating nursing from the practice of

The creative challenge

medicine, yet caring, as a concept, remains elusive. It is argued (Stevens Barnum 1994) that the ambiguous term 'caring' has three discrete meanings:

1. The first has to do with taking care of, in the sense of tending to another. This tends to be expressed in physical acts to meet patient needs; this is care as an activity.
2. The second notion of caring has to do with a concomitant emotion or attitude that occurs in the nurse in relation to the patient. The nurse who cares is the one who has an emotional investment in the patient's well-being; that is, the nurse cares about the patient – here care is attitudinal. Because it is possible for a nurse to take care of a patient with a caring attitude, the difference between these two meanings may be lost. But it is possible for a nurse to take care of a patient's needs, using appropriate nursing skills, but still feel no real concern.
3. The third sense of care is that of caution, of being careful to do something correctly. This meaning often carries a sense of guarding against injury or accident; care has to do with precision here.

It is clear that all three senses can occur simultaneously. A nurse may take care of a patient, with a caring attitude and be careful to do things in a safeguarding manner. The word 'care' has precise meaning. It belongs to the intellect and the root is in 'sorrow'. Care is not akin to cure. It is more related to 'pathos' in that the feelings are touched. When one gives care the feeling is experienced, and responded to, by extending oneself toward another. Care is expressed in:

> . . . tending to another, being with him, assisting or protecting him, giving heed to his responses, guarding him from danger that might befall him, providing for his needs and wants with compassion as opposed to sufferance or tolerance; with tenderness and consideration as opposed to a sense of duty; with respect and concern as opposed to indifference. (Jolley & Bry 1992, p. 302)

EXTENDED MEANINGS OF CARING

Not all theorists have limited the common meanings of caring to three; Morse et al (1990) identified five conceptualisations of caring as:

- a human trait
- a moral imperative
- an affect

Creativity and caring

- an interpersonal interaction
- a therapeutic intervention.

From the caring as a human trait perspective caring is innate, part of human nature and essential to human existence but although all humans have the potential to care, this ability is not uniform. Writers such as Benner & Wrubel (1989) concur that caring is a 'basic way of being in the world' (p. 398).

Caring as a moral imperative sees caring as a fundamental value or moral ideal in nursing. For theorists such as Watson (1985) caring is the adherence to the commitment of maintaining the individual's dignity or integrity. Caring as affect emphasises that the nature of caring involves empathetic feeling for the patient experience whilst caring as an interpersonal interaction sees the nurse/patient relationship as the foundation of caring. Finally, caring as a therapeutic intervention describes caring actions such as attentive listening, patient teaching, advocacy, touch and technical competence, placing emphasis on adequate knowledge, and skill links caring directly to nursing work.

PARADIGMS OF CARING

In their review of nursing literature on caring Morse et al (1990) identified 35 authors' definitions of caring. Only a small number of these can be addressed here. Much of the debate has concentrated on eliciting caring as a distinct aspect of nursing (Leininger 1984, Watson 1985). These theories of caring are not compatible with compliance or subservience in relation to medicine and the care/cure dichotomy, but articulate a strong case for professional autonomous nursing with care and patient advocacy at its core.

Some theorists (e.g. Gaut 1986) have attempted to operationalise definitions of caring. Gaut considers care to be a distinct and central phenomenon of nursing. She uses an action description of caring concerned with methods of evaluating competencies required in caring actions and considers caring to be an intentional human enterprise. She states that the 'competency model of caring goes beyond the identification of just observable performative skills to include broader considerations such as intention, choices and judgements that underlie the performance' (Gaut 1986, p. 82). Here Gaut talks about care as nurse behaviour rather than about caring in its emotive form.

Using a similar perspective, Wolf (1986, p. 91) developed a 'caring behaviour inventory'. The ten highest ranked are:

The creative challenge

- listening attentively
- comforting
- being honest
- having patience
- being responsible
- providing information so that the patient can make informed decisions
- touching
- showing sensitivity
- showing respect
- calling the patient by name.

Here Wolf is identifying representative behaviours that give clues to caring or concern – what she calls attachment – indicating the nurse's emotional involvement.

Watson's 'theory of human care' is based upon her belief that 'caring is the essence of nursing and the most central and unifying focus for nursing practice' (Watson 1989, p. 33). Watson defines caring as a transpersonal value:

> In transpersonal human caring, the nurse can enter into the experience of another person, and another can enter into the nurse's experience. The ideal of transpersonal caring is an ideal of inter-subjectivity in which both persons are involved. This means that the value and views of the nurse, though not decisive, are potentially as relevant as those of the patient. A refusal to allow the nurse's subjectivity to be engaged by a patient is, in effect, a refusal to recognise the validity of the patient's subjectivity. The alternative to caring as inter-subjectivity is not simply the reduction of the patient to an object, but the reduction of the nurse to that level as well. (Watson 1989, p. 60)

Watson's emphasis on the psychological, emotional and spiritual dimensions of care are reflected in the content of her earlier list of theory content/process (Watson 1989, pp. 9–10), items which she calls carative factors (Box 2.1).

As Morse et al (1990) point out, several questions arise in relation to Watson's theory. First, there could be a broad gap between clinical reality and the nurse-caring process. Second, it may not always be possible to attain the depth of nurse–patient relationship required by Watson's theory. Third, it brings into question whether nurses really are nursing in situations where the caring relationship has not developed. Finally, as Barker et al (1995) have also pointed out, not all caring is nursing so has nursing the right to stake a claim to be the 'caretaker of care'?

Like Watson, another major care theorist, Leininger, views nursing through a changing world view. Leininger (1991) considers the

Box 2.1 Carative factors (adapted from Watson 1989)

- Formation of a humanistic–altruistic system of values
- Instillation of faith–hope
- Cultivation of sensitivity to one's self and to others
- Development of a helping–trusting relationship
- Promotion and acceptance of the expression of positive and negative feelings
- Systematic use of the scientific problem-solving method for decision making
- Promotion of interpersonal teaching–learning
- Provision for a supportive, protective and corrective mental, physical, sociocultural, and spiritual environment
- Assistance with the gratification of human needs
- Allowance for existential–phenomenological forces

patients' world especially in the sense of the culture in which they reside. In her sunrise model she takes an anthropological perspective, looking at how the individual is influenced by their culture. Her main objective is to take the patient's world as given and to care accordingly, not seeking to reinterpret this world or its meanings. Leininger asks how patients' perceptions of their world then impacts on their health: 'All human cultures had some forms, patterns, expressions, and structures of care to know, explain and predict well-being, health or illness status' (Leininger 1991, p. 23). She holds that care is not isolated and sees culture and care as virtually indivisible and identifies three modes of culturally congruent care:

- cultural care preservation or maintenance
- cultural care accommodation or negotiation
- cultural care re-patterning or re-structuring. (Leininger 1991, pp. 41–43)

Leininger's model has been criticised on the grounds that it requires an extensive knowledge of anthropology and that it is abstract. However, Leininger was one of the first theorists to alert nurses to the need to consider cultural values and practices that influence patterns and meanings of care.

SCIENCE OR ART

It has traditionally been accepted that nursing is based upon both art and science (Abdellah et al 1960). The art of nursing is closely tied to the realities of the practice situation and is aesthetic and expressive in nature. The science of nursing is empirical and instrumental in nature based upon careful systematic research. Benner & Wrubel (1989) state that violence is done to caring when the distinction between the expressive and the instrumental role is separated in practice. The expert nurse combines these two roles.

Benner (1991) develops her theory of care by listening to what nurses say about their work and their experience. By analysing nurses' narratives she finds that for nurses it is important to 'know' the patient; for Benner, engaged knowledge of the patient and the family is the basis of proper care. Following Dreyfus & Dreyfus (1980) she expresses the difference between novice and expert behaviour. Benner is particularly interested in how we come to 'know' the patient, a process which she regards as highly intuitive. Benner describes a concept, which she calls skilful comportment, that values subjective experience over objective procedures. Benner & Wrubel (1989) build on this conceptualisation, pointing out how nursing and other caring practices have become devalued in a highly technical culture. Western society values autonomy, individualism and competitiveness but such a society does not always recognise that technological breakthroughs such as organ transplants are rendered dangerous without the context of skilful compassionate care. The dominant view of knowledge in the western tradition tends to stress abstract, theoretical knowledge at the expense of local, specific, practical knowledge and expert clinical judgements in particular clinical situations. This has led to nursing becoming at best paradoxical and at worst devalued. In order for both nursing practice and theory to flourish, there is a need to acknowledge and examine care both as science and as art.

COGNITION, INTUITION AND CREATIVITY

Ways of knowing has long been the subject of debate within nursing theory. It is clear that both cognitive abilities and intuition play a part in nurses' ability to care for people. Four patterns of knowing have been identified in nursing: empirical (the science of nursing), aesthetic (the art of nursing), personal knowledge and ethics (Carper 1978). It is the identification of such patterns that alerted scholars to the idea that science alone will not answer many significant questions in the discipline of nursing.

Such patterns have never been regarded as discrete or static. White (1995) for instance, added a fifth dimension – sociopolitical knowing – which is considered an essential pattern for understanding

Creativity and caring

that may evolve from all other patterns of knowing. This pattern focuses on the broader context for the caring processes. It includes organisational, cultural and political processes that influence both patients and nurses. For nurses to be innovators in both policy and practice in the current health care climate it is clear that a grasp of this fifth dimension is essential.

Patterns of knowing include both theoretical and practical knowing. Savimaki (1994) distinguishes between these two but allocates them equal significance. Theoretical knowledge includes the basic values, principles and conceptions of nursing. Its goals are to promote thinking and understanding of the discipline of nursing. Its base is intellectual and it is organised into many of the assumptions, concepts and models with which we are familiar in nursing. Practical knowledge, however, is not organised in the same way, partly because parts of this knowledge are not yet articulated and it may be that the artistic, as opposed to the scientific, dimensions of nursing practice are not even amenable to total articulation. Practical knowledge is achieved through personal and collective means and by reflection. Personal knowing is arrived at through one's own practice, reflection and synthesis and through integration of the art and science of nursing with practice. An example of this integration leading to creative caring is given in Application 2.1, which describes the way in which a night nurse, in the midst of the high technology which is required in a paediatric postoperative setting, showed warmth and compassion by quietly sharing her own painful experiences.

Moch (1990) identifies three components of personal knowing: experiential, interpersonal and intuition. Knowing through intuition is when knowing is achieved without the explicit use of scientific reason. It is knowing without knowing how. It could be argued that when nurses use intuition to know, they open themselves up to allow sensing and understanding of the patient's responses. Intuitive knowing, whilst previously neglected, is now seen as a component in clinical knowing, thus providing a basis for care. Nurses are now encouraged to let that inner voice surface, to believe in it and to trust it as a useful source of knowledge in the creative human enterprise of caring, an enterprise that requires aesthetic knowing that is imaginative and creative, allowing the knower to be engaged and interpretive.

REFLECTION AND CREATIVITY

Closely related to intuition is reflection, which provides nurses with another way of generating knowledge. Reflection is the throwing back of thoughts and memories in cognitive acts in order to make sense of them and to make contextually appropriate changes if they are required. Taylor (2000) states that it is the use of both a rational and an intuitive process which allows the potential for change. She suggests that there are three main kinds of reflection:

- technical
- practical
- emancipatory.

They are categorised according to the kind of knowledge they involve and the work interests they represent. All forms of reflection provide processes whereby everyday life events can be looked at carefully and sorted into systematic patterns, issues and values. Technical reflection is based on rational, deductive thinking and allows the generation of empirical knowledge. Practical reflection leads to interpretation for description and explanation of human interaction. Emancipatory reflection leads to transformative action, which seeks to free nurses from taken-for-granted assumptions, which potentially limit them and their practice. All three types of reflection can be facilitated through creative expression and in turn can generate autonomous, creative nursing care.

CHALLENGE TO CREATIVE CARING

Motivating factors and qualities required to be a good carer are implicitly in the mass of literature on the topic. Nurses must be compassionate, competent, confident and conscientious. Traditionally, caring was epitomised by efficiency, physical hard work, routine and order. Nurses were expected to be compliant, discreet and responsible. Before 1980, research rarely dealt with the concept of care or the nature of caring. Since then a new vision of the nature of caring in nursing has emerged, but how relevant is it when set against the time constraints and resource limitations of modern nursing? The nursing literature acknowledges the universal nature of caring and seeks to identify professional competencies associated with caring rather than isolating motivating factors and the qualities required to be a caring nurse. Emphasis is placed on the development of relationships through which caring work evolves. The interactive nature of the caring relationship is seen as essential. Yet the time the nurse spends with the patient and their family, especially in acute settings, may be severely limited. Even in community settings there may not be time to build up relationships over a long period of time. The response of the health visitor in Application 2.1 demonstrates the creative use of time to provide care.

Person-centred approaches to care, with emphasis on facilitated self-care, the patient as consumer and patient education are all amenable to a care philosophy. Facilitated self-care, that is those processes which allow individuals and families to take responsibility and to function effectively in developing their own health potential, requires nurses to use their knowledge, experience, affective elements and feelings as well as reflection. Knowledge alone may encompass the areas described in Box 2.2. However, the important factor here is how the knowledge base is organised and how the nurse shares important and complex ideas in a way that is meaningful.

As the dividing line between care and cure becomes less clear we may question the fit of care and cure as the appropriate boundary between medicine and nursing. As governments apply pressure to improve the cost-effectiveness of health delivery, attention has been focused on the benefits of moving some areas of health care work and responsibility from expensive to cheaper health care providers, in particular, from doctors to nurses. There was real concern that such policies might erode nursing autonomy and undermine its sense of professional identity, so impoverishing the quality of patient care (Williams et al 1997). On the other hand, such new dimensions to role and work might enable nurses to achieve greater autonomy and an ability to bring their values to bear on a wider range of health services. Williams (2000) points out that research in this area has explored the policy drivers and economic ramifications of this shift but few have reflected on how ideas, values and beliefs are being challenged. In her study of primary care, Williams found that both doctors and nurses valued ideas about

---

Box 2.2 Types of knowledge

- Content/subject matter knowledge
- Process and relationship structures (problem solving)
- Technical methods (skills, proficiency) and professional theory (philosophy, models and frameworks)
- Care organisation (primary nursing, care plans)
- Care contexts (hospital, community, rural/remote)
- Care aims, purposes and outcomes (promote wellness, restore health, prevent further deterioration, assist to death)
- Characteristics and identification of self-carers

care, holism and compassion but the way in which these core values were interpreted and treated differed significantly between medicine and nursing.

The rise of evidence-based care presents a challenge to the nursing values of care, holism and compassion, and hence to creative caring (Shorten & Wallace 1997). As managers and administrators seek to control nursing actions, to limit caring time and to require concrete, measurable outcomes, how can nurses reconcile these demands with care that may not have quantifiable outcomes other than patient satisfaction? All of the examples of creative caring given in Application 2.1 could not be categorised as being based on scientifically based research findings. Nursing may still have the central dilemma of being [committed] to care in a society that refuses to value care (Reverby 1987).

As stated earlier, a view of what it is to be human grew out of the mechanistic model of the 17th and 18th centuries. In nursing, as elsewhere, technology has been adopted in stages until it has reached the point where it is accepted as a means of enhancing life. The widespread use of computers and other technology in nursing practice, research, education and administration reflects professional acceptance. As assimilation of technology promotes value changes, emphasis may be placed on quantity rather than quality, or knowledge may be viewed as a source of power, and such possibilities create a serious challenge to nursing. Use of technology may result in dehumanisation, loss of privacy and breaches of confidentiality. Increased use of machines may lead to decreased human contact and interaction. Alternatively, a proactive response to technology by nurses may ultimately support caring in nursing. Increased knowledge and skill will enable nurses to use technology more efficiently and appropriately and to incorporate it into a care-based practice.

Caring can best be accomplished by a concerted effort at the integration of appropriate philosophies and research findings; nursing's evaluative processes such as quality assurance schemes; application of systematic approaches to nursing such as the nursing process within models of nursing; and a keenness to utilise new techniques and labour-saving equipment such as computers and information technology, whether in the community or in a hospital context.

CONCLUSION

Many questions are yet to be answered about the nature of caring in nursing. Can a nurse care too much? Can nurses care for others without themselves being cared for? Does caring distinguish nursing from other professions (Smith 1999)? Caring cannot meet all patient needs – it does not achieve cure or arrest pathology but can cure be achieved without care? Morse et al (1990) pose the related question: Can a nurse provide safe practice without caring? It may be necessary to practise without care in the sense it has been discussed in certain contexts. It is argued that, in order to care, a nurse must be immersed in the patients' experience yet to inflict pain is often a necessary part of a procedure and a part from which the nurse is necessarily disembodied. If the nurse becomes detached from caring in such situations, how can caring retain its theoretical position as the essence of nursing (Radley 2000)?

Whilst strides have been made in the conceptionalisation of care, further development and refinement of caring are necessary. One important shift is the move away from nurse-focused theories of care towards patient-centred theory. Patient outcomes of caring need to be considered in order to enhance the utility of the concept of care in nursing. The question needs to be asked: What difference does caring make to the patient and their family? Does caring change the course of illness? If this is the case it deserves its reputation as the essence of nursing. If not, perhaps it is necessary to consider what else is essential to nursing.

It is clear from the brief review of approaches considered in this chapter that there are discrepancies among the various conceptualisations of care, especially between those who view care as intervention and those who view it as an interactive process. Ongoing debate and clarification must be valued, especially where further development can be applied in the actual practice of bedside nursing.

References

Abdellah FG, Beland IL, Martin A, Matheny RV 1960 Patient centred approaches to nursing. Macmillan, New York

Barker PJ, Reynolds W, Ward T 1995 The proper focus of nursing: a critique of the 'caring' ideology. International Journal of Nursing Studies 32: 4

Benner P 1991 The role of experience, narrative and community in skilled ethical comportment. Advances in Nursing Science 14: 1–21

Benner P, Wrubel J 1989 The primacy of caring: stress and coping in health and illness. Addison Wesley, Menlo Park, California

Carper BA 1978 Fundamental patterns of knowing in nursing. Advances in Nursing Science 1: 13–23

Dreyfus SE, Dreyfus HL 1980 A five stage model of the mental activities involved in directed skill acquisition. Unpublished report supported by the Air Force Office of Scientific Research (AFSC), USAF (Contract F49620-79-C-0063), University of California at Berkeley

Gaut DA 1986 Evaluating caring competencies in nursing practice. Topics in Clinical Nursing 2: 77–83

Jewson ND 1976 The disappearance of the sick man from medical cosmology, 1770–1870. Sociology 10: 225–244

Jolley M, Bry G (eds) 1992 Nursing care: the challenge to change. Edward Arnold, London

Leininger MM 1984 Care: the essence of nursing and health. Slack, Thorofare, New Jersey

Leininger MM 1988 Leininger's theory of nursing: cultural care, diversity and universality. Nursing Science Quarterly 1: 152–160

Leininger MM 1991 Culture, care, diversity and universality: a theory of nursing. National League for Nursing, New York

Moch A 1990 Nursing practice: high hard ground, messy swamps and the pathways in between. Deakin University Press, Geelong

Morse JM, Soldberg SJ, Neander WL, Botorff JL, Johnson JL 1990 Concepts of caring and caring as a concept. Advances in Nursing Science 14(1): 1–14

Peacock JW, Nolan PW 2000 Care under threat in the modern world. Journal of Advanced Nursing 33(5): 1066–1070

Radley A 2000 Health psychology, embodiment and the question of vulnerability. Journal of Health Psychology 5(3): 297–304

Reverby S 1987 A caring dilemma: womanhood and nursing in historical perspective. Nursing Research 36(1): 5

Sarvimaki A 1994 Science and tradition in the nursing discipline. Scandinavian Journal of Caring Sciences 8: 137–142

Shorten A, Wallace M 1997 Evidence based practice: the future is clear. Australian Nursing Journal 4(6): 22–24

Smith MC 1999 Caring and the science of unitary human beings. Advances in Nursing Science 21(4): 14–28

Stevens Barnum BJ 1994 Nursing theory: analysis, application, evaluation. Lippincott, Philadelphia

Taylor BJ 2000 Reflective practice: a guide for nurses and midwives. Open University Press, Buckingham

Watson J 1985 Nursing: nursing science and human care – a theory of nursing. National League for Nursing, New York

Watson J 1989 Watson's philosophy and theory of human caring in nursing. In: Reihl-Sisca J (ed) Conceptual models for nursing practice, 3rd edn. Appleton Lange, Norwalk, Connecticut

Williams A 2000 Nursing, medicine and primary care. Open University Press, Buckingham

Williams A, Robins T, Sibbald B 1997 Cultural differences between medicine and nursing: implications for primary care. A summary report. National Primary Care Research and Development Centre, University of Manchester

White J 1995 Patterns of knowing: review, critique and update. Advances in Nursing Science 17(4): 73–86

Wolf ZR 1986 The caring concept and nurse identified caring behaviours. Topics in Clinical Nursing 8(2): 84–93

Creativity and caring

Application **2:1**
Joanna Richards

A carer's perspective on professional caregiving

The creative challenge

Having a child with multiple disabilities has brought me into contact with a wide range of care professionals, all of whom support me in various ways in my caring role. Of all the very many encounters, there are a few episodes that stand out as having been particularly caring. It is these snapshots of professional care, viewed from my perspective as a parent carer, that form the focus of this short chapter.

When Saskia was born, I was very well looked after by an experienced midwife who stayed with me all the time, was relaxed and kind and nice to have around. But what remains with me, as having been the most valuable aspect of her caring, is neither her technical competence as a midwife, nor her calm efficiency in dealing with the birth of a baby with Down syndrome. It is the fact that every evening during my subsequent 4-day stay in the hospital, she came to see me and we had a chat and a cup of tea together before she started her night shift on the labour ward. And some weeks later she phoned me at home, saying she'd been thinking about us while she'd been back in Trinidad on holiday, and just wanted to know if everything was going well.

Saskia's first year was a traumatic time for all of us. A major surgical intervention intended to improve her quality of life resulted in irreversible brain damage. Such an overwhelmingly negative outcome poses an enormous challenge to those providing care, both professionals and family. Of all the many nurses we met during our 6 weeks in hospital, two remain etched in my memory as having been especially caring. One was the nurse who went against the medical opinion that 'these children don't feel pain' and insisted that Saskia be given analgesia. This nurse took on the role of advocate for my baby at a time when I was not in a fit state to speak out with sufficient force. The other was the night nurse who was there for me through the long, sad hours, as I struggled to reach out to my damaged child, by providing human warmth and compassion in a cold, high-tech world and quietly sharing with me still painful personal memories of a baby born with no chance of life.

Back home, it took time to adjust to the endless round of caring for such a profoundly disabled child. The frequent trips to hospitals and the many home visits just felt like an additional burden. I found it difficult enough simply getting through the days; having to talk to professional after professional seemed only to reinforce all the negatives. One day when Saskia was very poorly and it was taking hours to get her to feed, the health visitor called. Her refreshingly helpful response to the fairly dire situation was to direct her attention to Anje, my toddler, asking her if she had had any lunch. While the two of them were in the kitchen chatting away and finding something to eat, I remember feeling intensely relieved that for once I didn't have to put on the coping act of the polite chat and cup of coffee. Instead, I was being given the much-needed space just to be myself and to concentrate on what was most important to me at that moment.

For a long time, I found it hard to live fully in the present, as I was constantly referring back to how Saskia had been before the brain damage had occurred. The professional response to this was either to listen sympathetically without comment, letting me go on, or else to stop me in my tracks by abruptly changing the subject. The person who did most to help me move on was a young student nurse on her first placement. Saskia lay more or less motionless throughout the visit, quite unresponsive, and I started my usual piece about what a dear little poppet she had been before her operation. Without any hesitation the student interrupted me, saying cheerfully 'Well I think she's a dear little poppet now!'. That spontaneous remark helped me realise the importance of bringing all my positive feelings about Saskia into the present, not leaving them languishing in the past, in some hopeless 'if only' limbo.

Before writing about these experiences, I had thought no more about them beyond acknowledging that they remained in my mind as examples of professional caring that had really made a positive impact on me. On reflection, I can see that what the examples have in common is the fact that the person concerned made his or her own very individual response, over and above that which might reasonably have been expected of a competent practitioner. This accords very closely with the concept of creativity defined by the Oxford dictionary as 'showing imagination beyond routine skill'. I am sure there is no textbook that suggests that midwives ought to visit women in their own time, nor that nurses should go against what senior doctors say, or share intimate details of their private lives with patients, nor that health visitors should roll their sleeves up and get into the kitchen to make lunch for their clients. And you cannot teach the right thing to say in any given situation.

A carer's perspective on professional caregiving

Six Steps to **Effective Management**

Creativity in caring may not be something that can be taught, but it can certainly be facilitated. An important question that emerges from these brief reflections is whether the current climate of professional practice encourages such creativity to thrive, so that health care practitioners feel enabled to respond to individual need in ways that can transcend the mechanics of routine care.

Chapter **Three**

The changing professional role of the nurse

Sue Merrylees

- **Models and theories of professional activity**
- **Factors affecting professional socialisation**
- **Current challenges for the professional nurse**

OVERVIEW

This chapter looks at the changing role of the nurse and the new opportunities that nurses have in the 21st century. Taking many of the themes found in contemporary practice, the chapter explores the challenges, opportunities and some of the difficulties of professional life in nursing today. The concept of leadership is central to this discussion and in line with the overall aim of this text; modern leadership will be explored within the context of models of professional activity. Drawing on factors intrinsic to nursing and influenced by the wider issues in UK society, the concept of professionalisation is explored from the perspective of the individual practitioner. Some wider and more general issues that are pertinent to the nursing profession as a whole are also discussed.

INTRODUCTION

The chapter is set out in three parts: models, professional socialisation and challenges for the professional nurse.

Six Steps to **Effective Management**

Part 1: Models

Models of professional activity and how each impacts upon nursing activity are explored. The models used are drawn from a range of literature sources such as the recognised work of Moloney (1986) and the more recent work of Davies (1995). These are used to build a picture of the development of nursing practice becoming a professional activity. The questions to be addressed here concern the stage and maturity of the development of nursing as a profession.

- Can the models be applied to nursing?
- Can the degree of autonomy and accountability in contemporary nursing practice justify the term professional?
- Are nurses suitably prepared and rewarded for the high status associated with professional practice?

Part 2: Professional socialisation – the influence of occupational sociology

This part explores the influence of occupational sociology, highlighting some broad developmental issues, motivational factors and the experiences of individuals undergoing professional preparation. Key work with models, such as that of Melia (1987), is explored, together with issues such as gender and the image of nursing.

Part 3: Challenges for the professional nurse

Within the context of contemporary practice the conclusions from Parts 1 and 2 are then appraised in the light of some of the challenges that face the professional nurse in contemporary practice. Many questions are raised in this section and include:

- What is the impact on nursing of the quality agenda through the emergence of clinical governance?
- What is the role of the nurse in leading and developing services?
- How does the demand for a competent workforce impact on the development of nursing as a profession?
- Partnership working is a key feature of the modernisation agenda. How will this develop and how will the professional role of the nurse be affected?
- What will be the impact on professional roles when we move to a more inclusive way of working by putting users and carers at the centre of professional activity?

The creative challenge

34

- In terms of regulatory frameworks what effect will the changes being made to the Nursing and Midwifery Council (NMC) and the English National Board for Nursing, Midwifery and Health Visiting (ENB) have on the way the crucial issue of public protection is addressed?
- The development of evidence-based practice is a current buzz-phrase but what is the reality for the development of professional nursing practice?

In addressing these questions the future challenges for nursing begin to emerge.

PART 1: MODELS OF PROFESSIONAL ACTIVITY

The definitive explanation of what constitutes a profession leads to the same difficulty that nurses encounter in trying to define concepts such as caring and kindness – a virtually impossible task. There has been extensive work within this sphere and an overview of the definitions concluded by recognised authors is useful. Moloney (1986) in her book *Professionalization of Nursing* offers an appraisal of the early definitions of profession such as the work of Carr-Saunders and Wilson who defined profession by the amount of knowledge that each claimed. They concluded that those professions that had lengthy and rigorous training periods with a great emphasis on knowledge ranked as true professions. Service to clients is another aspect explored by Moloney in her analysis of the development of professional activity.

Flexner (1960) in the classic study of social welfare supports the notion of intellectual activity but adds that another attribute of professionalism is internal organisation. Pavalko's (1971) *Sociology of Occupations* further explores this with a model that describes different dimensions, distinguishing between occupations and professions along a continuum of attributes that include a code of ethics and a system of internal monitoring.

Autonomy is another feature first flagged up by Flexner and the concept of autonomy as a professional attribute is well documented by other authors such as Davies et al (2000) who examined the issue of professionalism from an economic perspective and suggested that a profession required a gatekeeping process to limit the number of those entering into it in order to meet only the demand required. This is related closely to the notion of exclusivity of task that was described by Moloney (1986) in terms of being a 'monopoly of services'.

The changing professional role of the nurse

The social standing that is attached to an occupational group is a feature that is explored as part of sociological studies. Johnson et al (1995) discuss the functional importance of the activities of any profession in light of the rules of the society in which the profession is practised. This links to the status and importance attributed to this profession by members of that society. From the literature emerge strong themes representing the development of clear models of professional activity.

How each of these attributes of a profession interrelates is essential to understanding the concept of professional activity and how this may apply to the development of professional activity in nursing. This section provides a theoretical structure to the discussion of contemporary challenges such as autonomy, accountability, gatekeeping, specialist skills and knowledge, service to clients and status and remuneration.

Autonomy

Autonomy in decision making is considered to be one of the features of sophisticated practice within any profession. In exploring decision making, Topping (1999) looked at the outcomes desired by employers from students undertaking a programme of advanced practice preparation. The study showed that the ability to make independent decisions was an essential component of such practice. One of the issues for nurses has always been the link between decision making and the structures within which nurses work, an example being a community psychiatric nurse wishing to amend a care plan but having to wait for the CPA (care programme approach) meeting to be able to make such changes. Moloney (1986) highlights that a key factor within the decision-making process is having the authority to actually make decisions.

Boundaries

There clearly need to be boundaries within professional roles to allow decision making to become legitimised. In health care the boundaries may not always be clear and therefore spheres and levels of autonomy can be problematic. It can seem that autonomy is limited by a variety of explicit protocols and unwritten cultural boundaries. Historically, practitioners made some decisions when they had no authority but little choice, an example being nurses in learning disability services prescribing across-the-counter remedies for clients where there was no medical practitioner available to make such decisions.

This assumed authority was not legitimate. It could result in practice that was not only dangerous to the clients but left the practitioner vulnerable to disciplinary action. There are, however, clear examples of the role of the practitioner being extended and legitimised, such as how the role of the advanced practitioner in nursing emerged out of the debate on junior doctor hours (DoH 1995). It would appear that factors of professional boundaries needed to be reexamined as a result of resource and demand. This has led to the development of a nursing role that has extended beyond the usual but one that is clearly defined and usually supported.

Advanced nursing practice

Advanced nursing practice is becoming legitimised in terms of autonomy through the development of specific postregistration options such as nurse practitioner programmes that meet the outcomes of the UKCC (now NMC) descriptors for *Scope in Practice* (1997). The publication of the UKCC descriptors for *Higher Level of Practice* in 1998 allowed individuals to evidence and benchmark their professional activities against set standards for advanced practice. Advanced practice can be seen in many areas such as neonatal care with nurse-led services for the total care of babies including transportation and transfer to specialist units. Practice nursing is another area of developed practice with nurse-led clinics becoming a normal and accepted role in primary care.

Diagnosis

The authority to make a diagnosis is a key area of concern when discussing autonomy as it relates to a fundamental principle in decision making. It is complicated by the fact that diagnosis is limited, conceptually, to a medical issue. Nurses and other health care professionals are able to make diagnoses but these must relate to their own spheres of practice. A good example of this is seen in tissue viability where the assessment and diagnosis of the skin condition relate directly to the interventions undertaken by nurses. This involves the nurse using an evidence-based tool (e.g. Waterlow 1991) and using this to assess the status of risk in any individual. The nurse is then able to prescribe a series of interventions designed to minimise the effects of pressure on the person's skin.

The changing professional role of the nurse

Treatment

As well as diagnosis, the prescription of treatment is seen as a medical role. Medical treatment is only one aspect of patients' experience and the prescription of care and therapy involves other health care professionals. The development of practice based on the application of recognised models of intervention or treatment supports this endeavour. It also highlights a key professional function – the evaluation of evidence.

Risk management

Risk management is emerging as a concept in service delivery (Alaszewki 2000) and the ability to make decisions based on good risk management strategies offers health care professionals a positive way forward. Clear role definition may be seen as limiting professional creativity but the ability to view the nurse's role in-depth is one of the key strengths of the modern professional.

Accountability

Accountability forms one of the recurring issues for the modern professional. Accountability can be defined simply as giving a reckoning for one's conduct, performance or duty (UKCC 1992). Davies (1995) describes how the principles of accountability are universal within health care but that the parameters of accountability differ from job to job. Within this explanation accountability is seen to relate to competence, experience, knowledge, authority and responsibility.

Within health care the question has been asked 'are nurses too accountable?' (Tingle 1990). Due to the changing nature of employment, practitioners often find themselves accountable to a range of masters, each with different concerns. For example, a nurse working in a nursing home for a 'not-for-profit organisation' would be accountable to that organisation and also to the local health authority as the registration and inspection unit under the Care Standards Legislation (DoH 2001a). Nursing practice on a day-to-day basis tends to be guided by the rules of the employer, with concern for meeting the standards prescribed by the relevant professional body.

Accountability is an area of study in its own right; professional accountability in nursing has been governed by a sophisticated system of self-regulation administered by the Nursing and Midwifery Council (formerly the United Kingdom Central Council). Davies'

(2001) essay 'The demise of professional self regulation – a moment to mourn' explores the emerging agenda in health and social care regulatory frameworks.

Gatekeeping

Abbott (1988) highlights the concept of gatekeeping as a facet of professional practice. He describes it as the erection of social boundaries via entrance qualification, which leads a profession to command higher status and higher reward. Within health care, gatekeeping is achieved through a variety of mechanisms:

- the entry requirement for training and education
- the exit criteria for graduation from training and education
- criteria for entry to the professional register including personal attributes
- employment specification.

For nursing, the development of a professional role has occurred through a variety of factors, one of which is the move to higher education. Gatekeeping in nursing is problematic, as planning issues and the nature of the nursing workforce make it impossible to currently move the entry criteria in order to be in line with other university courses. This creates a mismatch between perceived academic desirability and the need to meet the demand for a nursing workforce. *Making a Difference – the Contribution of Nursing, Midwifery and Health Visiting to Health Care* (DoH 1999a) has redressed some of the issues of gatekeeping through the encouragement of the use of accreditation of prior learning and step on/step off stages for preregistration nurse training.

Specialist skills and knowledge

One of the most interesting aspects about an activity such as nursing is the way in which knowledge is synthesised. Many contemporary commentators describe the practice of nursing as being knowledge based. Roper et al (2000), in the development of their model of practice over the last 15 years, provide a good example of how nursing can be seen as having a unique knowledge base. However, as with many other practice-based professions, it must also be acknowledged that without the practice there would be no theory or knowledge. Nursing provides a real chicken-and-egg situation. The need for knowledge within nursing is necessary not only to gain legitimate recognition from others in health care and in the world of academia, it also serves a very practical purpose (Salvage 1985). However, if practice and theory are developed in differing settings, a theory/practice divide can be created and the development of knowledge can lose its relevance to the everyday practitioner. The transfer from schools of nursing to higher education marks the end of a transitional process from an apprentice-based preparation to a research-based focus and with it the thirst for legitimate knowledge becomes paramount.

But how to define nursing knowledge? Moloney (1986) describes the use of specialist skills and knowledge as being related to a monopoly of services and argues that for any activity to be considered professional the acquisition of specialist skills is essential. In the past nursing has had some difficulty in being able to fulfil this objective. The Committee of Inquiry into Nursing (DoH 1972) suggested that this was the result of nursing being fragmented in nature with too many points of entry and too many points of exit. Vestiges of this view remain today but there is a new optimism in the ability to define the outcomes of professional practice. The *Making a Difference* (DoH 1999a) agenda has been designed to assist in this process through the partnership working that is the essential stem of the policy and its implementation.

By definition the constitution of specialist nursing skills and knowledge is as difficult as defining nursing itself. Turnbull (1999) suggests that nurses should be more concerned by what nurses do than by what they are. This leads to a concern with the issue of competence. The modern professional is therefore inevitably a practitioner whose competence is underpinned by specialist skills and knowledge. The development of research in supporting health care practice is an essential component of the process of continuing to develop new spheres of skills and knowledge. Nursing finding a home in higher education adds currency to the value of the knowledge and skills base of the profession.

Service to clients

As a component of professional activity, the service that is offered to the client is central to the purpose of that profession. Described as being an ideology of public service and altruism, client experience has formed an entire subindustry within health care organisations. Concern for the quality of the service delivered has many of its contemporary practices rooted in the political changes of the 1980s and 1990s (Ham 1999). The introduction of the internal market, based upon a belief in consumer sovereignty, led to systems of

The creative challenge

quality assurance that fulfilled contractual obligations. Client experience underpinned these but the system also emerged from other factors in the health service:

- increasing complaints
- increasing expectations of the health service
- technological advances
- litigation leading practice
- awareness of rights.

Fulfilling the obligations that nurses have to consumers of health services is a critical aspect of professional practice, yet one which is often led by administrators not practitioners. Contemporary health care policy – *The New NHS: Modern, Dependable, A First Class Service, The NHS Plan* and the subsequent *National Service Frameworks* (DoH 1997, 1998, 2000, 2001d) – points towards a new challenge for health care professionals, putting service users and their families/carers at the heart of service delivery.

Status and remuneration

The move toward the enhancement of professional status within health care is linked to issues of wages and reward. Salvage (1985, p. 25) describes how 'Raising the profile of the professional status of nursing, educating nurses in universities, and encouraging or accepting the substitution of nursing for medical labour all fuel the demand for higher salaries that governments are naturally unwilling to meet'. For nurses, along with other health care professionals, there is a conflict between status in society and the rewards received. The historical notion of helping others as a charitable act has some credence with this argument. Some nurses feel that patients would become alienated when presented with this level of professionalism. Most health care professionals rightly feel that the status and remuneration they have do not match the role and responsibility in the service that they provide and the professional approach that is expected of them. New government initiatives announced recently with the advent of the nurse consultant are seen by the profession as a means of recognising the value of some nurses. The higher level of practice initiative (UKCC 1998) is designed to describe and recognise practitioners who function at an advanced level. What emerges from both the nurse consultant role and the higher level of practice initiative is the concept of benchmarking; this process allows practitioners to measure practice against excellent everyday practice. This has to be seen as a

The changing professional role of the nurse

positive move toward validating the concept of leadership, as nurses perceive it in terms of a modern professional.

Summary

This section has presented an overview of the facets of practice that distinguish a professional approach from other ways of working. Perceptions of the maturity of health care professionals against these facets will depend upon the experiences of the individual reader. Many of the issues described in this section will be elaborated upon but this is perhaps a point at which to reflect upon your personal stance in relation to the issues presented so far.

PART 2: PROFESSIONAL SOCIALISATION – THE INFLUENCE OF OCCUPATIONAL SOCIOLOGY ON CONTEMPORARY NURSING

Occupational sociology is the study of the cultural and societal issues of any given occupational group and there are extensive studies exploring this concept within health care.

Traditional images of the nature of nursing and the debate of science versus art have resulted in confusion in terms of the professional focus of nursing. They are some of the factors that have restricted the internal development of the profession of nursing and have influenced the way in which others see the role of the nurse. Other factors that cannot be ignored when examining the difficulties that nursing has in asserting its right to be recognised as a profession can once again be traced in some part to the historical legacies of the development of nursing.

Class issues

The first and perhaps the most pertinent factor can be traced back as far as the 'new poor laws' of 1832 and the very start of the notion of public welfare which came to the fore with the formation of the Charitable Organisations Society in the 1870s (Hills et al 1994). The development of any policy that affects public welfare can trace its roots to the issues that affect society in general at any given time. Hills et al (1994) describe how the new poor laws were significant in that they removed the effects of poverty from the private to the public domain. The relevance of this to the development of nursing is that once a problem is identified as a public issue, there is a recognised need for something to be done about it. The poor law amendments of 1832 allowed the distinction between the deserving and the undeserving poor. In the case of the deserving poor it became the responsibility of many a middle-class lady to take up the call of charitable deeds with this poor group of unfortunates. The effect of this was to place the notion of welfare firmly in the domain of the middle classes, an increasingly influential group in Victorian society. This resulted in an acceptance of the respectability of the vocation of nursing for the young middle-class lady. The idea of moral education is one which was firmly entrenched in this development, with the duty of one class to educate and guide another, less fortunate, class in the realms of moral and physical health (Dingwall 1988).

The influence of class on the development of nursing can be related to the number of nurses in each of the nursing specialisms. Adult nursing can be seen to exert the most influence because of the numbers of practitioners involved. The fact that the smaller branches of nursing have developed with a different perception of their class influence serves to reinforce the problems of fragmentation of nursing as a profession as highlighted by Briggs (DoH 1972). The issue of class is important to the development of nursing in that the need to be taken seriously was negated by the idea that the practitioners involved in nursing were somehow 'playing' at it (Dingwall 1988).

Traditional roles

Another inherited image problem is the traditional view of the nurse as a doctor's handmaiden. Although not directly related to the issue of class, the effects of this image have connotations in terms of the traditional role of the nurse and in particular the idea of subservience. The medical profession has itself undergone a gargantuan struggle in its search for professional identity. Although the legitimisation of medicine has been very successful, the dominant role of medicine in health care has had a detrimental effect on the ability of nursing to establish credibility in terms of its own professional identity. Nursing has traditionally been practised within a culture of a rigid hierarchy with the nurse being subservient to the doctor. Although current trends in health care provision have meant a reexamination of that hierarchy, the image remains. If nurses are to be able to embrace the challenges and opportunities presented through the modernisation agenda then the limiting effect that a rigid hierarchy places upon creativity needs to be addressed. This can be done through bringing together professional activities and building upon the confidence emerging from the opportunities for professional leadership that are integral parts of every nurse's role.

Gender

Gender is another factor that has played its part in the problems associated with the development of professionalism within nursing. Nursing today remains a largely female dominated profession. There is evidence to suggest that gender distribution across the hierarchies relates to inequalities recognised in the recent policy initiative *Opportunity 2000* (Department of Education 1998). This report suggests that whilst efforts have been made to address the issues of unequal pay and conditions for women, there remains fundamental division between the managers and the managed. The work of the Royal College of Nursing report on workforce trends (RCN 1995) would support this view when it suggests that whilst the nursing profession has an overall 87% female workforce, 67% of men hold managerial positions. The implications of this are explored in some of the work of Davies (1995) who suggests that there is a traditional inability of women to be taken seriously in the workplace. The image difficulties this creates has meant that nurses will always find it difficult to gain legitimate recognition as a profession and highly motivated and dedicated workers to perform to the level they wish. This whole area has been considered by the NHS Executive in its review on the recruitment and retention of nurses (NHSE/CVCP 2001), the report highlighting best practice in recruitment strategies and examples of areas where such strategies have not only resulted in more men entering the profession but also an increase in students from ethnic minority groups. The sum total of these factors points to a rather fragmented and undecided professional focus. Differences of opinion amongst nurse leaders and a general tendency to political naiveté also play an important part in the difficulties that nursing has had in achieving a clear professional focus.

Motivation

Motivation to join a profession can be used as an indication of occupational sociology factors. Within public service the feeling that one can make a difference to the lives of others is often a strong motivational force. Comparative studies within the social work profession find that social work students have a strong political motivation for entering the profession. Pearson (1973) contended that social work students were in some way political deviants; they explicitly rejected

The creative challenge

the normal values of everyday life and concentrated on giving and helping others. Within nursing this same strong need appears to be present although nurses tend not to share the same political views. Melia (1987) describes how the reality of the role and the process of socialisation – through what she describes as the 'doing nursing and being professional' phases of socialisation – often force practitioners to revisit motivation. In social work similar findings (Uttley 1981) point to an idealism/reality gap. The process of professional social-isation clearly impacts upon the development of nurses as professionals and nursing as a profession.

Within the notion of the modern professional the form of prepara-tion and the move to higher education will impact upon such devel-opment. The evolutionary process of the Project 2000 programmes to diploma, degree and into the implementation of the *Making a Difference* (DoH 1999a) agenda has been instrumental in determining the professional focus of the workforce. Nursing is now seen as a much more professional option in determining career choice. Research (Parker & Merrylees 2001) shows that whilst students have a commitment to caring and providing a better service to clients, they also need to have a sensible career structure with levels of progres-sion and reward.

PART 3: CHALLENGES FOR THE PROFESSIONAL NURSE

Some of the key contemporary challenges facing nursing in the 21st century that are central to the ethos of the modern nursing profes-sion include:

- the impact of the quality agenda and delivery of quality ser-vices through governance
- the demand for a competent workforce
- leading and developing services
- partnership working
- putting users and carers at the centre of professional activity
- the impact of changes in the regulatory frameworks
- the development of evidence-based practice.

The impact of the quality agenda and delivery of quality services through governance

Clinical governance became a buzzword in the late 1990s. Proposed as a central theme of the modernisation strategy within the NHS, the notion of clinical governance has arisen from the broader social concept of the redistribution of previously centralised tasks. Stenson (2001) describes how public government has been regenerated in the last two decades because of a shortage of central resource. Concepts of accountability and citizenship are strongly represented in current policy and these trends are reflected in the management of service quality within the NHS. Clinical governance has brought with it a new form of collective accountability with clear reporting mechanisms through both internal and external structures. Stenson (2001) considers some of these changes in relation to crime control when he talks about the everyday processes of public government being underpinned by consensus and academic survey (p. 236). In relating this to health care nurses are able to see the relationship to evidence-based practice as the underpinning feature of quality services. This is enacted through a system of self-critique.

Clinical governance means that current and future professional approaches to practice will always be open to scrutiny and audit. This relatively new concept for nursing practice is a significant change in the audit process and means that new patterns of clinical confidence together with new professional identities are emerging. Openness of this nature and an acknowledgement that errors do occur – and are there to be learned from – is also a new departure, bringing concern and fear initially. The concept of the learning organisation (Handy 1998) is one that nurses need to embrace if they are to capitalise upon the opportunities such cultures offer through systems of clinical governance.

The demand for a competent workforce

Jowett et al (1994) started a debate on professional outcomes of pre-registration training in their research on the implementation of Project 2000. Further review led to the opinion that Project 2000, whilst adequately preparing practitioners, had led to a generation of nurses who lacked practical competence and confidence on qualifying. The Department of Health examined the issues and the *Making a Difference* (DoH 1999a) agenda was born. This agenda is demanding in that, for the first time, some of the early criticisms of nurse education (lack of flexibility and step on/off points) have had to be addressed. However, it needs to be recognised that the collaborative approach to practitioner preparation is being undertaken in the context of contemporary care services where the other features of new professional ways of working dominate the agenda.

The concept of lifelong learning and flexibility in the design and delivery of both preregistration and continuing professional development is a key feature. Service and education appear to be developing a much more cohesive partnership. Examples of this working can be seen in the development of joint appointments such as lecturer practitioners. A commitment to sharing responsibility for the student experience is demonstrated, for example, through the appointment of practice placement facilitators, located in the clinical area with a role to support student learning.

Leading and developing services

As professional maturity develops (Davies 1995) there are significant changes in the development and implementation of the concept of leadership. Melia (1987) takes us through the structural and managerial development within the health service from the 1960s and 1970s and describes how these changes brought about a new idealism in terms of leadership within the NHS. Ham (1999) critiques general management and describes a machismo approach linked to performance and remuneration prevailing throughout the 1980s and 1990s.

The last few years have seen a growing interest in the concept of clinical leadership, although the cynical would argue that the demise of a career structure linked to management and pay, with the flattened hierarchy of the grading system, means that alternative forms of structure emerge. The concept of clinical leadership is one, however, in which nurses feel professionally confident. Award for this form of leadership emerges from the role of the nurse consultant and other advances linked to practice developments. The newly launched concept of the 'modern matron' (DoH 2001b) is a similar celebration of the role of the nurse as a strong clinical leader. Through the development of strong clinical leadership, nursing is able to become creative in its approach to the professional role. Leadership allows for and celebrates innovation. Award schemes such as the 'Nursing Times and 3 Ms' demonstrate a whole range of innovations in practice and education that are led and implemented by nurses.

For the everyday practitioner there are frustrations with the notion of clinical leadership; the nursing press talks about some practitioners feeling unable to relate to new patterns of leadership because of pressures and shortages. Nurses must therefore keep a balanced view of the opportunities that the new forms of leadership offer and continue to ensure that realistic models of professional

The chaning professional role of the nurse

activity underpin emerging forms of leadership. Leadership needs to be seen as an integral part of the role of the nurse, not as an additional activity to be done only when time and energy allow. The promotion of leadership comes at every stage of professional development and needs to be seen as a philosophical approach in terms of professional activity.

Partnership working

Section 31 of the NHS Act 1999 (DoH 1999b) has had a significant impact on the ability of service providers to pool resources for specific health and social care activity. Underpinned by a series of National Service Frameworks the trend and impetus within partnership working are set to become a key feature of professional life for many nurses. Multidisciplinary working is a key feature of all professional life within the NHS and other service provision; the real change is that nurses now have the means and the political drive to 'join up' approaches to service delivery. A key example comes from care management systems proposed under the learning disability strategy *Valuing People* (DoH 2001c). The opportunity to work with others as equal partners will impact upon the culture and confidence of the nursing profession into the future. To be equipped for such developments the repertoire of skills possessed will be augmented and developed. There are already leadership programmes where a key component is negotiation, such as The Royal College of Nursing Leadership Programme 2001. Skills of negotiation go hand in hand with the development of the role of professional advocate. Much has been debated about the role of the nurse as an advocate, suggesting that a nurse cannot be a true advocate for a patient or client. Within the newly emerging professional roles where partnership working is key, keeping clients' needs in focus is an increasingly sophisticated role for the nurse, as balancing the need for multidisciplinary working and getting the job done can leave the service user out of the equation.

Putting service users and their families at the centre of professional activity

Working with users and carers is a concept central to the modernisation agenda. Enshrined within the agenda is a demand that health care professionals treat service users and their families as equal partners in the care process.

The creative challenge

Twigg & Atkin (1994) expand upon early work with service users and reiterate that the care process inevitably leads to an imbalance of power within the professional relationship with patients and families. They describe how carers are often seen as co-clients in the process and that the views of both groups remain sadly neglected.

The advent of the Internet and access to information regarding the specific pathology of the patient means that patients often have a greater understanding of the condition than nurses credit. In some areas of care delivery the use of direct payment, for example the National Service Framework for Older People (DoH 2001d) and *Valuing People – A Strategy for People with Learning Disabilities* (DoH 2001c), means that patients, clients and their carers not only have a say but actually will be able to directly commission services.

For nursing, all of these developments represent some real cultural and practice changes and empowerment becomes a central theme. Once again the skills of negotiation come to the fore but linking these to philosophies of service delivery based upon empowerment will not be easy. One of the key challenges for providers of education at pre- and post-registration level is to acknowledge that there is a need to prepare practitioners for this new professional role.

The impact of changes in the regulatory frameworks

In a Department of Health commissioned review of the UKCC in 1997, the review concluded that the UKCC were more concerned with professional development than with the prime function of protecting the public. Davies (2001) takes us through the effects that adverse publicity has had upon other health care professions such as the exposure of the General Medical Council (GMC) to criticism. She argues that failures to protect the public have inevitably led to proposals for reform. The precise nature of these is yet to emerge.

Through the development of clinical governance, it appears that self-regulation has at one stratum become devolved to a local level; however, the general protection issues will lead to the development of a new regulatory framework.

Using evidence-based practice

Davies & Gomm (2000) offer the following evaluation of the challenges presented in using evidence-based practice. They say that

The changing professional role of the nurse

some may find the prospect as being 'practice by protocol', others may see it as impossible but hopefully even more may recognise and adopt the challenge of practising through research insight. However, most of the evidence presented through dissemination systems has to be seen as 'context dependent'. This means that to adopt an evidence-based approach the professional needs to have the skills not only demanded by the exploration of the evidence and research but also well-developed evaluatory skills in order to unpick and apply the evidence. The role of the new professional in nursing is underpinned by a commitment to lifelong learning. Fostered within this concept is a need to acknowledge and update skills in reading, interpreting and evaluating evidence.

The prospects for the development of professional roles through evidence-based practice are enormous, the concept of benchmarking supports such development and the *Essence of Care* (DoH 2001e) package gives some examples of such opportunities in terms of the development of specialist skills and knowledge.

CONCLUSION

The role of every practitioner is evolutionary and a process of learning. One of the key themes of recent developments is the notion of lifelong learning.

Current preparation of all practitioners is not just concerned with the knowledge, skills and attitudes for safe practice but also encourages nurses to think. Thinking is an essential component of creativity and it is through the development of systems where creativity is to be celebrated and not feared that nursing will undergo a professional renaissance. In the creation of a learning culture through the development of a commitment to lifelong learning, people who lead and develop services can foster a philosophy of creativity. Nurses are also taught to be responsible and accountable; factors that in terms of the modern and contemporary professional are essential qualities and attributes that should equip us for the ever-changing world of health care provision.

The development of nursing as a profession has in some ways been evolutionary and at times even revolutionary; nursing has reached a stage of professional maturity in terms of where it sees professional accountability and its role in the delivery of health care. Howeve, nursing is expanding into new and exciting roles and structures are emerging to support the development of creative and positive practice. Nurses as individuals need to grasp the nettle and then collectively contribute to the development of organisations and structures that allow new creative roles to emerge. There is a huge amount of talent and energy in the nursing profession, some of which remains untapped. Using this potential in a positive way will lead nursing through the next stage of professional maturity into a role that is confident, creative and celebrated.

References

Abbott AD 1988 The systems of professions: an essay on the division of expert labour. University of Chicago Press, Chicago

Alaszewski A 2000 Managing risk in community care. Baillière Tindall, Edinburgh

Davies C 1995 Gender and the professional predicament in nursing. Open University Press, Buckingham

Davies C 2001 The demise of professional self regulation – a moment to mourn. In: Lewis G, Gerwitz S, Clarke J (eds) Rethinking social policy. Sage/Open University Press, London

Davies C, Gomm R 2000 Using evidence in health and social care. Sage, London

Davies C, Finley L, Bullman A 2000 Changing practice in health and social care. Sage, London

Department of Education 1998 Opportunity 2000. Stationery Office, London

Department of Health 1972 Report on the Inquiry into Nursing, Chair Asa Briggs. HMSO, London

Department of Health 1995 Greenhalgh Report. HMSO, London

Department of Health 1997 The new NHS: modern, dependable. Department of Health, London

Department of Health 1998 A first class service: quality in the NHS. Department of Health, London

Department of Health 1999a Making a difference – the contribution of nursing, midwifery and health visiting to health care. Department of Health, London

Department of Health 1999b The NHS Act. Department of Health, London

Department of Health 2000 The NHS plan: a plan for reform. Department of Health, London

Department of Health 2001a Care Standards Legislation. Department of Health, London

Department of Health 2001b The modern matron. NHSE Circular HSC 201/10: Implementing the NHS plan – the modern matron. Department of Health, London

Department of Health 2001c Valuing people – a strategy for people with learning disabilities for the 21st century. Department of Health, London

Department of Health 2001d National Service Framework for older people. Department of Health, London

Department of Health 2001e Essence of care: patient focused benchmarking for health care practitioners. Department of Health, London

The changing professional role of the nurse

Dingwall R 1988 An introduction to the social history of nursing. Routledge, London

Flexner A 1960 An autobiography. Simon & Schuster, New York

Ham C 1999 Health policy in Britain, 4th edn. Macmillan, London

Handy CB 1998 Beyond certainty: the changing world of organizations. Harvard Business School, Boston, Massachusetts

Hills J, Ditch J, Glennerster H 1994 Beveridge and social security: an international retrospective. Clarendon, Oxford

Johnson T, Larkin G, Saks M 1995 Health professions and the State in Europe. Routledge, London

Jowett S, Walton I, Payne S 1994 Challenges and change in nurse education: an evaluation of the implementation of Project 2000. NFER, Slough

Melia K 1987 Learning and working – the occupational socialisation of nurses. Tavistock, London

Moloney M 1986 Professionalization of nursing: current issues and trends. Lippincott, Philadelphia

NHSE/CVCP 2001 Good practice in recruitment and retention of nurses. Stationery Office, London

Parker J, Merrylees S 2001 Why become a professional? Presentation to East Yorkshire Learning Disability Institute (EYLDI) Conference, University of Hull

Pavalko R 1971 Sociology of occupations and professions. Peacock, Itasca, Ill., USA

Pearson A 1973 Social work as the privatised solution of public ills. British Journal of Social Work 3(2): 209–227

Roper N, Logan W, Tierney A 2000 The Roper–Logan–Tierney model of nursing based on activities of living. Churchill Livingstone, Edinburgh

Royal College of Nursing 1995 Report on workforce trends. RCN Publications, London

Salvage J 1985 The politics of nursing. Heinemann, London

Stenson K 2001 Crime, control, social policy and liberalisation. In: Lewis G, Gerwitz S, Clarke J (eds) Rethinking social policy. Sage/Open University Press, London

Tingle J 1990 A duty of care. Nursing Times 86(30): 60–61

Topping A 1999 Sapiential authority: a qualitative study examining chief and nurse executives' perception of advanced practice. RCN Research Conference, Edinburgh

Turnbull J 1999 Learning disability nurse – victim or culprit. Journal of Learning Disabilities 4(3):

Twigg J, Atkin K 1994 Carers perceived: policy and practice in informal care. Open University Press, Buckingham

UKCC 1992 Code of professional conduct. UKCC, London

UKCC 1997 Scope in practice. UKCC, London

UKCC 1998 Higher level of practice. UKCC, London

Uttley A 1981 Why social work – a comparison of British and New Zealand studies. British Journal of Social Work 11(3): 329–340

Waterlow D 1991 Reproduced by permission in Redfern S, Ross P (eds) (2000) Nursing older people. Churchill Livingstone, Edinburgh

Application 3:1

Ginny Collings

Making a difference with residents instead of for them: a health improvement initiative in Bournemouth

The need for a community-based health improvement project arose following a review of health visiting services in Boscombe, near Bournemouth. As part of the review we, as practitioners, identified the importance of providing a service that linked directly to the expressed needs of local residents. The existing service was based on normative need and professionally led but was having little impact on the health of local residents. Ideas for change were discussed and support was given to consider what changes could be made within current resources.

We started by holding a public consultation day, which was advertised via all agencies and the local evening newspaper and radio station. A leaflet and poster were produced and widely circulated to invite local people to a series of workshops to be held in a local community centre. We hired a healthmobile bus and arranged for it to be located in the local shopping centre from 8.30 am to 4 pm for one day during half-term week when the precinct was busy with local families. The day was supported by staff from local, statutory and voluntary agencies, including:

- two healthmobile employees
- three health visitors
- one community development officer
- four complementary therapists
- four midwives
- three local residents
- two community nurses
- the community arts manager

Six Steps to **Effective Management**

- an area manager for community nursing
- three students
- two health promotion specialists
- one professional footballer
- three local businessmen.

Of those who visited the bus, 340 received direct consultations from staff, a leaflet inviting them to attend community workshops and a questionnaire asking them what could be provided in the area to improve their health and well-being (84 completed questionnaires were returned on the day). Around 60 children were asked about their health and 30 entered a competition based around healthy eating.

There was wide public support for the idea of a healthy living centre to give people a chance to be involved in their own health and the health of their community. Ideas given on the day about health needs of local people included:

- affordable healthy eating choices
- help with losing weight and staying fit
- activity/exercise for the elderly
- child care support
- targeting the problems associated with social isolation
- alternatives to existing health care.

With support from line management, attempts were then made to set up a multiagency steering group. This was a difficult phase and we soon found ourselves in a political jungle and becoming rapidly aware of the many different agendas. Discouraging months were to follow with meetings and discussions about a healthy living centre for the area that offered a wide range of facilities. Around this time the area was designated a public health action area and a management committee was formed but it still felt as though we were going round in circles as various agencies battled over power bases, priorities and political agendas. When a lead agency was appointed to head up the healthy living centre bid we decided to pull out and concentrate on the services local people had said they wanted, reasoning that if some facilities were set up in response to expressed needs, public confidence would be encouraged and we would be seen to be doing something in response to our public consultation day.

UNIVERSITY INVOLVEMENT AND THE BOSCOMBE TEAM

At this stage the Institute of Health and Community Studies (IHCS) at Bournemouth University became interested in our work and aware of our frustrations. They offered to support three health visitors working as project coordinators over three sites: Boscombe, Townsend and West Howe (Boscombe and West Howe are public health action areas). They also gave us practical support with office equipment and administrative help as well as advice and research support.

Bournemouth University joined forces with the local communities in these three areas to develop a successful, innovative health improvement programme. Bournemouth University (IHCS) and Bournemouth Primary Care Trust jointly fund the project which has also gained the backing of regional interprofessional education funds as well as human and physical resources provided by local stakeholders. It is also central to the healthy living centre bid in this area, which has now been successful.

The Boscombe team is made up of residents, volunteers, university staff, local family workers, private business staff and statutory agency representatives. The project is based on health improvement through empowerment, community development and social inclusion. The work combines research, education and practice development. It targets local health needs and service priorities. The project contributes to health improvement work in the following areas:

- public health action to build capacity and support social inclusion
- the needs of children and vulnerable young people
- family health
- mental health
- coronary heart disease prevention.

The project has many strengths, not least of which is its multiprofessional approach and its provision of student placements for a variety of disciplines (nursing, social work, community development). The project provides community-based learning opportunities for students via a multidisciplinary arena for experience and application of theory. The students gain experience of working with local agencies and private business and have the opportunity to work alongside residents to develop the project further.

Everyone involved in the project has a shared vision of how to improve the health of local people, particularly those living in deprived areas. This vision is underpinned by the recommendations within the Acheson Report (1998) which addressed inequalities and poverty in relation to health. The project was designed in response to the weight of scientific evidence which supports a socioeconomic explanation of health inequalities. This evidence traces the roots of ill health to factors such as education, income and employment and the material environment as well as lifestyle.

The three project coordinators also practise as health visitors within their localities which has given them an intimate knowledge of the community and the issues that affect health. It also enables the project to gain the most from their strong existing professional networks.

Making a difference with residents instead of for them

Six Steps to **Effective Management**

The project has several research projects attached to it and benefits from the university's support. There are currently three studies being undertaken in Boscombe: an investigation of older people's eating habits while living at home, partnership working to prevent coronary heart disease, and an evaluation of the exercise component of the project itself.

The project currently offers various services for local residents as outlined in Box 3.1.1.

THE EXERCISE GROUP

The 'Bums and Tums' group was set up in response to local residents, requests for cheap, accessible exercise opportunities with crèche facilities. Sessions are held in the local community centre. They are suitable for all levels and cost £1 per session, which includes crèche provision. Two local residents who trained to be instructors are now confidently running and developing the classes and four others have been involved in the session as administrative support workers.

The sessions are fun and informal and health professionals are available for advice and support. Residents have found them to be socially rewarding and an opportunity to get physically fit. The crèche, run by social service-supported workers, caters for children aged between a few weeks and 5 years. Comments about the 'Bums and Tums' sessions from local residents and from one of the instructors can be found in Boxes 3.1.2 and 3.1.3 respectively.

FAMILY LUNCH

Access to cheap, healthy food was one of the priorities highlighted by residents during the public consultation day in October 1997. The first planning meeting for the food project held in July 1999 comprised health visitors, family workers, a local restaurant owner,

---

Box 3.1.1 Services for local residents

- Easily accessible exercise and crèche facilities for local families (the cost is £1 per session)
- A weekly lunch provision with opportunities to learn new skills and access cheap, healthy food
- Involvement with the planning for a 'walk-in advice centre' and the development of a community information newsletter to meet the needs of local residents
- A variety of specialist skills in public health, child and family health, education and research

Box 3.1.2 What local residents say

- To be honest 2 years ago I never imagined that I would have the opportunity to exercise that I have today. This is all thanks to the 'Bums and Tums' classes that I began when they started in Spring 1999. To explain my situation, I am a very busy mum who looks after two young children aged 4 years and 18 months and also works 22 hours a week, mainly in the afternoons. I can't drive and have no family living in Bournemouth who can watch the children or give me 'some time for myself'. The classes began at an ideal time for me, my daughter was just 4 months old and I was ready to tone up my now flabby muscles.

- My child care is split between myself and my husband meaning that as soon as he comes in from work I have to leave to start my shift, subsequently the only way I would be able to exercise would be if the classes provided a crèche. Secondly as I am unable to drive, the classes would need to be within walking distance or else I would be looking at a dreaded bus journey! Finally the classes would need to operate within an affordable budget. With a young family we simply can't afford the luxury of expensive health clubs.

- 'Bums and Tums' fulfilled all these criteria for just a pound. It gives me the opportunity to exercise, meet other mums and give me a well-earned break away from the kids! It has also been a wonderful chance for my children to mix with others and to benefit from the company of other adults. In conclusion today I couldn't imagine life without my weekly 'Bums and Tums' and I feel lucky that in Boscombe we have such a brilliant facility provided for us.

- I began attending 'Bums and Tums' because I had been to aerobics previously and had enjoyed the class. I was told about the classes by my health visitor and realised that it would also be an opportunity to put my son Tai in the free crèche for an hour and have some time to do something for me. It also gave me the chance to meet other mums, which was what I needed. I thoroughly enjoyed the classes and it gave me something to look forward to every Friday, as it was the only real time I had for me. When the classes expanded to both Wednesday and Friday I began attending twice weekly.

dieticians and residents. A draft for consultation highlighting the rationale of the project together with aims and proposed method was considered, with the Boscombe Family Drop In being proposed as a venue. Subsequent meetings were arranged with families to find out their views. It was agreed to start a lunch club in October 1999

Making a difference with residents instead of for them

> **Box 3.1.3** What the resident instructor says
>
> ● After a year I was approached about training to be an instructor and I jumped at the chance. Not just for the chance to teach, but also to give something back to the group of people that had given me so much. Since starting at 'Bums and Tums' I have changed as a person. I have gained in confidence immensely and it has helped me learn to communicate with people, which I found so hard before. I now teach the Wednesday class and I have found so much support and encouragement from everyone and I feel truly close to everyone. It is such a relaxed and comfortable atmosphere that people can come along and not feel self-conscious because it's not a room full of skinny women in leotards. We are normal women who just want to keep fit and live a healthier lifestyle. My fitness has improved immensely and I can relay that back to the women that when I first attended I could do about five sit-ups and now I'm teaching the class. I believe that it has benefited me greatly. I love it and it's more than just an aerobics class to me.

charging £1 for a meal with children eating free. The first lunch saw 18 adults and 14 children enjoying a delicious meal ably cooked by our volunteer chef assisted by residents. Since then we have continued to provide a wholesome cheap lunch that can be replicated by families and on average 12 families sit down together with family workers, health visitors, students and researchers. There have been opportunities to learn more about food hygiene, nutrition and organisation. Various topics have been raised over mealtimes such as faddy eaters, food allergies, temper tantrums as well as housing, relationship difficulties and coping with stress. The project has potential to contribute to the needs of some local families as a learning tool but also as a provision of cheap healthy food. There is the opportunity to enjoy a family setting around the meal table as well as learn new skills and increase confidence with food preparation. Three residents have just successfully completed a basic food hygiene certificate with the local Environmental Health Officer using the lunch preparation as a learning base.

OASIS

In November 1999 an 'information and advice' group was set up as part of the healthy living centre bid to concentrate specifically on investigating the information and advice needs of the local community. OASIS (One Stop Access to Support and Information Services) will provide information resources under one roof and offer a range of information, advice and advocacy services to improve quality of life/health and well-being of the community. The multiagency team continues to meet on a regular basis and some funding has already been secured. It is planned to have students from the university involved with OASIS.

TEACHING AND LEARNING

The Boscombe Project has been able to make contributions to the teaching programmes at local family centres and university as well as having the opportunity to present at conferences with local residents. Working alongside residents has meant that we have been able to identify learning needs and facilitate opportunities. Residents have asked advice on training prospects and volunteering opportunities and we have been able to supply information about local courses and support them through these. Two residents have trained to be 'exercise-to-music' instructors after attending a course run by the YMCA, which incorporated first aid and included cardiopulmonary resuscitation training. The project supported them financially by accessing funds from various agencies and with child minding arrangements, support, advice and encouragement. Two more residents have been involved in administration support and have gained confidence in basic skills of organisation and preparation for the exercise class. One of these residents has developed her confidence and self-esteem through working with us and is now taking a certificate in welfare studies on the links between postnatal depression and exercise. We have a male chef working with the lunch project. He is a local resident and churchworker and has been a tremendous support to the work.

FUTURE DEVELOPMENT PLANS

In the future the project team is aiming to gain physical space for their work which includes space to provide exercise and nutritional facilities to the local communities in these three areas. We aim to offer opportunities for local residents to be involved in service planning and development and to continue to consider what will make a positive difference in people's lives and how we can help to make it happen. However, our main focus for the project will remain exploiting this chance to be proactive and reflective and really working in partnership with residents.

Reference

Acheson D (chair) 1998 An independent inquiry into inequalities in health: a report. Stationery Office, London

Making a difference with residents instead of for them

Application **3:2**

Sally Patrick

The Slough Walk-in Centre: an example of autonomy in nursing practice

Today is a very exciting time to be a member of the nursing profession. There are an increasing number of innovative projects extending the nurse's role. These projects are moving boundaries and questioning traditional roles; the walk-in centres are leading the way.

The prime minister, Tony Blair, announced the plan to introduce primary care walk-in centres on 13 April 1999. They were to be 'nurse led and to deliver convenient, accessible services that respond to modern lifestyles'.

As project manager/lead nurse of the Slough NHS Walk-in Centre I have taken on many roles during the last year. I have project managed a new service and been in sole charge of the budget for the building, purchasing of equipment, installation of systems and employment of staff, both nursing and administrative. Building networks and establishing relationships have also been part of my remit and I have been responsible for all clinical aspects within the Walk-in Centre (WiC).

Slough was chosen as a site for a WiC because of its shortage of GPs – at the last count ten whole time equivalent (wte) posts – and also a 50% vacancy rate of district nurses. None of the GPs is accepting patients on to their lists and therefore all patients are being allocated by the local primary care agency. Slough has a 40% ethnic population and an increasing number of asylum seekers.

I first heard that Slough had been successful in its bid for a WiC at the end of 1999 while managing a drop-in medical centre for university students in Oxford. Prior to this I had worked in general practice for 10 years and had successfully obtained my BSc(Hons) in Health Studies and Nurse Practitioner Diploma at the Royal College of

Nursing. I was appointed to the post of project leader in April 2000 with the remit that the WiC was due to open in 3 months.

PROJECT MANAGEMENT

My role was ill defined when I took up the post and I found that there was really only me to push the project forward. I was named the budget holder and it was my responsibility to ensure that the WiC was delivered within budget.

I had a copy of the Department of Health's guidelines to set up a WiC, including minimum standards, and this was to be my bible. A joint development group had been formed prior to my appointment; this had been meeting regularly to try to formulate what the WiC would do. It soon became clear that if the Slough facility had any chance of opening on time we needed to stick with the NHS Executive's minimum services list for a WiC.

BUILDING

The Chest Clinic premises at Upton Hospital had been allocated for the project and, along with the WiC, a GP practice and a walk-in dentist were to be co-located. The Chest Clinic, however, was not due to relocate until the beginning of June, less than 1 month before we opened! Hence it was necessary to start some of the building work while they were still in situ. This took place at weekends while they were closed. During May 2000 the GP practice pulled out of the project, which enabled me to enlarge the space for the WiC and to push for greater disabled access and improved conditions for the nurses.

RECRUITMENT

As part of a pilot our opening hours had been determined by the Department of Health and were 0700–2200 hours on weekdays and 0900–2200 hours at weekends and on bank holidays.

We had estimated a maximum of 97 visitors per day, so excluding myself 6.2 wte nurses had been budgeted for. This would allow for two nurses per shift and one nurse working 1100–1900 hours to cover for breaks.

The first round of interviewing was very disappointing and only two wte nurses were appointed. This would not allow the WiC to open at the beginning of July. After consultation with the Primary Care Group, Community Health Trust and the South East Regional Office of the NHS the opening was delayed by 2 months to the beginning of September 2000. Again this enabled me to push for improved accommodation.

The second round of interviewing was far more successful and another 4.2 wte nurses were appointed. Two were qualified emergency nurse practitioners; the others were experienced A&E and practice nurses. Experience was imperative as nurses employed at the WiC would be working as autonomous practitioners and had to be aware of their limitations as well as their capabilities.

WiCs were planned as nurse-led services but to keep the GPs on board it had been decided to have a GP on site from 1900–2200 hours on weekdays and 1400–1800 hours at weekends. These GPs were supplied by the local out-of-hours (OOH) cooperative and employed by the WiC. These doctors would see only those patients whom the nurses were unable to deal with and who were not registered with a local GP.

The GPs stayed for 3 months and during that time saw only 13 patients. After the GPs left the WiC established stronger working relationships with the local surgeries and the out-of-hours cooperatives.

PATIENT GROUP DIRECTIONS

In August 2000 modification and amendments were made to the Medicines Act 1968 and Patient Group Directions (PGDs) became legal. This meant that nurses and other named health professionals could administer and supply medications without having formal prescribing qualifications.

I believed that if the WiC was to be successful it would be necessary to have certain PGDs in place to complete consultations or lose our patients to other health providers. The Trust pharmacy was very short staffed and an independent consultant pharmacist was employed to produce the PGDs. These can be found on the Internet as an example of good practice (http://www.groupprotocols.org.uk).

The Drugs and Therapeutics Committee approved all of the PGDs and those for antibiotics were agreed by a microbiologist. A comprehensive list of possible treatments for the most common presenting complaints (infections of throat, ear, eye, skin and urinary tract) was drawn up. Emergency contraception was another important PGD as Slough has the highest rate of teenage pregnancy in Berkshire. The opening hours of the WiC would make emergency contraception more accessible. We now have 40 such PGDs in operation.

The WiC is situated at the entrance to an old community hospital in a deprived area of Slough with very little security. After consultation with the local police force I decided that the strongest pain relief to be kept on site would be ibuprofen 400 mg.

Strategically placed on the outside walls of the WiC are signs indicating that nothing stronger than aspirin is kept in the building. This has, I believe, stopped any undue attention from the local narcotic abusing population.

SYSTEMS – COMPUTERISED RECORDS AND THE PAPERLESS OFFICE

The WiC team had an information technology (IT) specialist and in consultation with her and our local IT manager we decided to install a system called ADASTRA. This is a very robust system, easy to use and reliable. It enabled us to note the patient's details, a record of the consultation, any medication supplied and to fax the information to the patient's GP at 0200 hours.

In line with Caldicott and the Data Protection Act we have taken all possible precautions to keep the WiC systems secure. We have a 'safe haven' where the fax is kept and it has restricted access. I therefore clean my own office!

RELATIONSHIPS

There had been discussion before opening about what our minimum age for treatment would be. After considerable thought and meeting with other WiCs I decided that our minimum would be 2 years of age. We would see the under-2s and advise but no treatment would be supplied.

I had several meetings with representatives from our local A&E who were sceptical about what the WiC could achieve. A referral protocol was, however, established and numerous other relationships have been formed:

- the local eye unit
- minor injury unit
- orthopaedics
- ear, nose and throat

but direct referrals to specialties are not yet available. Everyone has to go through A&E.

X-ray was available on site but only on weekdays between 0900 and 1700 hours and a radiologist only visited twice a week to read the X-rays. The local A&E had already stated that if anyone needed to be X-rayed then it would be better to send them there as we would not be plastering. We find this works very well as the numbers we refer for X-ray are relatively small and the cost of an on-call radiographer would be prohibitive.

The Slough Walk-in Centre: autonomy in nursing

The local GPs were on the whole not supportive of the idea of a walk-in centre and thought that it would increase their workload as did the GP out-of-hours services.

Links were established with the local pathology department to ensure that they would accept specimens from us. The WiC only requests microbiology specimens and the results are sent both to us and to the patient's GP.

TRAINING

The nursing and administrative staff started work 2 weeks prior to the WiC opening on 4 September 2000. Their induction programme is outlined in Box 3.2.1.

Ten months after opening more than 20 000 patients had been registered. Attendance figures are increasing by approximately 10% per month and in November 2001 more than 3300 patients attended. Our average daily attendance figure is 115.

I am currently recruiting more nurses and administration staff. There is an antenatal clinic once a week. The community mental health team started a weekly clinic for the administering of depot neuroleptic medication in September 2001 and a walk-in dental clinic opened in January 2002.

Our relationship with the GPs and out-of-hours cooperative is improving as they see the benefits of our service. We are getting more referrals and the results, as can be seen above, are distinctly encouraging for the future of both the project in Slough and those around the country.

In September 2001 we went live with a new computer system, the NHS CAS system which has been installed in all the NHS Direct centres. The system needs development to make it suitable for face-to-face consultations as at present it is for telephone triage. However over the next few years it will enable patients to have consistency in the care that they can expect to receive wherever they go for advice.

Box 3.2.1 Induction programme for nursing and administrative staff

- Resuscitation
- Emergency contraception
- Child protection
- Mental health
- Computer training
- Pharmacy
- Drugs and alcohol team
- Clinical governance
- Data protection

The creative challenge

One continuing problem is the recruitment, retention and provision of suitable training for the nursing staff. This is being slowly addressed and hopefully as word spreads about what an exciting and innovative service we are more suitably skilled nurses will want to join us.

The roles that I have performed since coming into post are many and varied. They have made me engage with multidisciplinary agencies and negotiated tasks for which I had no experience or training. It has given me the opportunity to create a service which, although having clear guidelines from the NHS, is unique for Slough. Hopefully it will give the residents, visitors and commuters to Slough a primary care service that is more easily accessed.

I believe that my nursing background and professional development have enabled me to practise autonomously and to be creative in leading the Slough NHS Walk-in Centre.

The Slough Walk-in Centre: autonomy in nursing

Section **Two**

CHANGING RELATIONSHIPS IN HEALTH CARE

OVERVIEW

The focus of this section is on some of the significant changes that involve relationships. There are three main areas addressed: nature and purpose of leadership, negotiating for organisational change and making sense of collaboration.

The chapter written by Ann Ewens on leadership presents a way of managing change and developing people who work in health and social care. Ann examines four models of leadership and makes the important points that leadership models must be constantly expanded and developed, that issues of power need to be differentiated and that influencing policy is a key to leadership.

The associated application addresses points made in leadership literature that educational programmes should reflect reality and student learning should focus on the workplace. The application illustrates how this is addressed in an educational setting where students are helped to unpick and make sense of their own practice.

In Chapter Five Colin Beacock argues that an in-depth exploration of the wider issues that influence the delivery of health care must be addressed. The social culture of the population for which the NHS was originally designed has been transformed. The population at large are better educated and prepared to be partners in care rather than the recipients of a hierarchical dynasty. Ethnic groups are no longer an insignificant minority but are integrated and valued members of our society. The influence of globalisation erases the acceptance of insularity at either a local or a national level. How then are managers and leaders to respond to the evolutionary challenges that are apparent? Negotiation is perceived as a central factor in a number of models designed to link theories to health care practice. These major concepts will be addressed in many of the following chapters.

Application 5.1 focuses upon an initiative within a multiethnic population in East Berkshire. This project illustrates how negotiation can lead to the development of new initiatives, through interdisciplinary collaboration and by working in partnership with community groups in order to promote healthy lifestyles. Prabha Lacey provides the reader with insights into some of the problems encountered, including the length of time and the perseverance required. A significant factor is that as some of the practitioners who were involved moved on the project also developed and moved successfully into a further phase.

In Chapter Six the main theme is collaboration. Elizabeth Howkins engages in a more in-depth evaluation of the strengths and the challenges that may face nurses when developing a collaborative approach to practice. The chapter sets out to make sense of the paradox of collaborative work. On the one hand this is seen as essential for patient-focused care and, on the other, a process that professionals find difficult.

Application 6.1 by Anne Owen provides an example of a project to introduce self-managed, integrated teams within a community health care trust by addressing the process of change as nurses move from being in a group to a team. Some of the difficulties associated with building a team are explored in this practice example. Anne found that professional identity really did matter to nurses and that they found that letting go some traditional roles and adopting new roles painful. Facilitator support is vital to the change process.

Chapter **Four**

The nature and purpose of leadership

Ann Ewens

- Why leadership now?
- What is leadership?
- Styles of leadership
- Styles of leadership – implications for nursing

- Leadership in nursing
- Developing leadership in nursing

OVER VIEW

This chapter on the nature and purpose of leadership comes at a time of great change within the health care system. The 'old order' of the NHS as a highly hierarchical and controlling organisation is reducing. A new organisational culture is emerging based on the development of social networks within and across health and social care (Ferlie & Pettigrew 1996). Social relationships in this new era will be of great importance; people are no longer willing to be told what to do. Professionals and patients wish to participate in decision making about how services are to be organised and delivered. Working in partnership with all stakeholders will be the prominent style of the future.

Managers in the NHS have been primarily concerned with managing resources and maintaining stability (King & Cunningham 1995). This managerialism was the dominant style of the NHS but is no longer suited to the needs of a network-style organisation. The NHS of the future will be based upon cooperation, collaboration and interagency working. The importance of interagency working and partnerships in the future delivery of health and social care means that a more facilitative culture needs to be created. Leadership is aimed at providing this through its focus upon managing change and developing the people who work within health and social care.

INTRODUCTION

This chapter examines the changing model of leadership taking place within the NHS and explores the implications of these changes for nursing. Part 1 explores the issue of why leadership has become a current focus for attention within health care. The NHS is facing some major challenges in the 21st century including demographic, cultural and organisational changes. If the NHS is to rise to these challenges then effective leadership will be needed.

Part 2 considers how the term 'leadership' is understood. Indicators of leadership provide a useful way of recognising leadership when it occurs rather than any one definition. Styles of leadership are then explored in Part 3, including transactional, transformational, renaissance and connective leadership. A shift from the old 'transactional' style of leadership towards styles better suited to a rapidly changing environment will be the key to securing an effective health service in the 21st century.

The implications for nursing of different leadership styles are explored in Part 4. The emphasis in the literature on 'transformational' leadership offers an ideal opportunity for nurse leaders to emerge using already well-developed skills such as the ability to communicate effectively. However, the less well known renaissance and connective styles also have much to offer nursing, particularly in terms of policy development and interprofessional working.

Part 5 explores leadership in nursing, addressing the question: Why will leadership improve patient care? If leaders develop interpersonal relationships involving listening to both patients and staff, nurses will begin to feel respected and valued and respond by providing higher quality care. Finally Part 6 considers the role of management and education in developing leadership in nursing. Managers have a responsibility to create and support a learning organisation, while educators have an opportunity to develop nurse leaders.

PART 1: WHY LEADERSHIP NOW?

The timing of this book is no accident. Health care is facing a number of challenges in the 21st century, all of which will require effective leadership. Good leaders will be needed to help people change and innovate to meet these challenges. Three main challenges are highlighted, all of which have some significance in terms of the development of leadership within health care:

- demographic changes
- cultural changes
- organisational changes.

Demographic changes

The demographic map of the UK in the 21st century shows a marked trend towards an older population (Chapman 1996, Sofarelli & Brown 1998). The significance of this trend is that the demand for health care will rise because older people often require more services (King & Cunningham 1995). As the population ages, this leaves fewer adults of working age who can provide care services, either formally or informally. Recruitment into professional care roles is already under strain and this pressure is likely to increase.

The challenge facing health care, however, is not only how to provide enough services for a 'sicker' and older population but also how to ensure that the older population also means a healthier population (Chapman 1996). This will require the NHS to shift its focus from being a 'sickness' service towards being a 'health' service (King & Cunningham 1995). Successful health care organisations of the future will focus on serving the community through health promotion and illness prevention (Trofino 1993).

The development of different types of service will be required; innovative ways of delivering both primary and secondary health care services must be found. Primary health care can no longer afford to define itself in terms of general practice; a much wider community focus will be needed. Public health and community development will need a greater profile if a healthier population is to become a reality. Health centres must continue to expand in terms of the diversity of services offered. It is no longer feasible to view the GP as the only significant provider of primary health care.

Secondary care services are no longer able to meet demand and every winter hospitals face a new and more urgent 'bed crisis'.

The nature and purpose of leadership

New ways of organising secondary services must be found. Centres will need to be developed where people will come to a 'high-tech' environment for their day surgery and be cared for back at home by the family and primary care services. A&E services will have to be separated from inpatient services with direct access to residential care beds for the elderly and vulnerable.

Changes in how services are to be organised and delivered will require new and creative ways of thinking. People who have vested interests in keeping the status quo will need to be inspired to make changes and adapt to different ways of working. This is particularly the case with professional groups who can often become self-serving and keen to maintain their power bases. Leaders with vision for the development of new services will be essential. These leaders must be able to work with different professional groups, recognising their individual and group needs. Leadership, rather than management, is what will be required because the future will be about managing change.

Cultural changes

The value base of society has changed since the NHS was first set up. Despite the return of a Labour government in 1997 many of the principles of the free market established during the 1980s and 1990s remain and no less so than within the health care environment. Personal choice as an inherent value is now ingrained into the fabric of society. The general public has increasingly become a discerning consumer of health care and people today want to know they are getting high quality care (Chapman 1996, Trofino 1993).

Through the availability of advanced communications systems such as television and computers, people now have a better understanding about their health and their expectations of health care services are greater (King & Cunningham 1995). The challenge for the NHS is to provide patient-focused services that allow for patient choice whilst also offering a high standard of care (Chapman 1996).

Health care professionals will need to accept that users of services will often be better informed about their own care needs and that the main focus for professional activity will be to assist people in making choices from the options available. To achieve this, health care professionals will need to be able to work from a reliable evidence base (Chapman 1996, King & Cunningham 1995) and be able to work in a flexible and dynamic way (Sofarelli & Brown 1998) in partnership with service users (Chapman 1996).

Leadership in this new consumer-orientated environment will be a crucial factor in helping to reorientate the delivery of health care from that of the service provider to the service user. Health care services have in the past been professionally dominated and have often served the needs of the professions rather than the public. For example, from my own district nursing experience in the late 1980s and early 1990s it was not considered a good idea to give a patient a set time for a visit. The district nurses' time was seen to be of greater value than those using the service and the patient was expected to remain indoors and available.

Leaders can, through working ethically and valuing their followers, inspire them to examine and be aware of the value base from which they are working. In the past managers have worked from a different stance more akin to the 'do as I say and not as I do' approach. This has not motivated professionals to provide the best possible care but good leadership has that potential.

Evidence-based practice is a much used term but how professionals change their practice towards this goal is less well articulated. Leadership has a significant role to play. Through supporting and developing followers, a leader can motivate them to take on the responsibility of ensuring that the right thing is done to the right people at the right time.

Furthermore, good leadership can create an environment in which learning is valued and making mistakes are seen by leaders as opportunities to learn (Sofarelli & Brown 1998). This will create an environment where people will take risks, do things differently and be willing to be guided by the hopes and aspirations of the service user.

Organisational changes

Traditionally leadership within the NHS was based upon professional hierarchies and the positions held within the organisation (King & Cunningham 1995, Sofarelli & Brown 1998, Trofino 1993); this was the case until the 1980s.

A review of NHS management by Sir Roy Griffiths (Department of Health and Social Security 1983) introduced general management to the NHS, breaking the monopoly of power held by the professions (Butcher 2000). This challenge to the leadership of the NHS by the professions was seen to be necessary by the government who wished to make some radical changes to how health care was organised. Leadership by the professions was viewed as constraining in that professionals tended to protect their own interests and

The nature and purpose of leadership

resist making changes. In the 1990s general management was used as the method to bring in a 'market' culture to the NHS, making professionals more accountable to consumers (Jones 2000).

However, in the 1990s the desire for a more market-orientated health service led to a competitive culture, far removed from the NHS foundation of equal access to health care for everyone which was not dependent upon income or situation (Jones 2000). The internal market created by the 1990 NHS and Community Care Act and subsequent policy reforms brought with it unequal access to health care. Patients registered with GP fundholders were able to secure services quicker and NHS Trusts found themselves fighting for business rather than working together in a collaborative way. After 18 years of a Conservative government trying with limited success to reform the NHS, the election of a Labour government in May 1997 brought with it an opportunity for a review of the NHS.

The review (DoH 2000) claimed that a return to the old order was not going to meet the new challenges facing the NHS. Likewise, the internal market, having initially shown promise, was inherently weak through its creation of a competitive culture in what should essentially be a public service. It was recognised that the shift taking place towards primary care should continue, with the NHS becoming a 'health' and not an 'illness' service (King & Cunningham 1995). Furthermore, with a strong political mandate to support and improve the health service the importance of the public as health care consumers was apparent.

A 'third way' was envisaged involving a rejection of both the professional dominance of the past and the more recent competitive approach of the market culture (Davies et al 2000). The future vision for the NHS is one of a strong primary care base, supported by a modern secondary care service, not through competition but through collaboration and cooperation. The NHS cannot work alone in tackling health issues. It is now recognised that inter-agency working between health and social care is essential if people are to have their complex care needs met. The key to the future will be the development of social networks (Ferlie & Pettigrew 1996) crossing agency boundaries and the development of working partnerships between professionals and service users and between health and social care.

Effective leadership in this new context is essential. It is no longer possible to rely on the authority of managers to bring about the radical changes that will be needed to realise the vision held for the NHS. While management is primarily concerned with running organisations, it will be leadership that is able to transform and change how health care is delivered (Bowles & Bowles 1999).

Leaders will be needed to form alliances and build partnerships throughout both the health and the social care sector. Leaders with a vision for how new services can be developed will be required if the demographic and cultural challenges outlined earlier are to be met. Leadership is about managing change (Posner & Kouzes 1988) and this will be the key to transforming the health care system.

A role for managers still exists and the service will still need to be organised and run well. Leaders will not necessarily be managers; however, a good manager may well be a leader (King & Cunningham 1995). Leaders will be the ones to determine what services need organising and through leadership this will be done in collaboration and cooperation across different agencies, different professions and with the user at the centre.

PART 2: WHAT IS LEADERSHIP?

In the past no distinction was made between the terms 'manager' and 'leader', both being viewed as synonymous with the other (Trofino 1993). Managers were viewed as the leaders of the NHS and this reflected the strong hierarchical nature of the NHS where power and authority were determined by the position a person held within the organisation. This lack of clarity about leadership, however, is no longer tenable: changes taking place in the NHS have created a new environment requiring management and leadership to be separated out as concepts and understood more clearly (Sofarelli & Brown 1998). Some of the differences between leaders and managers are set out in Box 4.1.

Sofarelli & Brown (1998) state that it is hard to define leadership precisely but that when summing up the differences between managers and leaders they write that managers are concerned with 'legitimate power and control' while in contrast leaders are concerned with 'empowerment'.

Distinctions began to be made between these two different concepts as it was recognised that the NHS was overmanaged but underled (King & Cunningham 1995). The functions of management were identified and seen to be different from that of leadership. The role of managers is to run organisations, while the role of leaders is to make changes (Posner & Kouzes 1988). According to Bennis (1990, p. 18) 'Leaders are people who do the right thing, managers are people who do things right', pointing out the fundamental difference in value base for the two groups.

It is with this in mind that the definition of leadership used in this chapter was chosen. The definitions of leadership are almost

The nature and purpose of leadership

> **Box 4.1** Contrasting the roles of managers and leaders (adapted from Sofarelli & Brown 1998)
>
> | **Role of the manager** | **Role of the leader** |
> | --- | --- |
> | Create stability | Be proactive |
> | Take control | Have integrity, an ethical |
> | Accomplish tasks | approach and sound principles |
> | Possess authority | Thrive on change, challenge the |
> | Hold power from their position | status quo |
> | Plan, organise and control human | Inspire followers |
> | and material resources | Have vision |
> | Enforce policy and procedures | Be willing to take risks |
> | Maintain hierarchical rule | Value people |
> | Put the organisation before | Develop relationships |
> | people | Communicate effectively |
> | | Not hold power through position |
> | | or authority |
> | | Empower others |

limitless (Lancaster 1999) and any decision about which definition is most appealing will be influenced by the beliefs and values held by the selector. For example, if you believe that leadership is an inherent quality born in some people and not others then a definition incorporating the idea of the born leader would seem reasonable. In contrast if you believe that leadership is something that is learnt and can be taught, you would be more likely to settle for a definition relating to the developmental aspects of leadership.

The evidence from studies looking at the idea that leaders are born or that certain personality traits are more likely in leaders does not exist. The idea that leadership is a collection of skills that can be taught and therefore learnt has also not been supported by research (Bowles & Bowles 1999, King & Cunningham 1995). According to Hurst (1997) and Cook (1999), both of whom carried out a literature review of leadership, there is much written on the subject but in the main it is opinion based with very few empirical studies.

Identified indicators that can be used to recognise leaders and leadership have been outlined in the literature. While a list of indicators may fall short of a definition it does provide clarity about what leadership is and what it is not. When an effective leader is recognised, the question is not: 'Is this person born a leader or taught to be a leader' but instead: 'What is it about this person that

Changing relationships in health care

Box 4.2   Indicators of leadership

- Leaders have followers and inspire them
- Leaders have principles and work in an ethical way
- Leaders are highly visible
- Leaders assume responsibility
- Leaders have vision and can communicate their vision
- Leaders thrive on change and are good at problem solving
- Leaders value people and facilitate the development of others

---

makes me know they are a leader?'. The answer to this question lies within the indicators of leadership set out in Box 4.2.

According to Drucker (1996) effective leaders will all behave in the same way and the questions they ask are: 'What needs to be done?' and 'What can and should I do to make a difference?' (Lancaster 1999). Leadership therefore is not about possessing traits or skills but is instead about an 'attitude that informs behaviour' (West-Burnham 1997). This is based upon an interactional view of leadership (King & Cunningham 1995) where leaders and followers are both engaged in a group process. Leaders need followers just as much as followers need a leader; it is a reciprocal relationship. Leaders – through communicating their vision, working in a visible and ethical way and by valuing the people around them – are able to inspire and motivate followers. Followers in response are able to rise to the challenges facing them because they trust and believe in the vision held by their leader.

PART 3: STYLES OF LEADERSHIP

As argued earlier, leadership is best viewed as 'interactional' involving both leaders and followers in a group process. King & Cunningham (1995) claim that this interactional approach can be displayed in two types of leadership: one type concerned with task accomplishment (transactional leadership) and the other with interpersonal relations (transformational leadership). These two leadership styles are the most frequently discussed within the literature (Bass 1985, Burns 1978). However, Cook (1999) in a literature review of leadership spanning UK, USA and Australian databases identifies two further leadership styles: 'renaissance' and 'connective'. Renaissance leadership involves empowerment and influencing health care policy. Connective leadership is the most mature of all styles and is a bridge between the transformational and renaissance styles.

The nature and purpose of leadership

Transactional leadership

In the past the style of leadership adopted within the NHS has not surprisingly reflected the hierarchical nature of the organisation and was based upon a 'transactional' model (Cook 1999). Leadership was viewed as being synonymous with management, no distinction being made between the two different concepts (Sofarelli & Brown 1998).

Transactional leadership involves maintaining the status quo of an organisation (Zaleznik 1977) and was well suited to the young NHS where stability was viewed as an important goal. Through planning, organising and controlling both human and material resources, leaders were able to achieve their primary task of accomplishing the goals of the organisation.

Leaders were expected to lead through the possession of power and authority from their position (Atwater & Bass 1994). Followers responded to the demands of the leader in this scenario in terms of exchange, i.e. services for a salary (King & Cunningham 1995).

Transformational leadership

This style of leadership as identified by Burns (1978) has subsequently been the most discussed within the literature. It is proposed by most contemporary authors in this field that transformational leadership is 'better' than transactional leadership (Alimo-Metcalfe & Alban-Metcalfe 2000, Footit 1999, NHS Executive 1999, Sofarelli & Brown 1998, Trofino 1993). However, Atwater & Bass (1994) warn that transactional leadership can be good in stable conditions, whereas a transformational style can cause disruption because it is aimed at change.

The argument for transformational leadership is strong in the present climate of the NHS. As argued earlier there are a number of challenges facing health care, all of which will require organisations and the people who work in them to undergo significant changes and the NHS Executive (1999) states that transformational leadership will be vital in achieving these changes. In the words of Sofarelli & Brown (1998, p. 203) 'Transformational leadership is a style which is ideally suited to the present climate of change because it actively embraces and encourages innovation and change'.

The indicators of leadership identified earlier in this chapter are taken from the literature about transformational leadership and they point to the interpersonal nature of this leadership style (King & Cunningham 1995). However, Bennis & Nanus (1985) describe four leadership competencies that are both comprehensive and well accepted within the literature:

- management of attention
- management of meaning
- management of trust
- management of self.

Management of attention

This involves the leader having a vision for the future. The leader is able to make connections so that people can see the 'big' picture while dealing with the micro level (McBride 1994). The leader ensures that followers have all the information that is required to help them work towards the shared vision and helps them develop their analytical skills in order to make their own decisions (Sofarelli & Brown 1998).

Management of meaning

The leader must be able to articulate and communicate the vision effectively. As Sofarelli & Brown state: 'To be effective, a leader must fulfil many functions, but one of the most important is the management of meaning and the effective articulation of their dreams to their followers in order to inspire them to accept and be committed to the vision' (1998, p. 204).

Management of trust

A relationship based on trust must be developed between leader and followers. To achieve this the leader must possess integrity, be honest, work ethically, be reliable and be highly visible.

Management of self

Leaders need to possess high self-esteem and have a good deal of self-awareness. This will give them the confidence and ability to encourage others, help them take risks and always be willing to learn. Leaders value learning both for themselves and others, viewing mistakes as opportunities to learn (Sofarelli & Brown 1998).

Transformational leadership is therefore an interactional process between a leader and followers. Its main strengths lie in its focus on the management of change and the empowerment of people within an organisation. The interpersonal relationship between

The nature and purpose of leadership

leader and followers is the key to this style of leadership. The relationship is viewed as collaborative in terms of everyone working towards a shared vision. The leader in this model leads informally by consensus rather than by gaining power and authority through position in the organisation.

Renaissance and connective leadership

Cook (1999) identifies two further styles of leadership in the literature: renaissance and connective. Little is written about either style but both highlight important issues that may be missing in discussions of transformational leadership. Renaissance leadership is a term used by Cook (1999) to describe a renewed interest in nursing leadership within Australia. Cook claims that nursing leadership has been lacking in Australia but that the present climate is one of turbulence and from this leaders are emerging. The focus of this leadership has been on influencing health care policy. Although Cook fails to develop his ideas further the issue of influencing policy is an important one.

Discussion about transformational leadership tends to focus upon the interpersonal relationship between leader and followers. Little attention is given to the issue of power and influence beyond the boundaries of this relationship. Transformational leaders do hold power and influence over their followers, albeit by consensus; however, this does not address the issue of power and influence at the policy-making level. Leaders will need to use persuasion in order to effect change at this level: 'Persuasion requires confidence, collaborative networks and mechanisms to ensure that views are respected by key stakeholders' (Cook 1999, p. 308). Leadership must include the leader having a function in influencing health care decisions at practice and policy level. This does not negate the role of transformational leadership but it will be important as this model is developed, both in the literature and within practice.

Cook (1999) also identifies connective leadership within the American context. This is described as a collaborative and persuasive way of working, with the main focus being upon building networks. Again the focus of the literature about transformational leadership tends to ignore the importance of networks in building alliances between different professional groups. The literature discusses leadership usually within the confines of a particular professional group rather than as an interdisciplinary or multiprofessional activity and the issue of the service user is often neglected. If leaders are to have influence at the policy-making level they will need to be effective at creating networks and working across a number of boundaries.

It is not proposed that either of these styles offers an alternative to transformational leadership but instead that they provide direction for leadership theory to expand and develop. Effective leaders will be transformational in their style but they will need to adopt an outward-looking, all-inclusive approach and not to be solely concerned with the development of their own group of followers.

PART 4: IMPLICATIONS FOR NURSING

The main leadership style experienced by nurses has been the transactional model. Doctors, managers and senior nurses have controlled nurses through the power and authority ascribed to their roles. Atwater & Bass (1994) believe that the transactional model is suited to stable conditions but argue that the current climate is one of change and therefore requires a different approach.

The transactional model has not served nurses well in that it has led to disempowerment and the stifling of innovation. Nurses have not had the opportunity to participate in the development of services; the emphasis has been on them taking a purely service provider role. Nurses with innovative ideas who wish to strive for excellence in patient care rarely found support and encouragement from managers or other colleagues. Instead a culture of 'mediocrity' has existed.

An action research study (Ewens et al 2000) reviewing the progress of community nurses after 1 year in specialist practice found this culture still firmly in place. The study showed the new practitioners felt demotivated and undervalued and the practice environment to be stressful and full of conflict. Nursing colleagues and managers had not provided them with support and encouragement for their new ideas but had instead felt threatened by them. During the study the new practitioners, senior community nurses and managers all talked about the practice culture being resistant to change and the prevailing view was one of 'keeping your head down'.

This lack of support and encouragement for nurses is symptomatic of an organisation run without effective leadership. The focus has been on running the organisation and getting the tasks done whilst ignoring the main resource – the people who work in it. Nurses are the single largest professional group working within the NHS and therefore constitute an enormous potential resource for improving and developing services. An organisation such as

The nature and purpose of leadership

the NHS which relies on the knowledge, skills and attitudes of its staff to provide high quality patient care is not ideally suited to the transactional model as its main leadership style.

Redfern (1999) warns that nursing criticises itself for lacking leadership but when leaders arise there is a tendency to go against their vision. For example, there has been a mixed response to the introduction of nurse consultant posts but innovations such as these should be viewed as opportunities (Bowles & Bowles 1999, Redfern 1999). The cynicism displayed by nurses and the lack of support given to nurses with a vision stem from working in a hierarchical organisation which made it difficult for nurses to gain confidence in decision making and to assert themselves (Trofino 1993), leaving nurses feeling disempowered and unable to support each other.

Transformational leadership offers an opportunity for nurses to break free from this negative approach, empowering them (Footit 1999) and lifting them to a higher level of motivation (King & Cunningham 1995). Despite the fact that nurses have had little experience of transformational leadership, as a professional group they are well placed to respond to the interpersonal nature of this style (Sofarelli & Brown 1998). Nurses exhibit leadership skills daily in their professional roles (King & Cunningham 1995, Salvage 1999) but strong clinical leadership has not been translated into organisational leadership. While nurses have been comfortable with their relationships with patients and other nurses this has not been the case within interdisciplinary teams or organisations (Dean-Baar 1998).

Transformational leadership offers nurses an opportunity to use professional skills such as communication and caring because the focus is upon the interpersonal relationship between leader and followers. Additionally Sofarelli & Brown (1998) state that nursing is an ethical profession and that the transformational leadership style is congruent with this. Nurses however need to believe in themselves and their own power (Dean-Baar 1998) in order to take on this style of leadership.

Transformational leadership is primarily concerned with the management of change (Sofarelli & Brown 1998) and nursing has experienced many changes (Chapman 1996, Cox 1996). Radical shifts have taken place within nurse education over the past decade and modern nursing practice is very different from that of the past, including considerable role expansion and increased autonomy (King & Cunningham 1995). Nurses must use the skills they already possess to bring their vision for the NHS into view and transformational leadership offers nursing an opportunity to do just this.

Changing relationships in health care

Leadership is about more than just relationship building and will involve nurses in developing strategies to influence decisions made at all levels in the organisation. If effective leadership is to emerge within nursing then there must be a commitment by the NHS towards accepting the contribution nursing can make at both practice and policy-making level (Legg 1996); likewise nurses must recognise their role beyond direct patient care.

The NHS has not been conducive to the progress of nursing, with nurses having experienced both gender and professional power struggles within the organisation (Dean 1996). The leadership literature has tended to ignore the issue of gender and when discussed has pointed to the different leadership styles adopted by men and women (Cook 1999). Men, it is claimed, adopt a more transactional style while women take on the feminine approach of transformational leadership (Lancaster 1999). Additionally it is proposed that men are seen as managers while leadership is considered a soft skill better suited to women (Wedderburn Tate 1996). At first glance this points to further support for nurses adopting a transformational style. However in the longer term this may allow the NHS to ignore the fundamental imbalance of power between men and women.

In the past nurses have been kept out of positions of power and authority and despite their large numbers have wielded little political influence (Trofino 1993). One consequence of working within a controlling organisation has been to 'disempower' nurses, leaving them an oppressed group. Nurses fear power because of the negative connotations it has for them (Kuokkanen & Leino-Kilpi 2000) and this makes it difficult for nurses to use their power to influence policy decisions. Kuokkanen & Leino-Kilpi (2000) argue that it will be essential for nurses to believe in their own power and state that transformational leadership will facilitate this because it involves an empowering process. Transformational leadership is therefore not a 'feminine' approach but it is a style well suited to liberating the oppressed, the underrepresented and those who feel unheard including nurses and service users. Future development of leadership theory should therefore explore the issue of power and ensure that the empowering process of the transformational model involves helping oppressed groups. A good leader will be someone who does not worry about the 'old boys' holding power but instead has a strategy for 'getting to the table' where decisions are made (Lancaster 1999).

A further limitation of considering leadership within the boundary of an interpersonal relationship between leader and followers is the lack of recognition given to the interprofessional and

The nature and purpose of leadership

interagency nature of service provision. It is essential to recognise the importance of social networks for the future of health care delivery. The connective style as discussed by Cook (1999) recognises the importance of leaders collaborating, persuading and influencing others through the development of networks. As Alimo-Metcalfe & Alban-Metcalfe (2000) state, leadership in the new millennium will involve 'connectedness' which they describe as having a closer sensitivity to the needs of a range of stakeholders both inside and outside of health care. Leaders will be required to work in partnership with others and barriers between agencies must be removed.

Salvage (1999) warns that nurses must not consider themselves as having a monopoly on caring and should be willing to work in partnership. As nurse leaders emerge it is important that they are committed not only to their own group of followers but also to developing networks and partnerships with service users and other professionals from both health and social care.

PART 5: LEADERSHIP IN NURSING

Why will leadership improve patient care? Leadership aims to improve patient care via a cohesive workforce (Malby 1997) by focusing on interpersonal relationships between leaders and followers. A key role for leaders is to listen to those around them, to hear what is being said and to turn the hopes and aspirations of others into a shared vision.

Leadership will firstly improve patient care through encouraging others to listen to patients. Leadership is an ethical, empowering process and the leader models a way of working with patients based on their own integrity and principles. Leadership is about helping oppressed groups to be heard and to have their views about how services are organised and delivered respected.

A nurse on a psychiatric ward provided an example of this after listening to a group of inpatients talk about the lack of dignity shown to them by the hospital. Working with the patients the nurse arranged for a 'special' meal to be organised in recognition of the patients' desires to be valued. The meal involved a nicely set table and well-presented food, which was to be served by the qualified staff and health care assistants. The nurse involved had to work hard at persuading managers to release the money involved in providing extra resources. The most challenging aspect was winning the support of the health care assistants who initially resented the idea of any of the staff 'serving' food to the patients. The nurse lis-

Changing relationships in health care

tened to the concerns of the health care assistants, acknowledging their difficulty in making this small yet significant change to their practice. Eventually it was agreed that a 'trial' meal would take place. The patients were very pleased to receive the meal and responded more positively to the ward staff. The health care assistants appreciated the more congenial attitude from the patients towards them. The nurse is now working towards looking at how patients and staff can work together in making the ward environment a better place to be.

Listening to patients is a very important part of providing high quality care but nurses also often feel that the organisation does not listen to or respect them. This has a negative effect upon their ability to provide good care through creating low motivation and poor morale. The culture of an organisation affects those working in it because they tend to model its values. When staff feel that they are not cared for, then they find it difficult to care for patients (Atwater & Bass 1994, Lancaster 1999).

On a recent leadership course one student shared a practice example of how she had left nursing because she did not feel valued and went to work for social services. While working for social services she was provided with supportive, high quality supervision which resulted in her feeling more motivated and respected for her contribution to client care.

Leadership can improve patient care through the development of leaders who will listen and, more importantly, hear what nurses have to say. If the culture of the organisation is not supportive, effective leaders work towards changing the norms (Atwater & Bass 1994). This is difficult because it involves challenging people and making them feel uncomfortable. Providing patient-focused care is often talked about but it is not always recognised how difficult it is to achieve. Change is difficult and challenging, especially when working with demotivated staff (Willis 1999). The introduction of the 'special' meal in the psychiatric ward was an example of how the nurse involved needed to overcome the initial resentment of the health care assistants and other colleagues. Good leaders will encourage their followers to reach for higher goals, will provide better care and will facilitate them in their own professional development.

Nurses enter into the profession to do a good job and provide high quality services. It is the pressures and conflicts within the organisation that often demotivates them. The role of leadership within an organisation is to empower those who work in it, allowing them to get on with the job they wish to do and although employers can influence care, individual nurses have more direct

The nature and purpose of leadership

impact upon how patients are cared for (Cunningham 1997). According to Cook (1999, p. 306) a nurse leader is 'a nurse directly involved in providing clinical care that continuously improves care and influences others'. Good leadership does improve patient care (Cook 1999).

PART 6: DEVELOPING LEADERSHIP IN NURSING

This chapter has argued that effective health care in the 21st century will require leadership. Nursing as the largest professional group has much to offer in terms of future service development. Nurse leaders will have a vital role in ensuring that nursing makes a full contribution towards this venture. Managers and educators involved with nurses are in a position to facilitate the development of nurse leaders who will be able to really change health care positively.

The culture of an organisation has a significant impact upon the working practices of the people in it and the manager has a role to play in creating what is termed a learning organisation (Sofarelli & Brown 1998, Trofino 1993). A learning organisation is one in which innovation and creativity are supported and valued (Alimo-Metcalfe & Alban-Metcalfe 2000) and where leaders are encouraged and allowed to flourish even if this means learning from mistakes (Sofarelli & Brown 1998). Nurses need to be prepared as strategic and critical thinkers (Trofino 1993) and this will only arise within a facilitative culture. Managers can create this culture by being committed to learning and education (Legg 1996) and through providing nurses with information, opportunity and support (Kuokkanen & Leino-Kilpi 2000). Studies have shown that where managers are flexible and willing to delegate power this correlates positively with increased autonomy, job satisfaction and commitment from nurses (Kuokkanen & Leino-Kilpi 2000).

As discussed earlier not all leaders will be managers but a good manager may well be a leader. Good managers are likely to work in a similar way to good leaders and a major aspect of their role will be concerned with the professional development of their staff. The government recognises the value of professional development claiming that this will be the way nurse leaders are created (DoH 1999). Nursing has undergone a radical shift in the training and education of nurses (Chapman 1996) and the move of nurse education into higher education has provided nursing with an appropriate environment for developing leadership (Cook 1999).

Bowles & Bowles (1999) state that educators are faced with a problem about how to support, develop and teach leadership because not enough is known. This neglects the consensus within the literature about transformational leadership. It is well articulated in the literature that leadership is focused on an interpersonal process between leader and followers and involves an empowering process. Nurses as an oppressed group can benefit from an empowering leadership style and this should be the guiding principle for managers and educators when considering professional development.

The liberating nature of higher education with its focus upon critical thinking and reflective practice offers nurses an ideal opportunity to develop both personally and professionally and will result in them feeling more valued (Footit 1999). It is stressful to be a change agent, leadership is not easy and leaders must have high self-esteem and self-awareness if they are to succeed. Higher education provides nurses with an opportunity to explore their beliefs and values and to become self-aware (Cook 1999).

Leadership development will require educators to take on and model the empowering approach of the transformational style. Didactic teaching in large lecture theatres may be able to transfer information about leadership theory to nursing students but this will not be the way nurses become leaders. Educators will need to develop programmes that are consistent with the values inherent in transformational leadership. Students need to experience an environment in which they are valued, inspired, allowed to take risks and required to learn from reflecting upon their own experience. Through this 'matching principle' of education and practice (Ward 1999) nursing students can learn to believe in themselves and their own power and this in turn will facilitate them in achieving the same in their colleagues. Leadership is a process not a product. Nurse leaders will need to be developed over time at all levels of the organisation. Managers and educators have a responsibility to provide the right environment for this development to take place.

CONCLUSION

This chapter has explored the nature and purpose of leadership. It has been argued that the NHS is changing from a hierarchical to a network organisation. A new, more facilitative culture is needed to support the development of partnerships between patients and service providers and between professionals across agency boundaries. Leadership will support this new culture through managing change and developing the people working within health and social care.

The nature and purpose of leadership

A number of changes are taking place that signal the importance of leadership including demographic, cultural and organisational changes. Leadership will facilitate the development of new services and help to turn the NHS from a 'sickness' to a 'health' service. Culturally society has become much more consumer orientated and leadership will support the reorientation of health care to being patient and not professionally led. The new NHS will be based on cooperation, collaboration and interagency working; leadership will enhance this through its focus upon building networks.

Attempts to understand the nature of leadership have failed to find a sole definition of leadership. The consensus within the literature points to support for the transformational model which is seen as an empowering process concerned with the development of an interpersonal relationship between leader and followers.

Four styles of leadership were explored: transactional, transformational, renaissance and connective. Transactional leadership is associated closely with management and leading through power and authority gained from position within the organisation. Transformational leadership is the most discussed in the literature and is considered more appropriate for contemporary health care because of its focus upon the management of change. Renaissance and connective leadership styles address some of the issues neglected in the literature about transformational leadership including the recognition that leadership involves influencing decision making at policy level and building interprofessional and interagency networks.

Nursing as an oppressed group has been marginalised in the past due to the dominant transactional style of leadership adopted in the NHS. Transformational leadership offers nursing an opportunity to take a lead by utilising their well-developed interpersonal skills. However, leadership theory needs to be expanded and developed. Power differentials need to be acknowledged and transformational leadership should be viewed as a style aimed at liberating the oppressed, including nurses and service users. The focus upon the interpersonal relationship between leader and followers needs to be widened to consider the importance of leaders in creating social networks across professions and agencies.

Transformational leaders in nursing will improve patient care through listening to both service users and nurses. When patients and nurses feel respected and valued, both groups will be able to make a full contribution to the development and provision of better services.

Managers and educators will have a significant role to play in facilitating the development of nurse leaders. Managers have responsibility for creating a learning environment within the workplace where creativity and innovation are encouraged. Educators also have a responsibility to provide nurses with a learning environment conducive to the development of creative thinking and innovation. Managers and educators need to match their style of management and teaching to the transformational model. Leaders will emerge when nurses feel valued and inspired to strive for excellence.

References

Alimo-Metcalfe B, Alban-Metcalfe R 2000 Heaven can wait. Health Service Journal October 12: 26–29

Atwater D, Bass BM 1994 Transformational leadership in teams. In: Bass BM, Avolio BS (eds) Improving organisational effectiveness through transformational leadership. Sage, London, pp 48–83

Bass BM 1985 Leadership and performance beyond expectations, 2nd edn. Free Press, New York

Bennis W 1990 Why leaders can't lead. Jossey-Bass, San Francisco

Bennis W, Nanus B 1985 Leaders: the strategies for taking charge. Harper Row, New York

Bowles N, Bowles A 1999 Transformational leadership. Nursing Times Learning Curve 3(8): 2–5

Burns J 1978 Leadership. Harper Collins, New York

Butcher T 2000 The public administration model of welfare delivery. In: Davies C, Finlay L, Bullman A (eds) Changing practice in health and social care. Sage, London, pp 17–29

Chapman G 1996 Leading today for tomorrow: the importance of nursing in the business of health care. Nursing Standard 10(24)(suppl): 3–5

Cook M 1999 Improving care requires leadership in nursing. Nurse Education Today 19: 306–312

Cox C 1996 Understanding leadership: challenges, changes and opportunities. Nursing Standard 10(24)(suppl): 6–7

Cunningham G 1997 Ward leadership. Nursing Standard 12(4): 20–25

Davies C, Finlay L, Bullman A 2000 Changing practice in health and social care. Sage, London

Dean D 1996 Leadership and you: planning for success. Nursing Standard 10(24)(suppl): 12–13

Dean-Baar S 1998 Translating clinical leadership into organisational leadership. Rehabilitation Nursing 23(3): 118

Department of Health 1999 Making a difference: strengthening the nursing, midwifery and health visiting contribution to health and healthcare. Department of Health, London

Department of Health 2000 The NHS plan: a plan for investment, a plan for reform. Department of Health, London

The nature and purpose of leadership

Department of Health and Social Security 1983 National Health Service management inquiry. Griffiths Report. HMSO, London

Drucker P 1996 Foreword. In: Hessenbein F, Goldsmith M, Beckhard R (eds) The leader of the future. Jossey-Bass, San Francisco, pp xi–xv

Ewens A, Howkins E, McClure L 2000 Fit for purpose: does specialist community nurse education prepare nurses for practice? Nurse Education Today 20: 1–9

Ferlie E, Pettigrew A 1996 Managing through networks: some issues and implications for the NHS. British Journal of Management 7: S81–99

Footit B 1999 Leading nurses into the future. Nursing Management 6(2): 23–26

Hurst K 1997 A review of the nursing leadership literature. Leeds Nuffield Institute, University of Leeds

Jones L 2000 Reshaping welfare: voices from the debate. In: Davies C, Finlay L, Bullman A (eds) Changing practice in health and social care. Sage, London, pp 8–16

King K, Cunningham G 1995 Leadership in nursing: more than one way. Nursing Standard 10(12–14): 3–14

Kuokkanen L, Leino-Kilpi H 2000 Power and empowerment in nursing: three theoretical approaches. Journal of Advanced Nursing 31(1): 235–241

Lancaster J 1999 Nursing issues in leading and managing change. Mosby, St Louis

Legg S 1996 The learning profession. Nursing Standard 10(24)(suppl): 10–12

Malby R (ed) 1997 Developing nursing leadership in Europe: a study of nursing leadership needs. King's Fund Management College, London

McBride A 1994 Transformational leadership. Nursing Outlook 42: 284

NHS Executive 1999 Leadership for health: the health authority role. NHS Executive, Leeds

Posner B, Kouzes J 1988 Development and validation of the leadership practices inventory. Educational and Psychological Measurement 48: 483–496

Redfern L 1999 It's tough at the top. Guest Editorial. Nursing Times Learning Curve 3(8): 2

Salvage J 1999 Changing nursing changing times. Nursing Times 93(5): 25–26

Sofarelli D, Brown D 1998 The need for nursing leadership in uncertain times. Journal of Nursing Management 6: 201–207

Trofino J 1993 Transformational leadership: the catalyst for successful change. International Nursing Review 40(6): 179–187

Ward A 1999 The matching principle: designing for process in professional education. Social Work Education 18(2): 161–170

Wedderburn Tate C 1996 Out of the trench: developing nurses' leaders. Nursing Standard 10(24)(suppl): 8–9

West-Burnham J 1997 Leadership for learning – reengineering 'mind sets'. School Leadership and Management 17(2): 231–244

Willis J 1999 Courage to change. Nursing Times 95(21): 2–3

Zaleznik A 1977 Managers and leaders: are they different? Harvard Business Review 3(55): 67–78

Application **4:1**

Ann Ewens and Elizabeth Howkins

The development of a leadership module

In this application a leadership module offered at The University of Reading is examined and the values explicit in the module are considered in terms of helping nurses to develop leadership skills. The interactive learning process that will be explained here was the basis of matching education with the reality of the workplace.

BACKGROUND

The rationale for the development of the Leadership in Health Care Practice module was the rapidly changing context of professional practice. It was recognised that a shift was taking place from traditional concepts of professionalism towards the creation of leaders who can work in creative and innovative ways. The stated aim of the module was to develop clinical leadership skills in nurses, midwives and health visitors who have responsibility for the management, education, development or supervision of others (University of Reading 2000, p. 9). But of equal importance was the implicit aim to help students believe in themselves, their power and their ability to effect change.

DEVELOPING THE MODULE

In creating an educational experience that would help develop leadership skills in the participants our first task was to consider what we both understood by the term leadership and what we knew from the literature in this field. We established that the most essential aspect of leadership was the interpersonal nature of the relationship where leaders develop themselves and their followers. We also recognised the negative effects of the traditional hierarchical style of leadership so often experienced by nurses. To address this aspect we decided to create a positive learning experience for the students, based on transformational leadership.

Our next step was to consider how we could translate the literature about transformational leadership into a lived experience for our students. Transformational leadership involves an interpersonal process. The leader establishes trust and respect from followers through working in an open and honest way, sharing information and by valuing them. We agreed that the module would focus upon process and not content. Many educational programmes start with what needs to be taught rather than what the students want to learn. Having established the need to concentrate on the learning process we set out some principles and student-led course outcomes that would ensure that our teaching approach reflected that of transformational leadership.

Principles

Each member of the module (students and lecturers) will:

● have an opportunity to contribute to how the module is run and what is taught
● have the right to be heard and have these views respected
● give a commitment to attend all the sessions and seek permission from the group for any absence.

This approach meant that unlike other modules the sessions could not be established beforehand. It was important however that the module participants were fully informed about our intentions, so prior to the module commencing a letter was sent welcoming the student to the module, explaining our intention to create a positive interactive learning environment, which would require their full attendance.

Because the main task was to mirror the process of transformational leadership, a format for the sessions was carefully planned, i.e. what would happen, when it would happen and who would be responsible for that part of the session. This tight organisation was considered necessary if the group was to 'gel' quickly and for a trusting relationship to develop.

The first session was different because of the need to establish the group. We started the session with a 'getting to know you' type exercise, followed by both of us setting out the aim of the module and our rationale for the teaching style adopted. We felt it was necessary to be completely open and honest about what the members were to experience.

Changing relationships in health care

To establish the egalitarian ethos embedded in our principles, members of the group (including ourselves) were asked to set out the group rules and to identify what we wanted to achieve. Thereafter we proposed that the format for future sessions should include a formal opening to our meetings, giving people time to tune into the morning's work. We acknowledged that students often rush to a course, then spend the first hour worrying about their children, the ward, the budget and other problems.

We then spent time exploring issues from practice and looking at implications in terms of leadership. After a break for coffee, the next session was on an issue identified by the group. This included a lecture by a guest speaker, or led by one of us. Each meeting was formally closed, giving everyone an opportunity to say how they felt about the session and how they wished the module to progress the following week.

WHAT THE STUDENTS SAID ABOUT THE MODULE

At the end of the module the students said that the whole experience had encouraged their ability to think strategically and to understand how change can be managed. They expressed time and again that their greatest learning was from the 'shared practice' sessions. These sessions were about their practice as it is now; it was real 'warts and all' but by analysing it they were able to identify leadership styles, their roles, their strengths and weaknesses and how changes could be or were made.

They acknowledged that setting up and facilitating adult learning throughout the module was extremely important. Because the learning environment was protected, safe, friendly and encouraging students felt valued and were truly able to learn in a manner that reflected transformational leadership. When asked how they knew they had learned about leadership and themselves, comments included understanding the importance of relationships in the process and not just having the knowledge.

REFLECTIONS ON THE MODULE

The style of teaching adopted for the leadership module provided an opportunity to mirror the values of transformational leadership but also to acknowledge the wider issues of networking and influencing policy which are prominent in other leadership styles.

The development of a leadership module

Our main focus for the module was to get the learning process to reflect the underpinning philosophy of our approach to leadership and let the rest emerge as the group developed and matured. Any concern that the content would be lost to the detriment of the process was ill founded. The students identified really pertinent issues for the taught input, including empowerment, power and authority and teamwork. The majority of the issues addressed in the literature about leadership emerged as a result of jointly planning the programme. The taught sessions addressed issues raised by the students and were therefore always relevant and useful.

The time spent exploring practice proved to be the most highly valued aspect of the module. Students were given an opportunity to have a practice issue analysed by the group. The person bringing the issue to the group gave a brief description of the event but then sat and listened for at least 30 minutes before contributing to the group discussion. One of us acted in a facilitation role for the discussion while the other was able to offer some analysis and explanation of the whole discussion.

Time and again the issues of valuing and respecting staff and of the leader being a highly visible, ethical practitioner were brought into focus. Where things had gone wrong, transformational leadership was seen to be missing. When things had gone well, this was usually due to a leader who had the qualities identified in the transformational leadership literature and was able to influence key people.

Commitment from us was a crucial aspect. Had we not taken our attendance and role as facilitators seriously then we would have lost credibility with the group. The students matched our high expectations of them and ourselves with an increase in motivation and attendance. Anyone wishing to miss a week, including us, needed to gain permission from the group beforehand and in return an effort was made to ensure that the absent member was given written and verbal feedback the next week.

CONCLUSION

Educators can become focused upon delivering programmes without considering the impact their approach has upon students. As educators we found that delivering a leadership module using the values underpinning transformational leadership empowering for both students and ourselves. Instead of concentrating on the content of our teaching it was highly motivating to spend some time thinking creatively about how we could make a difference to the learning experience. Nurses have very often being subjected to controlling environments that have in turn stifled their motivation and enthusiasm. Our vision was to break free from this, by mirroring in the classroom the type of leadership style we wished them to develop.

Evaluation of the module by the students endorsed this approach to learning about leadership and students went away feeling motivated and positive about their nursing roles, feeling that leadership was a reachable goal for them and that they already had many of the abilities of a good leader.

The final activity of the module was the development by the students of a ten-point survival plan for leadership as outlined in Box 4.1.1.

Box 4.1.1 Ten-point survival plan for leadership

1. Vision and the big picture
2. Creativity
3. Reflection
4. Relationships and teamwork
5. Celebration
6. Perspective
7. Momentum
8. Respect
9. Empowering
10. Nurturing

Reference

University of Reading 2000 Master of Arts/Postgraduate Diploma in Health and Nursing Studies. Course handbook 2000/2001, p 9

The development of a leadership module

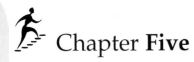

Chapter **Five**

Evolution or revolution: the place of negotiation in organisational change

Colin Beacock

- Drivers of change
- Legal and governmental influences
- Economic and demographic influences
- Sociopsychological influences
- Technological influences
- Organisational cultures
- Health inequalities
- Virtual organisations
- 'Modernising' agenda
- Models for negotiation
- Service democracy

OVERVIEW

This chapter is presented in two parts: the first considers how a range of change factors influence organisations and suggests models for the analysis of change factors in the operating environment of health care organisations; the second describes how these models for analysis can be applied within the context of the current 'modernising' agenda. Concludes by emphasising the potential of negotiation as a means for achieving change and for its use in designing democratic systems of organisational management and development.

INTRODUCTION

The need for negotiation in health and welfare services is born out of the fact that, in a democratic society, wherever change is being

Changing relationships in health care

implemented there will be a number of competing interests at play. The establishment of the NHS offers one example of how contrasting perspectives on a crucial social development gave rise to competing interests. Ham (1999, p. 4) describes how:

> the shape taken by the NHS was the outcome of discussions and compromise between ministers and civil servants on the one hand, and a range of pressure groups on the other. These groups included the medical profession, the organisations representing the hospital service, and the insurance committees with their responsibility for general practitioner services.

When social policy is developed and applied in an atmosphere of competition of this nature, there will always be winners and losers. Given that the NHS was planned as a crucial component of the Welfare State and was key to the postwar recovery of the United Kingdom, it is questionable whether or not such a competitive model of change management is conducive to social policy development. Ham (1999, p. 5) further states that:

> Willocks has shown how, among these groups, the medical profession was the most successful in achieving its objectives, while the organisations representing the hospital service were the least successful. A considerable part too was played by the civil servants and ministers. In turn, all of these interests were influenced by what had gone before. They were not in a position to start from a blank sheet and proceed to design an ideal administrative structure. Thus history, as well as competing interests, may be important in shaping decisions.

If history plays its part in the process of decision making in our services, so does the British political system through its legislative machinery and prevailing political ideologies. As a result, organisations engaged in the provision of welfare in the UK have undergone persistent, if not consistent change since the establishment of the Welfare State in 1948. Commenting upon the nature and effect of political influences on organisational change, Handy (1995, p. 13) considered how:

> Over the last ten years, this process of change has accelerated violently. Under Thatcher and Reagan greed was good . . . but there is a curvilinear logic in the universe. Prosperity can not last forever. Empires and organisations flounder. The world must be reinvented. We can now be certain only of uncertainty. And to plan for the future we must learn to think differently.

Reference to Thatcher and Reagan illustrates the influence which political ideologies, electoral systems and even individual political personalities can exert on welfare organisations and helps identify

Evolution or revolution: the place of negotiation

the place of politics in effecting organisational change. Yet politicians and their ideologies are but one of a range of factors which influence the process of change and thereby the development of policy in organisations of any nature.

This chapter is set against a service in which service users, patients and a variety of provider agencies in both the state and independent sectors have an increasing role to play as stakeholders.

PART 1: KEEPING IT SIMPLE – THE ANALYSIS AND UNDERSTANDING OF CHANGE FACTORS

If one of the tasks of management is to establish meaningful systems of communication in complex services, then those systems need to be simple and understandable. If people involved in health and social care services are to feel that they are partners in change, rather than victims of it, then it is essential that they are able to identify and understand the factors that are driving change in our services. One mechanism that meets the criteria of being simple and understandable – yet meaningful – in the analysis of change factors in organisations is the political, economic, social and technological (PEST) inventory which offers a useful, simple guide for the analysis of the causation of change in the operating environment of organisations.

As a development of this model, Bowman & Asch (1989) identified four main environmental factors that influence organisations:

- legal and governmental influences
- economic and demographic features
- sociopsychological and cultural influences
- technology

and which impact at operational and strategic levels. If negotiation helps to achieve change, analysis of how these factors influence the operating environment can assist organisations in clarifying where change is coming from. If, as Handy (1995) suggested, we could only be certain of uncertainty, it is essential that organisations develop shared visions of their future and their potential in order to survive. It appears necessary for organisations to change and learn at a rate that is at least equivalent to the rate of change in their internal and external environments, if they are to prosper. Analysis of the triggers for change which Bowman & Asch (1989) have established, and their influence upon contemporary services, reveals the complexity of the issues involved.

The rule of the land – legal and governmental influences

Reflection upon recent political history enables an appreciation of how health care organisations have been influenced by these factors. These organisations have been affected by both direct legislation pertaining to health care policy and indirectly through a range of policies that affect the environment within which they operate. The era of Thatcher and Reagan saw the rise of monetarist systems of economic management and a political dogma which gave rise to the introduction of internal markets in the NHS. Whilst the period of government since the Labour victory at the 1997 election has seen a declaration of intent to expunge all trace of markets in health care, many of the vestiges of markets remain into the second term of Labour administration. Indeed, where private finance initiatives are concerned, the concept of private capital in public services appears to be stronger than ever. Reform of the NHS has been a central part of governmental policy and this has directly impacted upon the processes and structures of health care management in the NHS and independent sectors. The 'modernisation' agenda in health and social care has seen a wholesale restructuring of services. The effects of devolution across the UK have further compounded the effects of reform in such a way that there are four distinct, and in some ways separate, policies on reshaping the health and social care services in the countries of the UK. However, whilst the detail and systems of reform vary, the key factors which underpin the reforms, as laid down in the government document *The New NHS: Modern, Dependable* (DoH 1997), included 'partnership'. 'Partnership' is perceived in the modern, dependable NHS to be the means by which professional barriers can be broken down and a more inclusive form of management, which encourages participation by all stakeholders, may be developed. This approach has significant influence over the status and nature of negotiation in the health care system and speaks to a need for greater engagement by all participants in the processes of change. The challenge for managers and all other participants in this process is to produce a mechanism for negotiated change which capitalises upon the perceived benefits of partnership working.

If legislation is generally made by government, then the effects of devolution of authority to tiers of local, regional and national government is bound to have a substantial effect on the legislative process. However, the greater majority of law relating to health services has emerged from common law and has been built upon

Evolution or revolution: the place of negotiation

the case law system. The current development of an increasingly litigious society is having its effect in health care and has led to major change in health care organisations, particularly in terms of risk management and financial planning. Governmental influence is not restricted to pure politics.

Case law has an indirect influence upon the operating environment of a health care organisation, in that the judgement is usually in respect of individuals and organisations outwith the body involved, but creates precedence, which affects it. The effects of policy development across a broad range of governmental departments create similar indirect influences and the need for change in health care organisations. The consequences of shifts in policies for housing, finance, education and transport will create change pressures for health care organisations. In each of these circumstances, there is a need for inclusive forms of negotiation as part of a change management strategy so that the organisation can adopt a more responsive and flexible system and process of operation to meet the pace and volume of change in its operating environment.

Making the world go round – economic and demographic influences

Since the Industrial Revolution, shifts in population and the effects of poverty in society have had an impact upon the development of society and the health of its citizens. Fraser (1973) considers that the Industrial Revolution was relatively successful as a social process because the shift in population from an agrarian society was not accompanied by a rapid rise in population. Consequently, poverty, as a product of this industrialisation, was not as intense as it was in 19th century Ireland, nor in 20th century India. Nonetheless, the relationship between poverty and population shift, as a key demographic change, is exerting influence upon modern health care policy makers, most especially because of the inequalities that have developed at regional, national and global levels. In reviewing the Report of the Working Group on Inequalities in Health (1980), Whitehead (1988) concluded that there were significant health factors which pertained to variations in demographic and economic factors in the UK at that time, as outlined in Box 5.1.

As a factor for creating organisational change and within which to conduct the process of negotiation, economic and demographic factors evolve in themselves. The effects of advances in transport and communications have led to an appreciation of the global context of health care provision. Demographic shifts have established

Changing relationships in health care

> **Box 5.1** Inequalities in health – demographic and economic factors
>
> - Lower occupational groups have been found to experience more illness which is likely to be chronic and incapacitating
> - Owner–occupiers tend to have lower rates of illness and death than local authority housing tenants
> - The unemployed have much poorer health than those with jobs
> - Although women have lower mortality rates than men at all stages of life, there are variables in marital status, employment, presence of children within the home and occupational class within the female population
> - Areas suffering social and material deprivation have been found to have much poorer health profiles and the gap between the health of the rich and that of the poor is greatest in the north

patterns of migration, unforeseen by previous generations, and an awareness of disease patterns and the effects of poverty upon a world-wide scale.

In recent years, the effects of 'globalisation' and the growth of health inequalities between ethnic groups, nations and continents have been of concern to the World Health Organization (WHO). Reflecting upon the present levels of inequality that exist between the developed world and third world countries, the WHO (1999, p. i) considered that it was essential that people had access to health services. The WHO also considered that those services must have the capacity not only to improve the health of the individual but the system by which they are delivered must also be capable of reducing social inequalities, which contribute to ill health.

On the basis of this argument, establishing equitable health care is as important as the setting up of services in themselves. There is an implication that the process of health care, where it recognises the need for equality of opportunity, can have an enabling capacity that inequalities can only serve to impede. There is a correlation, therefore, between the economic benefits derived from the provision of a health care service and the inclusive nature of that service. However, the need to establish more inclusive systems of health care, whereby the process could generate this kind of secondary benefit for the national economy in terms of a healthier population, was impeded by factors described by the WHO (1999, p. 3), including:

- too low an expenditure by governments on health care as a part of gross national product
- distribution of services in most countries is in favour of the 'better-off'

Evolution or revolution: the place of negotiation

- the process of health care delivery is profoundly anti-poor and anti-illiterate.

As a result, inequalities between countries have become accentuated. Opportunities for negotiation are limited when inequalities are so pronounced and the development of an organisational culture appropriate to health care is a secondary consideration in these circumstances. The degree of the inequality currently faced by health care providers is summarised by the WHO (1999, p. 3): 'Unacceptable and growing disparities in health between rich and poor countries, rich and poor people, between women and men, are the main characteristics of human kind at the start of this millennium'.

If there is a place for negotiation in the process of organisational change it is surely most relevant where there is direct conflict. Poverty and inequalities on the scale described by the WHO are sufficient to cause social disruption and even war.

Let there be light: understanding organisational cultures and relationships – sociopsychological and cultural influences

As we become an increasingly multicultural society and a more global community, the impact of the variety of beliefs, attitudes and values that confront our welfare services becomes increasingly complex. Our ability to comprehend the views and beliefs of other ethnic and racial groups is crucial to providing a socially appropriate service. Being sensitive to the cultural needs and aspirations of consumers is only part of the work that needs to be undertaken to produce a system of health care in which negotiation can fulfil its potential for creating and accommodating change. It is essential that the organisation is able to analyse and understand the component parts of its own culture and the values, attitudes and beliefs that exist within its internal systems if it is to anticipate and respond to change in a manner that is truly inclusive. Furthermore, in much the same way that one of the products of equality in health care provision is a societal sense of well-being, understanding the culture of an organisation can help to raise the morale of its workforce through inclusive systems of change management. Whilst not always easy to measure, morale is a very fragile commodity and maintaining high levels of morale is essential if an organisation is to become flexible and adaptable.

The relationship between the various systems and structures of organisations was considered by Homans (1952) who concluded that an organisation is made up of three operating environments:

- the *geographical* environment, i.e. the organisational layout and physical structure of the organisation
- the *technological* environment, i.e. the plant, machinery and skills of the workforce
- the *cultural* environment, i.e. the values, attitudes and beliefs of the employees

each of which could be considered to be of relevance to the development of the organisation in terms of change processes.

Homans (1952) observed that whereas the geographical and technological environments within an organisation were very concrete concepts, organisational culture was an abstract concept and had many variables associated with it. Not least of these variables was what Homans termed the difference between 'formal' and 'informal' cultures. He offered an example: whereas the stated aims, values and vision of the organisation might be encapsulated in a formal company mission statement, the impact of that statement on the attitude of workers on shopfloor might be minimal. This would be especially so if the priorities of the company were not shared by the workforce, where their informal values were geared to individual and small group priorities. This might mean that whereas the company had a formal priority to maximise profits by creating products in the most cost-effective manner, the workers might have an informal priority to maximise individual income and protect employment. Collectivisation and organisation of labour through trades unions allow these two apparently conflicting values to be expressed as separate values of organisations involved in the process of negotiation through a rational system of internal politics. Where no such structures and systems exist, there is the potential for the informal priority of the workforce to become internalised and subsumed into the general culture of the employees. Consequently, the effect is for a distance to grow between the formal management culture of the organisation and the informal values of the workforce, giving rise to an internal political milieu within the organisation, which is neither rational nor productive. Dissonance and disaffection can become the products of conflict when no attempt is made to accommodate or adapt opinion through a process of negotiated change. If the distance in perception between management and workforce is too great there is no opportunity for the members of that workforce to put alternative concepts or formalised proposals. Where consultation is perceived to be a token exercise, there is a strong probability that the informal cultural norms will inform the majority of opinions and attitudes adopted by the workforce. In these circumstances there is little

Evolution or revolution: the place of negotiation

opportunity for managers to influence the thinking of the work-force. They have no prospect of shaping the informal culture through a process of negotiated change, or of achieving collective learning.

If both the internal and external political environments have a major influence in organisational development, and the need is for organisations to seek alternative systems of learning if they are to survive in increasingly complex theatres of operation, what mechanisms and principles might enhance change management?

One way forward is to analyse the constituent parts of the organisational culture, most especially the differing 'formal' and 'informal' elements of that culture. Hofstede (1984) conducted a large-scale study of organisational culture in more than 800 subsidiaries of the computer giant IBM. He identified four crucial and consistent components of organisational cultures, considering them to be cultural features of organisational behaviour and describing them as:

- *Power–distance.* This mechanism described and quantified the interpersonal power and influence of the boss and subordinate, when perceived by the weaker of the two. It was found to be a crucial determinant of how an organisation could promote change and the systems used for enabling growth.
- *Uncertainty avoidance.* Whereas current management theory considers matters of 'risk', Hofstede described the tendency of organisations to try to manage uncertainty by the use of technology, rules and rituals. He found that 'bad' rules may arise out of differences in values between those who made them and those who have to follow them. 'Good' rules could set energies free for further developments and were not perceived as being constraining.
- *Individualism.* The degree to which staff are valued and enabled to act as individuals, accepting responsibility and promoting creative problem solving was found to be determined by a number of features, as well as social norms. Employee educational levels, organisational history and subculture, organisational size and organisation were all found to be key characteristics.
- *Masculinity.* Hofstede found that organisational development, where it stresses openness and expression of emotions, represented a counter-culture in the modern business world of the early 1980s. That world fitted more readily with traditional masculine rather than feminine values. If a more open and expressive form of management is being established by an

organisation, this aspect of organisational behaviour and culture cannot be ignored.

An analysis of organisational characteristics offered by Schein (1986) considered that priorities for consideration in determining organisational culture should include:

- *Observed behavioural regularities within the organisation.* The manners of address and acknowledgement of formal protocols of the organisation were perceived to be of great importance, especially where they give rise to unnecessary bureaucracy or rigidities.
- *Social values and norms of the employees of the organisation.* These are of high relevance where issues of religious belief and personal standards in behaviour are powerful and are informing the thinking of the workforce.
- *Dominant values of the organisation.* This feature is most especially important if it is in direct conflict with the commonly held values and norms of the workforce.
- *Formal philosophy of the organisation.* The respective value of this feature depends upon the degree to which employees and consumers can relate to and respect its stated content. *Arbeit Macht Frei* (work creates freedom) was the stated philosophy of the Auschwitz concentration camp!
- *Informal rules for 'getting on' in the organisation.* The unstated rules by which a person gained promotion or recognition for performance within an organisation were crucial to the development of organisational culture. Corruption and inequality were found to be serious inhibitors to the development of an open, productive organisational culture.
- *Physical layout and environment.* The commitment of the workforce and the nature of their informal culture are affected by the physical layout and aspects of the organisation from which the employee draws immediate benefit. This includes the quality of the working environment, terms and conditions of employment and systems of rewards and remuneration.

Whilst other models exist for the description of behavioural characteristics of organisational culture, those offered by Hofstede and Schein have a relevance based in the reality of everyday work and practice. Any practitioner or manager in health and social care will recognise such behavioural characteristics as: How accepting is the chief executive of the benefits of cultural analysis? What are the informal and formal elements of the organisation that will have to 'come on board' with the idea before it can ever see the light of

Evolution or revolution: the place of negotiation

day? How will you make the project come to life? No matter what the issues concerned, consultation, negotiation and compromise will feature at various stages of the planning and implementation of the project, as they do in almost all aspects of democracy in organisational governance.

If one accepts that Homans has illustrated the fundamental concepts of internal organisational environments, then the works of Hofstede and Schein are probably best utilised, at the individual level, as a tool for determining strategies for implementation of a plan of action. Equally, they also form a system of reference for trying to understand the complexities of external organisations. This is a crucial aspect of organisational management but all the more so when political policies are promoting either direct competition or cooperation through partnership.

Vorschprung durch Technic? – technological influences

As evidenced by the influence of global issues, technology has served to radically alter the operating environment of health care organisations. It has also served to alter the expectations of consumers of health care who are becoming increasingly aware of the potential impact of information technology solutions on the types of service they are offered.

If there has been a revolution in information technology it has come at a price and one of the costs has been registered in terms of the greater inequalities that have been established in global health care. The advances in rich countries have naturally outstripped those of the poor and as access to information for decision making becomes more readily available and as technology-based treatments become ever more advanced, it seems logical that those inequalities will increase in scale. The general trend of growing inequalities is of concern for the United Nations General Assembly (2000, p. 11) who have stated that:

> the unprecedented opportunities opened up by globalisation also need to be harnessed in aid of the eradication of poverty, full employment, inclusion, equity and long-term social progress espoused by the World Summit for Social Development.

In terms of plant, techniques and health care interventions, new technologies have revolutionised working practices in health care. In terms of knowledge management, there are greater opportunities for the sharing of acquired knowledge. If one does not have access to new technologies or the skills to use them, then the effects on personal and organisational performance can be to accentuate the vulnerability of individuals and organisations.

In terms of effecting change in the NHS, *The New NHS: Modern, Dependable* (DoH 1997, p. 20) foresaw some specific developments which could be achieved through the use of information technology (Box 5.2).

The document further states that there will be a set of robust safeguards to ensure confidentiality and privacy. This illustrates one of the ethical dilemmas that can develop when technology advances at a rate that makes it difficult for organisational (or social) policies to keep up. In utilising these forms of technology, there is an ongoing need to gain the acceptance, permission and trust of a range of individuals and groups. This adds to the view that negotiation has to become an increasingly important element of organisational behaviour and that the need for skilled negotiators at all levels of the organisation is an essential part of workforce planning.

Collectively, the political, economic, demographic, cultural, sociopsychological and technological factors that drive change in a modern health care organisation are complex. The means for responding to them can be equally complex and the systems employed by health care organisations in modern societies have become equally complex. Health care organisations depend heavily upon the autonomy of practitioners for maintaining services and must recognise and value that autonomy, if they are to generate a learning culture where change is an integral part of routine function. Henry & Fryer (1995, p. 112) describe how:

Box 5.2   Effecting change through information technology

- Making patient records electronically available when they are needed
- Using the NHSnet and the Internet to bring patients quicker test results, on-line booking of appointments and up-to-date specialist advice
- Enabling accurate information about finance and performance to be available promptly
- Providing knowledge about health, illness and best practice to the public through the Internet and emerging public access media (e.g. digital TV)
- Developing telemedicine to ensure specialist skills are available to all parts of the country

---

Evolution or revolution: the place of negotiation

the postwar years in western culture began to see a trend towards much greater awareness of civil rights, which has imposed itself in all areas of life, not least amongst organisational communities. The emphasis on rights links closely to the notion of autonomy and encourages more participation in and greater responsibility for decision making processes in both the professional and managerial fields. It follows that the same principles of freedom and liberty should apply to any professional group.

In recognising and accepting these principles, it is incumbent upon the organisation to provide mechanisms that can cope with dispersed systems of working where technology has established new ways of working and where the traditional role of the boss as 'overseer' is no longer valued. Handy (1995, p. 211) has no doubt about what is the crucial commodity as organisations become more 'virtual': 'The trust is the rub. Virtual organisations are built on trust. This should be good news, because it is cheaper and more pleasing to trust people than to regulate, control and inspect them'.

Handy (1995) goes on to describe the factors that are crucial to an organisation in which trust is an essential feature of organisational culture, i.e.:

- selection of recruits, their placement and promotion
- how many people can we know well enough to trust? (Handy considers 50 to be the maximum and this must have implications for the size of work units)
- there is an increasing need for members of the organisation to communicate but that meetings do not need to take place in offices or in office time
- common goals, visions and values really matter and there has to be something greater as a target than making invisible shareholders even richer if an organisation is to achieve the trust of its workforce
- trust requires such high levels of commitment and awareness that it is impossible to trust someone who has let you down. If trust fails, regulation and inspection have to be reintroduced.

The more complex the influences which affect change in an organisation, and as that organisation becomes more dispersed and practitioners increasingly autonomous, the greater is the need for trust between stakeholders. What is required, therefore, is a model of change management that recognises and values its dependence upon trust and integrity within the organisation.

PART 2: TAKE YOUR PARTNERS FOR THE WALTZ – LEARNING TO DANCE TO A NEW TUNE

Shifts in political leadership create alternative operational philosophies in nationalised industries, such as health care. These alternative philosophies generate change in both statutory and non-statutory organisations. An example of how shifts in political philosophy affect changes in health care has been the effect of the election of a Labour administration in 1997 after 18 years of Conservative Party governance. Whereas UK working practices and legislation governing the arrangements for labour and workforce resources have been increasingly driven by directives from the EU, health and social care are still primarily driven by central government principles. The effects of UK devolution have served to create alternative perspectives in each of the four countries, but general trends and philosophies in health and social care are consistent with governmental policy.

Whereas political ideology of the recent past has propagated the idea that 'greed was good', contemporary political philosophy appears to be promoting the view that 'a problem shared is a problem halved'. The key to the current directions in management of health and social care in the UK have been guidance and legislation produced in response to 'modernising' strategies in the NHS and social services.

One of the main policy drivers has been the NHS Act 1999 (DETR/DoH Joint Unit 1999) in England, not least Section 31 of that Act, which enables the creation of 'pooled budgets' and lead commissioning by a single agency for the provision of health services that were previously the exclusive responsibility of either the NHS or local authorities. Given that there were few health care services provided by local authorities, the outcome is principally a shift from NHS to local authority management of a range of services for client groups. In trying to determine the underpinning political influence behind this development, one need look no further than the letter to staff-side representatives which accompanied the consultation on the proposed guidance for the enactment of Section 31 of the NHS Act. Entitled 'Modern partnerships for the people', the letter states:

> People want and deserve the best public services, which will protect and improve the health of their families, themselves and their communities. It is the responsibility of Government, local government and the NHS to ensure that those justifiable expectations are

Evolution or revolution: the place of negotiation

met. People care about the quality of the services they get – not how they are delivered or who delivers them. We all need to make sure that service quality does not suffer because of artificial rigidities and barriers within and between service deliverers.

As if to reinforce the point about abolishing artificial barriers and rigidities, the consultation paper had been prepared by the 'Joint Unit' which had been established by the Department of Health and the Department of Environment, Transport and Regions, demonstrating a cooperative structure within the civil service, which had not previously existed. Clearly, political factors within the operating environment are driving services and their management towards an increasing degree of cooperation and consensus. What was being illustrated in the letter from the Joint Unit was a political principle that was developed within the White Paper *The New NHS: Modern, Dependable* (DoH 1997), which laid down six key principles as outlined in Box 5.3.

Evidence of a shift towards a more consensual and inclusive style of management of public institutions is clearly demonstrated within this approach to service strategy development. Furthermore, the process of quality monitoring that will underpin this approach to creating a new NHS, i.e. 'clinical governance', is based upon an inclusive form of management of risk and decision making that depends upon the achievement of negotiated outcomes and accepted change. The subsequent effect upon management styles should produce an organisational culture in which openness, individual accountability and collective responsibility are acknowledged as priorities. Nonetheless, a by-product of these reforms will be restructuring and organisational reconfiguration.

Box 5.3 Six key principles of *The New NHS* (DoH 1997)

- A service which is genuinely 'national' and where inequalities in quality and access are abolished
- Increasing 'localisation' of control and responsibility for services
- The breaking down of organisational barriers and forging stronger links with local authorities to promote 'partnership' working
- Increasing 'efficiency' through cutting bureaucracy and targeting expenditure on patient needs
- Ensuring that 'excellence' was at the centre of decision making across the organisation and that quality of care was a paramount consideration for decision makers
- Increasing openness so that 'public confidence in the NHS could be restored'

Changing relationships in health care

The human elements of the service come to the fore in these circumstances and the means by which mergers and reconfiguration are managed – especially where different agencies with separate cultures, values systems and histories are involved – is crucial to the ultimate success of the emerging organisation.

A systematic approach to achieving negotiated change

In order to capitalise upon the opportunities created by a move to a more open and consensual style of service management, health care organisations need to establish systems which enable learning and promote collective responsibility and individual accountability. If that is to be achieved through an approach which is cost-effective, the processes involved will need to be sustainable and ensure the continuing provision of high quality practitioners, managers and educators. Health and social care organisations will need to adopt organisational development plans which recognise the need for succession planning that promotes positive negotiated change as a central part of formal and informal culture. In so doing, the task of generating leadership is crucial.

To establish systems for generating leadership, an organisation needs to develop clear understanding of its prevailing cultures and relationships and to have identified and explained, with the workforce and stakeholders, the key change factors affecting it. From that baseline a model for democratic communications in a process of change can be developed (Fig. 5.1).

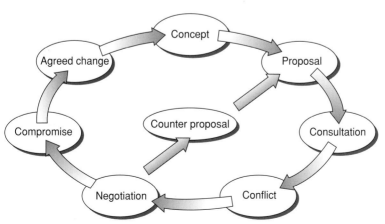

Figure 5.1 Democratic style of organisational change

Evolution or revolution: the place of negotiation

Taking a 'concept' as the initial stage of the change process, this cycle acknowledges that competing interests and triggers for organisational change exist, both within and outwith the organisation. Triggers may arise as a result of external or internal pressures but their effect is formulated as a concept. It is when that concept is offered for consultation across a range of groups with varying, sometimes competing, interests, that conflict arises. At that stage negotiation is the process through which compromise and acceptance can be reached. That may require a new cycle of concept formation to be undertaken and alternative or counter-proposals to be formulated but the ultimate outcome is compromise, agreement and acceptance.

The cycle can only operate effectively and compromise can only be achieved where there is an acceptance of the rights and values of partners in the process, either as practitioners, stakeholders or employees. Commenting on the nature of management in nursing and the products of effective leadership, Manthey (1997) considered that morale is the single most important determinant for the quality of patient care and questioned how nurses treat each other.

Manthey (1997) then went on to describe a model for developing leadership in the nursing workforce (Fig. 5.2). Recognising the fragility of morale in a process of managed change, Manthey suggested that this model can further develop the concept of sustainable, negotiated change whilst enhancing leadership qualities in the health care workforce. The generation of theories and proposals through the articulation of expectations is encouraged, as is negotiation arising from that articulation. In operational terms, adaptation of this approach would build upon models of quality development and monitoring which encourage group discussion and the articulation of views in a non-judgemental environment. Through a process of negotiation, leadership depends upon indi-

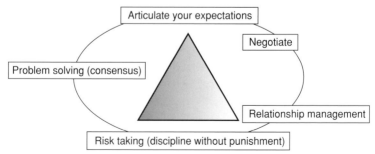

Figure 5.2 Ways of developing leadership capability in the workforce

viduals being able to subscribe to an agreed outcome and an accepted plan of action.

Manthey additionally emphasises the need for relationship management and a system of risk taking which does not utilise punishment as a means of discipline. To promote problem solving and the removal of recrimination or punishment, leadership must be exercised through collective, as well as individual, acceptance of responsibility. Agreements on parameters and ground rules give rise to a form of contract, which acknowledges the expertise and accountability of individuals and can include patients or service users. These characteristics must become part of the organisational culture if members of the organisation are to be enabled to generate new ideas and new ways of working with existing or new problems.

As a final stage, Manthey (1997) suggests that the outcome is a consensual form of problem solving which equates with an agreed and accepted outcome. Furthermore, the model can be cyclical and constitutes a sustainable means for generating leadership characteristics, problem solving and change management through a culturally valued method that utilises negotiation to advance the expectations of consumers and providers.

Whereas negotiation is central to Manthey's model, the nature and purpose of negotiation and its place in management practice require further explanation if that process is to be recognised and valued.

From words to action – negotiation in practice

In seeking to describe negotiation, Kennedy (1992, p. 1) said:

> Negotiation is the process by which we pursue the terms for getting what we want from people who want something from us . . .
>
> Negotiation is a synonym for trading; for exchanging things that we have that others want, for things we want from them. Implicit in every negotiation is the statement 'Give me some of what I want and I will give you some of what you want'.

and went on to suggest that negotiation was but only one means for getting what one wanted and that persuasion, coercion, giving in, problem solving, instruction and arbitration were all equally valid strategies for achieving that goal.

Kennedy (1992, p. 4) suggested that the appropriate times to use negotiation were:

- not always
- when you are given no choice

- when we need the consent of others
- when it is the only way to get what we want
- when the outcome is uncertain
- when the stakes justify our time and effort.

It can be argued that wherever a patient has the right to refuse consent to treatment, the practitioner must negotiate their right to practise. It is essential, therefore, that nurses form close allegiance with consumers of health care if they are to achieve their maximum effect in the process of negotiation. By adopting the role of advocate for patients' rights and by engaging with the process of governance as practitioners, nurses can gain a level of influence that has far greater effect than if they are simply representing their own position. As a means of achieving mutual empowerment, Moloney (1986, p. 302) suggested that:

> How skilful nursing is in developing creative partnerships and interaction with consumers will affect the rapidity with which nursing develops as a profession. To develop interaction, consumers should be kept informed about nursing's contribution to health care, the social significance of its services, and how it has been categorised as a semi-profession, despite its long struggle to achieve professionalism.

From these analyses, it appears evident that the process of negotiation and negotiation skills are regular features of modern nursing practice. In a service where patient empowerment and clinical governance are of ever-increasing importance, the task for managers and practitioners alike is to recognise and harness these features as a part of a change management process.

Adapting Manthey's (1997) work can give rise to a model for negotiated change in health care organisations. To produce long-term benefit, the status and meaning of negotiation must have relevance to all parties involved in the process of care and its management. To achieve this end, the operational methodology depends upon close working relationships between commissioners of services and providers of welfare services and the education and training that supports them. The status and potential of service users, patients, practitioners and managers in a more inclusive system of care, where negotiation gives rise to more dependable and incremental change, is determined by their capacity to generate improving quality and value to the organisation and the society it serves.

Even so, there are situations where the place of negotiation is to assist in overcoming the problems created by organisational change. The benefits of analysis of change factors, understanding

Changing relationships in health care

organisational culture, appreciating personal accountability and acknowledging one's own role in determining the future are put to the severest of tests when merger and reconfiguration proposals are presented. More than any other group in health care, managers have been, and will continue to be, affected by organisational change. Collective consultation and negotiation on the part of employees is the most public form of response to merger proposals in health care services. However, representation of the interests of managerial staff involved in this form of change is characterised by more discreet consultation, whereby the individual may well seek assistance in negotiating their own outcomes, rather than professional representation. In achieving negotiated outcomes for groups and individuals, representatives need to develop a model of reference which recognises the need for negotiated settlement for individuals and groups, and which has application to managers and staff-side representatives (Fig. 5.3).

By enabling workers to understand the issues that relate to themselves and the organisation in which they are employed and then helping them to acknowledge the factors involved, the representative or manager can help employees outline a prioritised set of possible solutions for their problems. Having acknowledged these factors, and building upon personal strengths and opportunities, the affected individuals are able to accept a more proactive role in achieving outcomes through negotiated solutions. By developing an action plan with a range of options, they are enabled to exercise a form of leadership when potentially they are feeling at their most disempowered and vulnerable. As a means for helping a range of stakeholders to contribute to change processes, and to make the fullest responses to consultations, the model is equally adaptable and enabling.

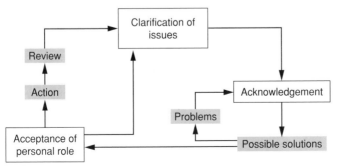

Figure 5.3 Model for assisting employees in merger situations

Evolution or revolution: the place of negotiation

CONCLUSION

Negotiation, then, is far more than simply a mechanism for achieving consensus management or personal goals. It is a mechanism by which to develop leadership skills and to enhance accountability and autonomy in the health and social care services. As a means for achieving sustainable growth and development, the very process of negotiation is an essential component of organisational development, through which shared learning, common understandings and communications can become an established feature of the organisational culture.

As a part of the process of managing change in complex, multi-agency systems of care, negotiation offers an opportunity to create partnerships and shared responsibilities that cannot be achieved through more directive and exclusive systems of management. But it is essential that organisations understand and can recognise the drivers for change which exist in their operating environment and that they develop strategic approaches to working with them. Equally, organisations that do understand the key elements of their own culture can also develop flexible and sustainable change programmes far more readily than those that do not.

References

Bowman C, Asch D 1999 Strategic management. Macmillan, London

Department of Health 1997 The new NHS: modern, dependable. Department of Health, London

Department of Health and Social Security 1980 Inequalities in health: report of a research working group chaired by Sir Douglas Black. HMSO, London

DETR/DoH Joint Unit 1999 Modern partnerships for the people. NHS Act 1999, Section 31: New flexibilities. Consultation document. Stationery Office, London

Fraser D 1973 The evolution of the British Welfare State. Macmillan, London

Ham C 1999 Health policy in Britain, 4th edn. Macmillan, London, p 4

Handy C 1995 Beyond certainty. Hutchinson, London, p 13

Henry C, Fryer N 1995 In: Henry C (ed) Professional ethics and organisational change. Arnold, London, p 112

Hofstede G 1984 Cultures Consequences Sage Publications, London

Homans G 1952 The human group. Churchill, London/Philadelphia

Kennedy G 1992 The perfect negotiation. Arrow, London, pp 1, 4

Manthey M 1997 Creative healthcare management. Workshop presentation, Nuffield Institute/Doncaster Royal Infirmary and Montague Hospital NHS Trust

Changing relationships in health care

Moloney M 1986 Professionalization of nursing – current issues and trends. Lippincott, Philadelphia, p 302

Schein EH 1986 Organisational culture and leadership. Jossey-Bass, San Francisco

United Nations General Assembly 2000 A/ac.235/25. United Nations, Geneva, p 11

Whitehead M 1988 The health divide. In: Townsend P, Davidson N (eds) Inequalities in health. Penguin, London

World Health Organization 1999 Health: a precious asset. World Health Organization, Geneva, pp i, 3

Evolution or revolution: the place of negotiation

Application **5:1**

Prabha Lacey

Setting up an Asian Women's Health Promotion Group in East Berkshire: how health and social care providers worked with service users to provide a service they wanted

This application describes how a multidisciplinary project team set up an Asian Women's Health Promotion Group in a town in East Berkshire. The team used a combination of methods to set up the project, including face-to-face interviews with clients and professionals, observational analysis and use of health promotion theories. Set up in March 1996, the group continues to run.

HOW DIFFERENT AGENCIES CAME TOGETHER

In 1994 six joint locality teams were formed to reflect the local authority structure in Berkshire. Senior managers from the health authority and the Family Health Services Authority (FHSA) were selected to work on the locality teams. Each team was to look at a specific issue relevant to their locality's population using techniques such as health needs assessment and population profiling as well as deprivation scores and socioeconomic profiles of the locality. A comprehensive profile containing aspects of the above data had been prepared for each locality to assist with this process.

118

Changing relationships in health care

COMPOSITION OF THE TEAM AND SELECTING THE PROJECT

This local team was made up of personnel from Berkshire Health Authority, Berkshire FHSA and local social services. The team followed guidance from the Public Health Medicine representative who had experience of health needs assessment, epidemiology and other public health skills. At the first few meetings the team discussed projects that could be realistically handled. It was decided to concentrate efforts on looking at the local ethnic population. At the time of the project (1994) this was the third largest identified ethnic population in Berkshire, the majority of whom were centred in one area of the town and tended to be registered with one local general practitioner who spoke a variety of relevant languages. Once this population had been identified the locality team set about planning how their needs could be met.

A meeting was set up with the local health visitors attached to the surgery to find out their views on this group of the population. The health visitors dealt mainly with the Asian women who attended the baby clinic at the surgery. They had an interpreter who worked with them in the surgery and also accompanied them on their visits. Problems arose with communicating information to the women and it was agreed to look at how this could be addressed.

PILOT SURVEY

The FHSA had funding available to carry out patient satisfaction surveys in a general practice setting. It was decided to carry out a survey of local Asian women who attended this surgery to find out their views on health. A budget for this work was secured from the FHSA and the survey was undertaken in March 1995. A skilled multilingual Asian researcher was employed to interview the women in the surgery and, if they agreed, a subsequent interview was carried out in their home. Of the 20 women contacted, 16 agreed to be involved in discussions at the clinic and, of these, 9 agreed to a further interview in their home. The majority of the women came from Pakistan and all of them spoke Punjabi. The survey found that the majority of women wanted regular provision of health information in a format that they could understand. In addition they also wanted an enhancement of explanation of referrals and diagnosis. As a result of the survey some small changes were made to the surgery, which included the provision of new seating and the purchase of television monitors with a video recorder for the waiting areas. A social worker was also provided to attend the baby clinic to advise and help the clients, using the interpreter with translations.

Setting up an Asian Women's Health Promotion Group

119

NEXT STEPS

Further interviews were carried out with the health visitors and their interpreter and members of the local social services team. These interviews revealed that the health visitors had also undertaken a survey of their Asian client group and had ascertained the health-related topics the women wanted to see provided in a format they could understand. In addition the interpreter was willing to undergo training as a Health Education Council, Look After Yourself (LAY) tutor to provide exercise and health-promotion-related activities for the women. As a result of these findings it was decided to seek funding to provide videos in Punjabi for use in the surgery waiting room and a suitable LAY training course for the interpreter.

SEEKING FUNDING

With the involvement of the local GP and the health visitors, a bid for funding from the Health Authority Joint Development Fund was put together with the aim of providing professional health promotion advice and activities at the surgery and in women's homes. The health visitors and other associated health professionals would organise a diary for health promotion events at the surgery. Different themes identified by the GP and health visitors would be used in association with videos in relevant languages, which would be played in the surgery waiting rooms. A different health promotion topic would be tackled each month. Primary care personnel involved would include the health visitors, practice nurse, the Community Health Promotion Department and the FHSA representative. Evaluation would take the form of follow-up surveys of the women to see if there had been any changes since the last survey undertaken by the locality team in March 1995; for example, had the women noticed any benefits from this service; had the GP seen a reduction in the numbers of patients wanting routine health promotion advice? The project was planned to start in September/October 1995 at a cost of £2000, split as follows:

- £1000 for the LAY training to include travelling and associated costs
- £1000 for audiovisual aids and literature to support the health visitors' programme.

The bid was submitted to the Health Authority in August 1995 but was deferred on the grounds that this service should be available from the local health promotion service. However in September 1995 the Health Authority asked for a brief outline of the benefits of the project to be resubmitted to their committee. The resubmitted proposal cut the cost of the bid to £1500 and this was agreed by the Health Authority in October 1995.

PLANNING THE PROJECT

Twelve videos in Punjabi were purchased to play on the video recorder in the surgery waiting room on topics listed by the health visitors, who arranged for monthly information to be displayed in the surgery to complement the videos. Although details of the LAY courses for the interpreter were obtained from the Health Education Council, due to a change in circumstances the interpreter was unable to undergo LAY training. The project bid was readdressed and the locality team decided to continue to work with the health visitors and social services personnel attached to the surgery to develop the project further.

REVISITING THE PROPOSAL

The Asian Women's Support Group in the area run by social services was heavily oversubscribed with a large waiting list of women wanting to attend. The social services Children and Families Centre (CFC) in the nearby town was interested in setting up a women's group in their area to complement the existing support group. They wanted the new group to be open access and available to women of any age. Following meeting with the CFC the locality team arranged to work jointly with the Centre and the health visitors to set up a local Asian Women's Group. A multidisciplinary project team was formed consisting of:

- two social workers
- two health visitors and their interpreter
- two personnel from the CFC
- one representative from the locality team.

Two members of the project team from the CFC had to leave due to changes in circumstances and were not replaced. However, this did not stop the project from progressing and regular progress reports were provided to the Children and Families Centre.

OBTAINING ADDITIONAL FUNDS

At this time another project under FHSA control finished early and the Health Authority agreed to transfer surplus funds of £600 to this project. In addition the roles of the original locality team changed in

Setting up an Asian Women's Health Promotion Group

that the FHSA member now became part of the Health Authority with a duty to undertake project work in a primary care setting. This meant that it was possible for them to take charge of the project as part of their main duties.

STARTING THE NEW PROPOSAL

At the first project group meeting a start date of 1 March 1996 for the formation of an Asian Women's Health Promotion Group was agreed. Targets that the group would set out to achieve are outlined in Box 5.1.1.

Box 5.1.1 Targets for the formation of an Asian Women's Health Promotion Group

- Provision of health-related information through the use of an interpreter
- A comfortable, women only, community environment for Asian women and their children
- A fixed weekly meeting to take place on a Friday afternoon between 1 pm and 3 pm during term time
- Provision for children to be looked after so that the women would not have any distractions
- Evaluation of the project using observational analysis each week followed up later by a questionnaire

---

Every member of the team was allocated a task to be completed by the next project team meeting. Everything was discussed and actions clearly documented. Subsequently a room was hired in a local parish centre which was within walking distance of the surgery. It was decided to use the parish centre because the entrance was in a separate area away from the church and it was felt this would not offend religious sensitivities. Use of a kitchen was also included in the price. Records were kept of all spending related to the project.

PUBLICITY

The Asian researcher who had undertaken the initial survey was commissioned to design the publicity for the group and the initial designs were tested at the surgery with the women. Using this method was essential to get the women involved in the project and to see it as an extension of the survey. Publicity in the form of posters and leaflets was designed to reflect different styles of dress appropriate to the community and depicted Asian women and children. The women felt happy about the publicity and a final design was agreed. To ensure good cooperation the publicity material was displayed at a full practice meeting for approval, before being colour printed for maximum effect and distributed at various points in the local community. These included the outpatient departments of the local hospital, local schools, local pharmacies, social services offices and local GP surgeries. In addition leaflets were handed out by members of the project team at their work locations and to other colleagues. All these activities were coordinated by the Health Authority representative. Toys for the children to play with and baby changing equipment were also purchased, plus tea and coffee making sundries for use by the group.

GOING LIVE

The project started on 1 March 1996 as planned. Women and children did attend and the atmosphere was informal with no pre-set agenda. Members of the project team who were present asked the women what sort of activities they would like to undertake. It was stressed that these sessions were for their own use and it was up to them to tell the project team what they wanted. The women suggested activities such as dancing, exercising to music, watching Indian films on video and learning about health-related topics.

Using this information, flexible weekly sessions were planned. These took the form of a 30-minute talk by a health professional, with a discussion, followed by leisure activities. The leisure activities usually took the form of singing, dancing to music and playing an Indian drum, which had been purchased for the group. There was no age restriction in order to encourage women to attend with family members. After the group had been established for a few months a supervised crèche was set up. Evaluation was carried out using observation of group behaviour and changes in the group over time. Numbers attending the sessions were also monitored to see if numbers fell or rose over a period of time.

For the first few terms most of the project team members attended the sessions, then a rota was organised. The interpreter was the catalyst at all the meetings, as she was fluent in several languages and was able to mix freely with the women and translate the proceedings for them. In addition she was able to encourage the women to take part in the different activities. It should also be noted that from the very beginning members of the project team who

Setting up an Asian Women's Health Promotion Group

attended the meetings participated with the women in all their activities. This was essential to ensure that they were not seen as onlookers or people trying to tell them what to do.

This method of hands-on activity seemed to work well with the women whose initial fears about the group were soon overcome when they found they could have fun and also learn things at the same time. Some of the women came with their husbands at first so that the project could be checked out. The interpreter and the project team members welcomed any visits and were happy to discuss the group. Using these methods the project soon started to receive publicity and BBC local radio and the local newspapers did interviews about the project. In addition other professionals found out about the group and were keen to use it to put forward their messages. Themes such as domestic violence were discussed with a specialist woman police officer using the interpreter. The local Citizens Advice Bureau also gave a talk about their work and as a result set up a monthly clinic for the women. The local college became aware of the group through one of the publicity posters and recruited women for their English for Speakers of Other Languages (ESOL) course.

EVALUATION

Rigorous evaluation of the project was not possible due to lack of funds. The Health Authority representative carried out weekly observations and noted that the women changed over time and became more relaxed. They also began to participate in the activities and to tell the interpreter what they wanted. Again due to lack of funds it was not possible to monitor the referrals at the surgery to see if the provision of health promotion advice by the GP had been reduced.

CONCLUSION

At the time of writing the project is still in existence. It has received support from the local community trust, social services and the local authority who have provided additional funding to keep the group running. A liaison group has also been set up to coordinate activities through these agencies and the project team, which now consists of the health visitors and the interpreter and two volunteers (formerly from social services and involved with the project from the start). The interpreter (who has now undergone training as a LAY tutor and provides an extremely popular exercise session for the women at the start of the meeting) now runs the weekly sessions. The group has organised social activities such as outings to the river

Changing relationships in health care

and a local wood, a first birthday party and celebrations for various festivals.

The project was able to start due to the presence of an individual who had the time to organise members of the project team without interfering with their current practice. In addition the project team members were all willing to participate in a hands-on way at the group sessions. The women trusted the team members and knew that the environment was safe, confidential and friendly. Women and children of different ages have attended and there appears to be a core group of about 8–10 women who attend regularly.

To make a project such as this work a catalyst is required. The key things to consider are time to undertake research around the idea and committed project workers. If the project workers do not feel enthusiastic about the project it will be difficult to start. The enthusiasm has to be there at the beginning and everyone involved has to feel part of the team. Seeing the women change over time as the group developed was one of the most rewarding factors. They now feel comfortable about expressing themselves and will tell the interpreter what they want to do. In addition they also organise themselves to provide food for the celebrations and for outings. Health promotion messages (e.g. healthy eating and exercise) continue to be delivered. The group is part of the community and has integrated itself into other activities.

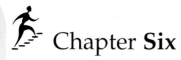

Chapter **Six**

Accepting the surfing challenge: making sense of collaboration

Elizabeth Howkins

- Paradox of collaborative work
- Patient focus on care needs collaborative approach
- Professions find collaborative work difficult
- Collaborative process not an end in itself

- Blurring of professional boundaries, not a generic worker
- Unequal power relationships
- Need to learn skills to work together

OVERVIEW

This chapter sets out to make sense of the paradox of collaborative work: on the one hand seen as essential for patient-focused care and, on the other, a process that professionals find difficult. But professionals have to find a way to manage the paradox. The main focus of the chapter is to examine a variety of issues that explain the nature of collaborative work and present ways to support collaborative practice.

INTRODUCTION

Nurses and other health professionals are expected to work with other professions and agencies to plan and deliver health care. There is nothing new in this, it has been part of health policy and

126

service expectation for 20 years or more. The difference today is that partnership between health and social care has become a priority under the Labour government (Poxton 1999, p. 1). New policies (DoH 2000a) and organisational structures should ensure that cooperation and collaboration become a reality, rather than just rhetoric. In addition there are attempts to change the organisation of nursing, to flatten the traditional hierarchical structure by encouraging teamwork and to move the value base of the NHS from competition to collaboration.

The desire, the need, the imperative for collaborative work can be compared to waves coming up a beach with the incoming tide. The waves keep coming, nothing stops their advance up the beach, no amount of castle building, hole digging or elaborate canal systems can stop their progress to the high tide mark. The incoming tide is something that has to happen, it is part of nature and the oceanic ecological system. The complexity and sophistication of modern health care means that to provide cost-effective and high quality health care, professionals and agencies need to work collaboratively. No one agency can meet the needs of individual patients and clients; like the inevitability of the incoming tide, the requirements for collaboration will continue and increase. By understanding the collaborative process, knowing why it is difficult, why it demands a lot of effort and why there are so few intrinsic rewards should help nurses to make fully informed decisions about their involvement in collaborative work. But to return once more to the metaphor of the incoming tide, nurses could decide to build their castles above the high tide mark and stay isolated in their own discipline; alternatively they could invest in a surfboard and enjoy the challenge of surfing on the incoming waves – perhaps a more challenging option, but they would at least be strategically placed to participate in a shared approach to health care.

However there is a dilemma: the care services need to 'build relationships with professionals in other agencies and teams' (Payne 2000, p. 1) to be in a position to provide a quality service for patients with complex health needs. Although there is a lot of rhetoric about teamwork and collaborative work being a good thing there is little evidence 'to substantiate the view that collaboration leads to an increase in quality of care' (Leathard 1994, p. 7) for patients and service users. Underlying this dilemma is a paradox: collaborative work in health care is an expedient in providing a flexible and responsive service to meet patient needs – but the very people delivering the care, i.e. nurses and other health professionals, find the process 'fraught with difficulties, problems, misunderstanding and conflict' (Howkins 1995, p. 66). Evidence

The surfing challenge: making sense of collaboration

abounds on the reluctance, failure and effort (Pietroni 1992) put into trying to promote collaborative work in the health service. To live with this paradox is unsettling and disturbing, because it means balancing two opposites and would appear at face value to be a recipe for disaster. It is here that Charles Handy's (1994) work on paradoxes is so helpful. He argues that as societies mature, become more complex and more turbulent they in turn have more paradoxes. He says there is no one theory to explain everything, there is no one order, but a need to learn to live with the paradoxes, accept the contradictions, minimise inconsistencies and work with the turbulence. He sums this up nicely in the following words:

> Paradoxes are like the weather, something to be lived with, not solved, the worst aspects mitigated, the best enjoyed and used as clues to the way forward. Paradox has to be accepted, coped with and made sense of, in life, in work, in the community and among nations. (Handy 1994, p. 18)

The intention in this chapter will not, therefore, be to try to resolve the paradox of collaboration but to accept it and to find ways in which health professionals themselves can manage it and learn to surf. Important to the discussion is the acknowledgement that interprofessional collaboration is not an end in itself, but a means to an end. The chapter will explore some of the issues that surround collaborative work, including teamwork and interprofessional education but from the nurses' perspective. The main focus will be to make sense of the paradox of collaboration, to examine the nature and purpose of collaborative work and to find ways to support collaborative practice.

The chapter is in four parts:

1. How past and present policies and traditions have shaped collaboration, including a section on the policy context shaping collaboration.
2. The organisational and professional response, including structures, language differences, unequal power relationships and ideological differences and role confusions.
3. Working together: the concept of collaboration.
4. Education for collaborative practice, including a discussion on interprofessional education and the framework needed to develop the education process necessary for collaborative work.

PART 1: HOW PAST AND PRESENT POLICIES AND TRADITIONS HAVE SHAPED COLLABORATION

The notion of different professionals working together and agencies collaborating in the provision of care is central to health and social care policies (DoH 1997, 1998a,b,c, 1999a, 2000a). The NHS and community reforms have in the last 9 years had a common theme:

● the need for better teamwork at all levels of the social and health care services
● need for integrated care based on partnership
● greater coordination and cooperation between the statutory and voluntary agencies.

The New NHS: Modern, Dependable (DoH 1997) emphasises partnerships across sections, organisations and professional groups working in a new culture of openness and cooperation. Subsequent implementation (NHS Executive 1998) and a public health White Paper (DoH 1998b) support the government's 'third way' in health care, which incorporates the notion of partnership throughout the changes and is driven by performance and quality issues. The six principles underlying the changes (DoH 1998c) are outlined in Box 6.1.

Box 6.1 Six principles underlying *A First Class Service* (DoH 1998c)

● *To renew the NHS as a genuinely national service* – patients will get fair access to consistently high quality, prompt and accessible services across the country.
● *To make the delivery of health care against these new national standards a matter of local responsibility* – local doctors, nurses and other professionals who are in the best position to know what patients need will be in the driving seat by shaping the services.
● *To get the NHS to work in partnership* – this can be achieved by breaking down organisational barriers and forging stronger links with local authorities. The need of the patient will be put at the centre of the care process.
● *To drive efficiency through a more rigorous approach to performance.*
● *To shift the focus onto quality of care* – excellence is guaranteed to all patients and quality becomes the driving force for decision making at every level of service.
● *To rebuild public confidence in the NHS as a public service* – this service will be accountable to patients, open to the public and shaped by their views.

The surfing challenge: making sense of collaboration

The surge of interest spurred on by concern about quality and outcome in health care is addressed in *A First Class Service* (DoH 1998c) but this White Paper (along with other policy documents) states that this will be achieved by fostering multiprofessional working. The other key issue in the 'third way' to health care is patient-focused care – a reorientation of the health system towards the consumer, which is the main focus of the NHS plan (DoH, 2000a). The determination of the government to modernise the NHS includes a change of culture to embrace partnership working; to design a health service around the patient, not for the professions. The voice of patients and carers now has to be incorporated into effective measures on patient and client outcome. In the past professionals have got it wrong; they have not listened to the consumer voice which spoke of a service characterised by poor referrals, missed communication and budgetary disagreements (Tope 1998, West & Field 1995). The result was a fragmented service (Vaughan 1998) driven by professionals, not the patient and carer. The aim now is an integrated and coordinated service responding to the consumer's health and social care needs. Warner et al (1998) sum up this discussion:

> Government statements (DoH 1998a,b,c) concerning health service developments emphasise the need for a collaborative, people-centred approach to health service planning and delivery. (Warner et al 1998, p. 20)

The changing role of the patient and carer, i.e. the emergence of the consumer, requires a fundamental culture shift for nurses and other workers providing health care. The shift is from a paternalistic approach to one of partnership, an approach which potentially lends itself to teamwork. At the time of writing the Bristol Royal Infirmary Inquiry (2001) has just been published; it is a damning report on the scandal associated with between 30 and 35 babies who died needlessly between 1991 and 1995. One of the main recommendations was that the NHS must put patients at its core and they must be treated with respect. A theme which runs through the report is the amount of power held by a few, thus creating a club culture with no evidence of leadership or teamwork. The report goes beyond the inadequacies of the Bristol Royal Infirmary to address lessons for the whole NHS and to reiterate the blueprint for a patient-driven health service.

NHS policies promote collaborative work as a necessity for future health and social care but there remain real concerns, both for the patient and the professional.

PART 2: ORGANISATIONAL AND PROFESSIONAL RESPONSE

Neither agencies nor people choose to collaborate for altruistic reasons but only as a matter of survival of the organisation (Delaney 1994, Hudson 1989, Statham 1994). The reason organisations and agencies have to collaborate is because they do not possess all the necessary resources to attain their organisational goals. However, it is people who work collaboratively, not the system, so attention to the inhibitions and barriers voiced or experienced by professionals that shape and dictate issues around collaborative work should be addressed. They fall into four main areas:

- organisational structures
- language differences
- unequal power relationships
- ideological differences and role confusions.

Organisational structures

Anyone working in health and social care will be well aware of the organisational differences that have impeded such activities as joint working, developing partnerships and setting up multidisciplinary teams. But with the NHS modernisation agenda things are set to change: structures are being put in place to encourage integrated working across all health and social care agencies. The changes should address the past difficulties of each organisation having different planning horizons and budgetary cycles and thus facilitate a coordinated approach to patient care.

Primary care trusts (PCTs) have a responsibility to enter into partnerships with local social services, using pooled budgets to jointly commission services. It is also anticipated that new 'care trusts' will emerge out of PCTs to commission health and social care in a single organisation. The aim is to avoid 'patients falling in the cracks' between the two services and being left in hospital when they could be safely in their own home. Making the organisations receptive to patients' needs by bringing the systems together makes sense and should help both staff and patients. The secretary of state for health, Alan Milburn, summarised the systems failures of the past and the challenge the NHS now faces to adopt a whole systems approach:

The surfing challenge: making sense of collaboration

Six Steps to **Effective Management**

All too often staff feel that they have to fight the system rather than work with it to get the care that patients need. The GP who has to spend hours on the phone trying to find a hospital bed for their patient. The junior doctor in A&E who has to spend hours trying to get their patient from casualty to ward. The ward sister who has to spend hours trying to arrange the discharge of their patients. The challenge for the NHS now is to re-engineer its services, by tackling these systematic weaknesses, so that the right patient can get the right care at the right time by the right person with the right skills. (Right Hon. Alan Milburn MP, Harrogate Management Centre Conference, 18 May 2001)

At a grassroots level the change from primary care groups to PCTs should improve the communication between practice nurses, doctors and community nurses as they will all be working for the same PCT. Community nurses and practice nurses have had different employers and contractual agreements. Practice nurses were usually employed by GPs but other community nurses were usually employed by NHS trusts. Although practice nurses saw themselves as part of the community nurse team they frequently could not participate in team meetings and nursing plans, as this activity was not seen as part of their contract. The opportunity to work together to improve patient care is now supported by these structural changes.

Language differences

Pietroni (1992, p. 7) states that the difficulties encountered in interprofessional work may be more to do with 'lack of knowledge of each other's language and not necessarily, as portrayed in much of the literature, as the result of personality clashes, power struggles and role confusions'. Language and the meaning of words used by professionals can, and does, cause confusion. All professions have their own special language; it is one of the ways of ensuring that the knowledge of the professional group remains distinct and special to that group, thus protecting the profession. However, it puts up barriers between professionals, with each group struggling to understand the other with varying success.

A practice example offers insight: Eileen Korczack, a district nurse, worked for Hampshire County Council Social Services Department for a year and found the greatest stumbling block was language and meaning. She writes:

As a multiagency group, although we thought we were talking about the same issues, very often we were not. We either used the same words to mean quite different things, or we used very different words but found we were all talking about the same thing. (Korczack 1993, p. 6)

An example of how misunderstanding can arise and result in conflict is nicely illustrated by Ovretveit (1993) in a conversation over the much-used term 'attachment'. He writes:

> I witnessed a furious argument between a GP and a nurse manager about whether health visitors should be attached to the practice. The GP meant 'have the same patients as the practice'; the nurse manager understood 'under the direction of the GP'. Perhaps it would follow that having the same clients would mean that GPs would direct health visitors more than they did at present, but we were not able to discuss this. The discussion deteriorated when the GP argued that he was accountable and ultimately responsible for the patient. (Ovretveit 1993, p. 5)

The illustrations could be extended across all professions but this offers some insight into how the use of different words and meanings are a substantial barrier to communication between professionals, clients, carers and voluntary agencies.

Unequal power relationships

To collaborate means sharing across boundaries, achieving equal partnership and everyone having a voice. But the nursing tradition militates against starting from an equal playing field as nursing is a gendered occupation (Davies 1995) where women occupy positions of subservience.

The traditional view accepts that the doctor is all knowing and powerful, whereas the nurse is portrayed as caring, unselfish, obedient and submissive. The majority of doctors and nurses working in the UK have also been trained in the UK and thus comply with the hidden rules and agendas involved (Hallam 2000, Wicks 1998). They are part of the cultural ethos of the British class system which is based on status and unequal relationships. The process of learning to be a doctor or a nurse involves the sociological process distinctive to each professional group (Melia 1987, Menzies 1960, Wicks 1998). Medical students see themselves as scientists with a clear clinical mandate to use these skills to diagnose, treat and cure disease, whereas student nurses are discouraged from using their own discretion and initiative in planning their work. In Menzies' (1960) seminal work on nurses' levels of stress and anxiety she found that the nurses' lack of involvement in decision making caused them stress. The task orientation of nursing eliminated any involvement in decision making about patient care and thus left the nurses disempowered. The sex role which relies on the stereotyping of a female-dominated profession means 'nurses are doubly conditioned into playing a subservient role: first by society generally, and secondly by the medical establishment' (Warner et al 1998, p. 25).

The unequal power base between all professions has significant and far-reaching implications in understanding the process of collaborative work. The problem of power in relation to collaborative or teamwork is because there is a basic assumption that the process needs to be open, democratic and equal between people, when our society sometimes works in the opposite way (Payne 2000). Payne makes the point that power in teams can be 'oppressive against some members of a team or some service users' (Payne 2000, p. 141). If one person in a team uses power to meet the goals of financial imperatives or management issues rather than team goals agreed from a service-user perspective, then this can be seen as an abuse of power and oppressive to some members. The recent example of such an abuse of power by a few over the many was seen in the findings from the use of power by some of the doctors in the Bristol Royal Infirmary Inquiry (2001). The needs of the parents and children were largely ignored with disastrous outcomes.

The concern for power can also be positive in teamwork as it raises the issues of inequalities, imbalance of power and stimulates power sharing. It is the manner in which the inevitable conflict is addressed that shapes the success of the team. Using conflict in a team situation does not have to be destructive – it can in fact be the very catalyst that is needed to make the team move forward and be creative. The danger in teamwork is leaving issues of power hidden and unacknowledged.

The setting up of primary care groups and trusts (PCGs and PCTs) offers an excellent example of the inequalities in power and status between doctors and nurses. *The New NHS: Modern, Dependable* (DoH 1997) recommended a new model for primary care with GPs and nurses in the driving seats. The requirement for nurses to have a place on the boards of PCGs (NHS Executive 1998) offered them considerable opportunities to play a full and equal role in shaping plans for local health improvement of primary care (While 1999). But so far nurses have had to fight for representation with an unequal outcome: seven GPs to only two nurses on a board. In an embryonic study into workings of PCGs (Smith et al 1999, p. 55) it was found that nurses have been almost invisible in the PCG debate and 'have consistently played second (and more often than not third or fourth) fiddle to GPs'. There is therefore a need to provide stable and powerful mechanisms to support and champion those nurses elected to the boards (Parkin 1999) so that the power structures do not destroy the kind of cooperation needed for collaborative work.

The following is based on a story told by a nurse who was part of a team building workshop in primary care. Significant issues included how the nurses' and GPs' views of their working environment were idealised based on a mutually respectful collaborative working relationship, thus supporting the notion that professionals accept the ideal even if the reality is different. The nurses acknowledged that GPs were in a position of power, but the GPs did not feel that they were, nor were they aware of their authority over nursing colleagues. But there was evidence that the doctors were making key strategic decisions affecting nurses without feeling a need to include them in discussions. The nurses felt that the GPs dominated the decision-making process. The outcome of the workshop was to point to the many 'imbalances, tensions and difficulties in the development of working relationships between doctors and nurses in primary care'.

Doctors do enjoy a more powerful position than nurses and there are good reasons why nurses have failed to improve their status. Nurses today have an opportunity to be part of the micropolitics of health care. The new practitioner roles, the blurring of professional boundaries, unified regulation, joint education and new workforces are all part of the government's modernisation agenda and provide a great opportunity for nurses to embrace a 'new professional identity' (Gough 2001). A culture shift – a different way of thinking – is now possible. Pippa Gough outlined this plea in a speech on modernisation when she encouraged nurses to 'step out of old professional ways of being, thinking, doing'. To let go of old certainties and to view 'the world through a different lens' (Gough 2001, p. 9)

Ideological differences and role confusions

The future of health care planning and delivery is to be a collaborative, people-centred approach (DoH, 1998a,b,c, Warner et al 1998). The emphasis is on the 'user, patient and client need' to determine health strategy, not professional need. The shift has therefore been away from professional autonomy towards patient/public accountability. The benefits to the consumer have been one of the government's major arguments in defending the changes to the NHS and 'has hinged on the notion of quality' (Soothill et al 1995, p. 8).

In order to provide a service responding to public participation the traditional role of professions is challenged. It is no longer a nurse's job, a doctor's job, a physiotherapist's job or social worker's job. The starting point is the patient/client health need. These consumers hold a view about the service they expect, their health needs do not respect organisational boundaries, and neither do they want to fight their way through communication and organisational barriers to access care (Tope 1998). A reassessment and reevaluation of professional roles is necessary so that health professionals are equipped for the future. A relevant observation from a document on undergraduate medical education from the General Medical Council (1993) and quoted by Warner et al (1998, p. 21) is that:

> there is a redistribution of the tasks undertaken by members of the caring professions. The overlapping of skills and responsibilities, whilst not diminishing the distinctive role of the doctor, calls for mutual respect and understanding of roles and a capacity for teamwork.

This is not calling for the dissolution of professional identity but for a more flexible collaborative approach to work. However, there have been calls for a 'generic worker'. In a study carried out by the Health Service Management Unit at the University of Manchester (Schofield 1996), it was envisaged that the health service would maintain a core of staff but that most of the work would be contracted out to a flexible and changing workforce. Another study by the World Health Organization (WHO 1994) suggested that the notion of nursing and medicine as separate occupations could disappear. These findings would seem radical and there are strong arguments (Harries et al 1999, Poxton 1999) to retain and build on what is special and distinctive about individual professions and to help the professions work at the boundaries, so seeing a blurring of roles rather than generic roles.

Roles have begun to change in the last few years: doctors have had to become business managers, community nurses have taken on self-management through the introduction of integrated nursing teams (*see* Application 6.1). Nurses are now doing jobs once done by junior doctors, support workers are doing jobs previously done by nurses. Other professionals such as physiotherapists, radiographers and technicians are also taking on jobs traditionally done by other occupations. Carers are now carrying out quite complex medical tasks once only done by doctors and nurses (English 1997).

An example of the boundaries between doctors and nurses being swept away is found in a pioneering London cooperative 'Harmoni', the NHS Direct triage out-of-hours calls. It is an inter-professional approach that builds on the government's proposals for 'physicians' assistants' set out in the planning document *A Health Service of All Talents* (DoH 2000b). A GP in Harmoni, Dr Lloyd, says: 'Get rid of the labels of doctor and nurse. The concept of a general health worker with a portfolio of skills that match the job required has to be the way in future. Call me a clinical general-ist and I will be happy' (Jones 2000, p. 20).

Although quite revolutionary developments, these changes are not achieved without cost. The professional relinquishing their role can experience severe loss and may regret the march of time. The effect of the role change in primary health care has been studied from both a nursing and a medical perspective by Williams & Sibbald (1999). Issues addressed in the study included boundary changes in role substitution which could 'endanger uncertainty, resulting in an impulse for innovation or, in contrast, a retreat into the protection of profession' (Williams et al 1997, p. 10). The level of uncertainty was seen as having important implications for the future of primary care nursing. Williams & Sibbald (1999) argued that a needs-led service should prevail over inflexible role demar-cation and emphasised that professional identity does matter, say-ing that:

> where professional identity is challenged, demoralisation and a sense of diminished autonomy may, in turn, adversely affect the care given and compassion shown to patients. Its erosion should be a matter of concern to nurses, doctors and policy makers alike. (Williams & Sibbald 1999, p. 743)

The study of integrated nursing teams (Application 6.1) describes how changes to professional identity really do matter to the nurses. The changes associated with letting go of traditional roles and adapting to new roles can be painful. Working closely with nurses to help them acknowledge their fears over loss of role and prepar-ing them for new jobs takes time and effort. Changes to profes-sional roles are taking place and will continue; the dissolution of professional boundaries is unlikely (Rawson 1994), but blurring of roles a reality. The degree of change to nursing roles is exciting and offers nurses a real opportunity to change culture. Examples of job changes for nurses are outlined in Box 6.2.

This section on ideological differences and role confusions has addressed the difficulties that the professions may find in breaking

The surfing challenge: making sense of collaboration

> **Box 6.2** Examples of job changes for nurses
>
> - The introduction of nurse prescribing and its extension followed the recommendation from the government allowing many nurses to prescribe an extended formulary
> - The autonomous role of nurse practitioners who make diagnostic assessments in nurse-led walk-in centres
> - In many GP surgeries it will now be the nurse who first assesses the patient, not the GP
> - All across health care the number of posts for nurse consultants and specialist nurse practitioners are growing rapidly

down professional boundaries, working more flexibly, being less tribal and developing new roles. But in moving forward to create a new culture the emphasis must remain firmly on 'how the patient can be served best through new ways of working – not on shoring up old professional demarcations and engaging in endless turf wars' (Gough 2001, p. 9).

PART 3: WORKING TOGETHER: THE CONCEPT OF COLLABORATION

There is an imperative to work together in a variety of ways and at different levels. Practitioners, carers and clients need to develop partnerships so that joint care packages are agreed and implemented. Practitioners from the same organisation have to work with each other in teams and on joint projects. These can include setting up integrated care pathways, implementing a team approach to pain relief, introducing self-managed nurse teams or devising protocols on care of the older person living in the community. Interagency work is another level requiring joint planning, resourcing and organisation and might include hospital discharge policy, child protection strategy, health improvement schemes (HImP) and innovative schemes that attract government funding to set up Sure Start programmes.

In examining these various ways of working together, many different words have been used to express the types of work and approach required: partnership, joint care, integrated care pathways, teamwork, and multidisciplinary health promotion. Any attempt here at defining and explaining each term would inevitably oversimplify its usage and no doubt be very confusing to read. However, there is one word that has overarching meaning and

Changing relationships in health care

usage to the many activities associated with 'learning and working together' and that is the concept of collaboration.

Collaboration

Collaboration needs to be set in context. The NHS is trying to move from a hierarchical organisation based on competition to an organisation based on cooperation; a less hierarchical structure achieved through flatter management with an emphasis on a team approach. Kraus (1980) argued that the model based on coercion in the form of hierarchically induced and reinforced authority, found in most organisations and social systems in western society at that time, should be changed to an alternative value system. Kraus (1980, p. 18) states that collaboration 'has at its core, non-competing, cooperative behaviour and non-hierarchical structures and processes in organisations'.

To encourage a different value system of any organisation requires radical change, but for a traditional bureaucratic organisation like the NHS it will be slow. Changes in how the individual views the organisation and how the organisation views its employees demand a process of resocialisation, heralded as a solution to the health care problems of the future (Sullivan 1998).

Collaboration can simply be defined as working together for a common goal and with the increasing complexity of health care provision, collaboration becomes more important in coordinating work (Sullivan 1998, p. 4). Collaboration does have a second meaning: 'to cooperate with or assist usually willingly an enemy of one's country (Webster International Dictionary 1976, p. 443). Some writers (Pratt et al 1998) argue that the second meaning, which has traitorous connotations, gives the use of collaborative work a sense of ambivalence and so may decide against its use. However, Loxley sees the potential for conflict in the word as significant, saying: 'conflict is interwoven with interprofessional collaboration because there are deep-rooted social differences in the division of labour which has developed over the last 200 years in health and welfare services' (Loxley 1997, p. 1).

Collaboration is not therefore an easy option; working with people of different status, across different professions and within different organisations realistically demands maturity, sensitivity and excellent negotiating skills. Collaborative working is easy to extol but very difficult to achieve. Much has been written about the theory, but the practice and promotion of collaboration take place in the cut and thrust of daily living.

The surfing challenge: making sense of collaboration

Collaboration consists of a range of attributes which are described here in relation to nursing:

- shared planning
- decision making in a collegiate structure
- problem solving
- setting goals
- assuming responsibility
- accepting accountability (Baggs & Schmitt 1988, Clarke & Mass 1998).

The collaborative relationship is built up over time, on the basis of respect and trust between the nurse, client, carer and other professionals. The contributions all parties bring to the relationship must be acknowledged with the understanding that all roles are complementary. It is in this way that loss of role is most often experienced (Clarke & Mass 1998) by those participating in the collaborative relationship. Although the ideal of collaboration is based on sharing, cooperation and coordination, it takes place in practice which is neither ahistorical nor apolitical. The struggle to acquire scarce resources, to accept different work ideologies and work with people who have variable access to power requires determination.

Collaboration is costly because it takes time to build relationships, to understand all parties, to agree a goal and to establish a decision-making process. If a collaborative approach is to be used then it must be justified, not just seen as a universal panacea to meet today's complex health needs. Collaborative work cannot be ad hoc, it must be planned with each profession learning collaborative skills and being aware of its value base. The level of commitment is expressed by Sullivan (1998, p. 634): 'Collaboration is more than a practice; it is as well a set of values; a state of commitment; a state of being as well as doing'.

Working to make sure that health care practitioners feel supported and valued is vital in creating the right environment for a quality service. The process will be discussed in Part 4.

PART 4: EDUCATION FOR COLLABORATIVE PRACTICE TO PROMOTE WELL-BEING, GROWTH AND DEVELOPMENT

Collaborative practice in the form of teamwork needs nurturing and supporting if it is to achieve its full potential. Messages from previous research on teamwork (Poulton & West 1994) indicate that many initiatives to promote teamwork over the years have not always been implemented. The valuable contributions made in the reports of Cumberlege (DoH 1986), Edwards (1987) and *Working Together* (DHSS 1988) in regard to teamwork include the importance of understanding each other's role, the need for regular meetings, the need to make objectives explicit and to have a common purpose. These were common themes throughout the reports in the 1980s but still not always found in practice. The reports foresaw that improvements in the future for teamwork would happen through education, by shared learning and in-service training. In reality this has been slow to happen for a variety of reasons, which will now be discussed.

The traditional model of nurse education is to prepare nurses who are competent, safe and knowledgeable in their distinct field but the curriculum did not address the preparation of nurses to work with each other, across professional boundaries and between agencies. This position is not peculiar to nurse education; other health professionals are also prepared to become 'knowledgeable and skilled practitioners able to deliver health care services that are satisfactory, appropriate, and cost-effective' (Sullivan 1998, p. 428) but in their distinct fields only. Education has traditionally been grounded in each discipline. Becoming a professional involves learning the values, beliefs and attitudes of the chosen profession. Each practitioner and each group of professionals has unique and specialist knowledge which is not available to others because of the extensive specialist training undertaken. The development of professional status and its associated autonomy are fundamental aims of professional education, but these same processes are barriers to collaborative work. Although each discipline is well prepared for its singular contribution, all find their 'educational preparation a total mismatch for the complex, interactive world into which they graduate and practice' (Sullivan 1998, p. 428).

The assumption that health professionals are prepared to work collaboratively is misleading, they do not automatically know how to work in teams. Learning for collaborative practice is only just being addressed in nurse education. Nurses and other health professionals need to learn to work collaboratively, at both pre- and postqualifying stages. However, the process takes time and is fraught with difficulties. To be able to work collaboratively needs professional maturity, to be able to let go of some aspects of role and work at the boundaries. Professionals feel threatened if their identity is challenged. Fromm (1972) succinctly sums up the distinctiveness of professions and how any threat will be treated with suspicion, saying:

The surfing challenge: making sense of collaboration

Man . . . has a vital interest in retaining his frame of orientation. His capacity to act depends upon it, and in the last analysis, his sense of identity. If others threaten him with ideas that question his own frame of orientation, he will react to those ideas as if to a vital threat.

Understanding how to retain a frame of orientation to deal with other ideas and values can be challenging and even frightening. Professionals will retreat to what they know, where they are safe, thus increasing tribalism. A report into the expansion of nurse roles, *Exploring New Roles in Practice* (DoH 1999b), found that professional tribalism is likely to be heightened as nurses change and expand their jobs, rather than breaking down barriers between groups. Extended roles mean greater accountability and as doctors and nurses have different approaches to accountability and regulation, doing things previously done by the medical profession does not make a nurse a member of that profession.

The challenge for interprofessional education is substantial, as there is a need to acknowledge the essential contribution each profession makes whilst at the same time ensuring that nurses and other health professionals are prepared to work in the real world of integrated practice.

Up until the 1990s shared learning was the common term used to describe professional groups learning together but, as Ewens (1998) argues, from the mid-1980s debate was taking place regarding a more precise definition. The term interprofessional education (IPE) was gradually adopted, describing events where 'two or more professional groups learn together with the aim of promoting collaborative practice' (Ewens 1998, p. 28). The notion of aiming to promote collaborative practice is an essential aspect of any definition, because without it there would be 'no greater commitment than sitting students in the same classroom' (Ewens 1998, p. 27).

In 1987 the Centre for the Advancement of Interprofessional Education (CAIPE) was set up in the UK to bring together a network of individuals and organisations dedicated to promoting collaboration across different disciplines, professions and agencies to achieve service user-focused care. A survey of IPE initiatives (Shakespeare et al 1989) developed by CAIPE produced a working definition of IPE, using three criteria:

- the primary objective of the event is educational
- it involves participants of two or more selected professional groups
- participants are learning together within a multidisciplinary context.

What was missing from this definition was the degree of learning and change as a result of the IPE experience. Collaborative education includes action from the participants to change their 'ways of knowing and understanding' (Ewens 1998, p. 28) with the explicit aim of promoting interprofessional collaboration.

The work that best offers insight and clarity about the changes required in IPE was done by Gyarmati (1986, p. 34), where she identified the conceptual differences between the terms multidisciplinary and interdisciplinary. She argued that they are 'fundamentally different concepts, the first involves juxtaposition or simple addition, while the latter entails integration and synthesis'. Multidisciplinary work involves organising students in practice to address common problems but addressing them from their own professional background; it does not therefore affect the 'principles, methods and main concepts of each discipline, they remain unchanged'. The meeting point of the different studies is simply the common subject under consideration.

An essential characteristic of interdisciplinary education is to synthesise and integrate the constituent elements of two or more professions. Interdisciplinary teaching cannot consist of the mere transfer of concepts and principles from one discipline to another, nor in mixing different disciplines. According to Gyarmati (1986) the interdisciplinary approach concentrates on the bases of knowledge, while the multidisciplinary is concerned with the application of that knowledge. Much of the literature on IPE does not attempt to make this distinction, in fact it tends to assume a multidisciplinary approach. An interdisciplinary approach would involve professionals learning together in order to move to 'new ways of thinking, rather than simply sharing with each other a fixed and unchanging perspective' (Ewens 1998, p. 28). Collaborative education has to include new ways of thinking, thus interdisciplinary education is a useful concept in the debate.

Organising IPE that challenges the ways professionals work together, but in a manner that still values individual expertise and takes account of the real world of practice, must be carefully planned. If the participants' experience of IPE is threatening, they are likely to retreat back into the safety of their professional roles, thus increasing professional tribalism. If it is a pleasant experience but does not demand the participants change in any way then it has been a waste of time. If it does not take account of the real world of practice, does not allow participants to talk about the 'tangles' of their own work and begin to find ways to change practice and sustain collaboration then 'all that happens is that they slip back or

The surfing challenge: making sense of collaboration

143

they get very disgruntled or discontented, or leave or something' (Menzies 1988, quoted in Pietroni 1992, p. 14).

Turning an unsuccessful IPE experience into a successful one has been a useful learning experience for myself and a colleague at the University of Reading. After many years of running IPE study days for community nurses and GP registrars, which were resource heavy and received mixed levels of evaluation, we decided to plan a totally new approach, incorporating a simulated learning exercise based on a genogram (Howkins & Allison 1997). The day was an overwhelming success, has now run for 7 years and includes social workers. The reason for the success was the use of a client-centred approach, based in practice. The process was experiential, so participants had to be involved and the theoretical framework was problem-based learning (PBL). The principal aim of PBL is that the 'starting point for learning should be a problem, a query or a puzzle that the learner wishes to solve' (Boud 1985, p. 13). The problem is presented in the form of the 'Carter family'; many participants each year have said that they also have a Carter family in their practice and that it is the Carter family that shapes the day. Evaluation of the study day over 2 years produced the themes outlined in Box 6.3.

The participants found the experience challenging intellectually as they made sense of the chaos around the Carter family, presented in a manner that mirrored working in primary care. They were also challenged professionally as the mixed groups used their pooled experience as a rich resource in the problem-solving process. Many usually shy participants found themselves wanting to contribute in a situation where they would normally have remained silent. They then found their contribution valued which added greatly to their own self-esteem. The place of reflective learning was recognised by participants in that 'others have important and relevant knowledge to contribute and that allowing this to emerge is a source of learning for everyone' (Pietroni 1992, p. 62). By using this example of IPE it has been possible to show the essential links between the theory of collaborative education and practice.

Box 6.3 Study day themes

- The significance of a positive learning environment
- Personal and professional experience used constructively in the group activity
- Students in control of their own learning
- Intellectually challenging and relevant to practice
- Importance of reflection and debriefing

Although the education programme outlined was successful by IPE criteria, what is still not known is how any changes related to collaborative work may be sustained in practice. Helping the individual nurse to take IPE learning into practice needs the recognition that other support mechanisms must be in place to help the nurse to change and develop. Collaborative education has to address personal and professional preparation in the form of reflective practice, clinical supervision, personal development plans and educational programmes to provide a collaborative education framework for nurses and all other health practitioners.

Nurses can be exposed to various educational experiences such as the one described above, but if they do not have the professional maturity, the self-awareness, the insight to enable them to share and thus acknowledge others' expertise, know what strengths they bring to any situation, are confident enough in their role, 'to let go', they will not be able to work at the boundaries of care. The development of reflective practice and the introduction of clinical supervision play a vital role in supporting and sustaining collaborative work. The development of education for collaborative practice is about personal and professional development; these aspects cannot be separated.

This section on education for collaborative practice to promote growth and development cannot be complete without reference to the importance placed upon leadership by the policies set out in *The NHS Plan* (DoH 2000a) and the significance of leadership for nurses and nursing in *Making a Difference* (DoH 1999a). The educational issues are about nurses first transforming themselves in order for them to become transformational leaders and to enable others to change and cope. Transformational leadership is about having a vision, sharing this with others and then working in a collaborative manner to achieve the vision.

CONCLUSION

This chapter set out to make sense of the paradox of collaborative work. On the one hand collaborative work is an expectation for all health and social care professionals and is also seen as both good and necessary for the delivery and organisation of health care. But on the other hand professionals and agencies involved in collaborative work find that it is neither an easy nor a comfortable option. Professional identity, professional status and professional autonomy are all aspects that maintain professionalism but they are also barriers to collaborative work. Finding ways to work at the

The surfing challenge: making sense of collaboration

boundaries of the profession and the confidence to let go some aspects of the professional role is a necessary step towards collaborative work. It entails accepting that there is a paradox that has to be managed but not necessarily resolved (Handy 1994). Professionals should be encouraged to rethink their occupational purpose and be able to discover their most effective practice. A level of uncertainty and a certain amount of conflict and antagonism are the inevitable consequences of collaborative work but these are not usually the feelings that professionals like or expect to associate with working together. However, these uncomfortable feelings provide the essential triggers to creativity and thus change.

As this chapter has shown, the process of working together is not straightforward, it is difficult and threatening, but a process that presents real challenges to professionals as they work more with communities and service users. In the metaphor used at the start of this chapter it was suggested that nurses could learn to enjoy the challenge of the surf rather than stay isolated at the top of the beach. Managing collaborative work and rising to the challenge can be compared with our reactions on a beach as the waves advance with the incoming tide. On the beach a person has two main choices: to keep out of the surf or incoming tide, remain safe and secure above the high tide mark or, alternatively, to surf or at least jump the waves. Learning to surf requires effort, risk taking, determination, courage and hard work and jumping the waves may be just a bit less effort. The outcome should be a great sense of achievement, with the added fun and thrill of surfing with others who are all striving for the same goal. But not everyone will want or be able to surf the waves but they could have jobs in the backup team, as technician, first aider, life saver or driver. Some people may take up the challenge and create a new sport to enjoy the waves or even design a new type of craft which will be more efficient than the surfboard. The permutations are endless but enjoying the surf or supporting others to ride the surf is a shared goal and a collaborative activity.

The significance of this metaphor is about change. Constant change is the reality of health care; there will be no period of stability, so rising to the challenge of the surf can be compared with the continual and inevitable changes in the health service for all practitioners. By staying above the high tide mark, building individual castles will mean professional isolation and being an observer rather than a participant. Learning to live and accept as normal the changing world of health care is an exciting challenge for all health professionals.

References

Baggs J, Schmitt M 1988 Collaboration between nurses and physicians. Journal of Nursing Scholarship 20(3): 145–149

Boud DJ 1985 Problem-based learning in perspective. In: Boud DJ (ed) Problem based learning in education for professions. Higher Education Research and Development Society of Australia, Sydney, pp 13–18

Bristol Royal Infirmary Inquiry 2001 Learning from Bristol: summary and recommendations. Chair: Ian Kennedy. COI communications. Stationery Office, London

Clarke H, Mass H 1998 Comox Valley Nursing Centre: from collaboration to empowerment. Public Health Nursing 15(3): 216–224

Davies C 1995 Gender and the professional predicament in nursing. Open University Press, Buckingham

Delaney FG 1994 Muddling through the middle ground: theoretical concerns in intersectoral collaboration and health promotion. Health Promotion International 9(3): 217–225

Department of Health 1986 Neighbourhood nursing: a focus for care (Cumberlege report). HMSO, London

Department of Health 1997 The new NHS: modern, dependable. Stationery Office, London

Department of Health 1998a Putting patients first. Stationery Office, London

Department of Health 1998b Our healthier nation. Stationery Office, London

Department of Health 1998c A first class service quality in the NHS. Stationery Office, London

Department of Health 1999a Making a difference: strengthening the nursing, midwifery and health visiting contribution to health care. Stationery Office, London

Department of Health 1999b Exploring new roles in practice (ENRiP). Stationery Office, London

Department of Health 2000a The NHS plan: a plan for investment, a plan for reform. Stationery Office, London

Department of Health 2000b A health service of all talents. Stationery Office, London

Department of Health and Social Security 1988 Working together: a guide to arrangements for interagency cooperation for the protection of children from abuse. HMSO, London

Edwards N 1987 Nurses in the community: a team approach for Wales. Information Division, Welsh Office, Cardiff

English T 1997 Medicine in the 1990s needs a team approach. British Medical Journal 314: 661–663

Ewens AE 1998 The changing role perceptions of student nurses on integrated courses in community health nursing. Unpublished PhD, University of Reading

Fromm E 1972 The anatomy of human destructiveness. Jonathan Cape, London

General Medical Council 1993 Tomorrow's doctors: recommendations on undergraduate medical education. GMC, London

Gough P 2001 Change in culture and deprofessionalisation. Nursing Management 7(9): 8–9

Gyarmati G 1986 The teaching of the professions: an interdisciplinary approach. Higher Education Review 18(2): 33–43

Hallam J 2000 Nursing the image: media, culture and professional identity. Routledge, London

Handy C 1994 The empty raincoat. Hutchinson, London

Harries J, Gordon P, Plamping D, Fischer M 1999 Elephant problems and fixes that fail: the story of a search for new approaches to inter-agency working. King's Fund, London

Howkins E 1995 Community nursing: dimensions and dilemmas. Arnold, London

Howkins E, Allison A 1997 Shared learning for primary care: a success story. Nurse Education Today 17(3): 225–231

Hudson B 1989 Collaboration: the elusive chimera. Health Service Journal 99: 82–83

Jones C 2000 Breaking down barriers. British Medical Association News Review May: 18–21

Korczack E 1993 Preparing for joint assessment. Primary Health Care 3(2): 6–8

Kraus WA 1980 Collaboration in organisations all? Human Services Press, New York

Leathard A 1994 Going interprofessional: working together for health and welfare. Routledge, London

Loxley A 1997 Collaboration in health and welfare: working with difference. Jessica Kingsley, London

Melia K 1987 Learning and working: the occupational socialisation of nurses. Tavistock, London

Menzies I 1960 A case study in the functioning of social systems as a defence against anxiety: a report on a study of the nursing service of a general hospital. Human Relations 13(2): 95–121

Menzies I 1988 Containing anxiety in institutions. Selected essays vol 1. Free Association Books, London

NHS Executive 1998 Better health and better health care – implementing 'The new NHS' and 'Our healthier nation'. HSC 1998/021. NHS Executive, London

Ovretveit J 1993 Coordinating community care. Open University Press, Buckingham

Parkin P 1999 Managing change in the community 1: the case of PCGs. British Journal of Community Nursing 4(1): 19–27

Payne M 2000 Teamwork in multiprofessional care. Macmillan, London

Pietroni PC 1992 Towards reflective practice – languages of health and social care. Journal of Interprofessional Care 6(1): 7–16

Poulton B, West M 1994 Primary health care team effectiveness: developing a constituency approach. Health and Social Care 2: 77–84

Poxton R 1999 Working across the boundaries. King's Fund, London

Pratt J, Plamping D, Gordon P 1998 Partnership fit for purpose? King's Fund, London

Rawson D 1994 Models of interprofessional work: likely theories and possibilities. In: Leathard A (ed) Going interprofessional: working together for health and welfare. Routledge, London

Schofield M 1996 The future health service workforce: steering group report. Lilley Industries Creative Packaging Ltd, Basingstoke

Shakespeare H, Tucker W, Northover J 1989 Report of a national survey on interprofessional education in primary health care. CAIPE, London

Smith K, Dickson M, Sheaff R 1999 Second among equals. Nursing Times 95(13): 54–55

Soothill K, Mackay L, Webb D (eds) 1995 Interprofessional relations in health care. Arnold, London

Statham D 1994 Working together in community care. Health Visitor 67(1): 16–18

Sullivan TJ 1998 Collaboration: health care imperative. McGraw-Hill, New York

Tope R 1998 The impact of interprofessional education in the South West region: a critical analysis. The literature review. Department of Health, London

Vaughan B 1998 A bridge between acute and primary care? King's Fund News 21(3): 3

Warner M, Longley M, Gould E, Picek A 1998 Health care futures 2010: commissioned by the UKCC Education Commission, Glamorgan, Welsh Institute for Health and Social Care

Webster's Third New International Dictionary 1976 Merriam, Springfield, Massachusetts

West M, Field R 1995 Perspectives from organisational psychology. Journal of Interprofessional Care 9(2): 117–122

While A 1999 The jury is out on PCGs. British Journal of Community Nursing 4(1): 46–47

WHO 1994 Technical Report Series No. 842. Nursing beyond the year 2000. A report of a WHO study group. WHO, Geneva

Wicks D 1998 Nurses and doctors at work: rethinking professional boundaries. Open University Press, Buckingham

Williams A, Sibbald B 1999 Changing roles and identities in primary health care: exploring a culture of uncertainty. Journal of Advanced Nursing 29(3): 737–745

Williams A, Robins T, Sibbald B 1997 Cultural differences between medicine and nursing: implications for primary care. National Primary Care Research and Development Centre, University of Manchester

The surfing challenge: making sense of collaboration

149

Application 6.1

Anne Owen

West Berkshire Priority Care Service NHS Trust approach to self-managed integrated nursing teams

In January 1996, following a lengthy consultation process, West Berkshire Priority Care Service NHS Trust (WBPCS) implemented self-managed integrated nursing teams (SMINTS) through the Community Nursing Project, a pilot study which aimed to provide effective and efficient nursing care by devolving management responsibility and integrating the nursing disciplines of district nursing, health visiting and practice nursing. Nurses from seven large GP fundholding (GPFH) practices were involved with nurses from seven similar sized practices used as a control. An independent management consultant who was responsible for the nurses' anonymised evaluation oversaw the project.

This application describes the change process, the training programme, how the nurses moved from groups to teams, the role of the nurse facilitator and the evaluation of the project.

CHANGE PROCESS

The drivers for the change were initiated by GPFH who felt that nursing management costs were too high and that nurse managers were too controlling in their style. There was also a feeling that nurses could work more effectively if some of the traditional barriers between the disciplines were broken. The community nurses based at the practices concerned were questioned about their attitudes to nurse management and current working practices and the vast majority responded that they were in agreement with the GPs. This did leave a small number of nurses who were happy with the status quo and who were reluctant to commit to the project.

A project board, which met regularly throughout the project, was initiated and consisted of trust managers, a GP and a practice manager. Community nurses were involved in the subgroups that were formed to look at finance and personnel issues. A nurse facilitator was employed to facilitate the nursing teams and, coincidentally, a training and development advisor was appointed prior to the project commencing.

The aim of the project was 'to provide competent, confident nurses working as full members of the primary health care team providing a flexible, high quality service with the minimum of hierarchical restrictions'. Specific objectives relating to the main problems expressed by nurses and GPs were agreed within this overall aim (Box 6.1.1). Each objective was developed to have process, outcome and measure to aid the evaluation process.

Senior trust managers worked with the nurses to overcome their expressed fears by involving them in the project from an early stage including travelling to look at the management approach used by other trusts. There was also an 'away day' held to which all of the community and practice nurses were invited. At this meeting the nurses proposed the model of management that they would prefer – that is, a self-managed integrated nursing team (SMINT) with a nurse facilitator who could

---

Box 6.1.1 Specific objectives in providing effective and efficient nursing care

- To work as an integrated nursing team within the primary care setting
- To establish a nursing team that will be integrated into the practice, working in a way which is sensitive to the needs of the practice and the population it serves
- The training and development of nurses should be tailored and available according to the needs of the individual and with the needs of the practice
- To ensure that effective professional and specialist advice and support is easily accessible and available to nursing staff in the primary care setting
- The nursing team to have greater autonomy (managerially, administratively and financially) to function in a way that they can respond to the local needs of the practice and the population it serves

Self-managed integrated nursing teams

provide professional advice and support but not direct line management.

The nurse facilitator was appointed 1 month before the start of the project. She spent this time introducing herself to the teams and to the lead GPs and practice managers and liaising with the training and development advisor who was also recently appointed. Her role was to offer professional advice and support to the nursing teams, to deliver the training programme and act as a conduit for information from senior management to the teams and from the teams to senior management.

FROM GROUPS TO TEAMS

When the project first began, there were distinct groups of nurses at each practice. Although they referred to themselves as teams there were few common objectives or purposes which could be demonstrated and many gaps which were obvious. This was hardly surprising given the historical nature of divisions between nursing disciplines and the fact that they had never before been encouraged to work closely together as a team.

The nurse facilitator initiated meetings at each practice to which all nurses – health visitors, district nurses and practice nurses – were invited. At those meetings she encouraged discussion about the 'teams', their current communication processes and relationships with each other. This also enabled her to explore with them what their fears were, if any, about teamwork, integration and self-management. She was then able to work to minimise these 'resisting' forces rather than push the changes through. This was particularly important with the nurses who were reluctant to change. At all times she tried to be empathetic towards them without being patronising.

It was interesting that at this point, none of the teams raised any issues about poor communication, conflict or other relationship problems. However, the nurse facilitator was approached individually by nurses who expressed concerns about the way in which their team operated.

It was also very noticeable that there were obvious divisions between the health visitors, district nurses and practice nurses in the majority of the teams at the onset of the project. In one team, when the practice suggested that the health visitors and district nurses moved into one room, there was great consternation expressed by the health visitors about possible breaches of confidentiality when they were on the telephone to clients. They failed to see, initially, that being together would aid teamwork. However, in another team a joint office had proved to be very successful to the extent that an occupational therapist whose time had also been purchased by the practice moved in with the nurses and became part of the team.

The move towards integration

When the question of integration was raised and questions were asked about how the teams could work more effectively for the benefit of patients/clients, there was some resistance and preciousness about roles. In one team, the health visitors were willing to help the practice nurses with immunisations but were less willing for the practice nurses to help them with well baby clinics as they felt that this was inappropriate. This issue was only resolved after a long, open and frank discussion which involved some healthy conflict, overseen by the nurse facilitator.

One of the lessons learnt through the process of teambuilding was that conflict could be healthy for the team and that lack of this could have been hindering the process in the past. Another was that if the teams were to become true teams and not just groups of people who happened to work together, the nurses had to learn about each other's skills, knowledge and roles and to respect them. This was achieved through discussion, teaching and shadowing. In two of the teams it was also achieved by using skill mix to have a nurse who worked with the district nurses and health visitors thus learning more about the roles and encouraging discussion between the two disciplines.

The biggest disappointment in this movement towards integration was the lack of practice nurse involvement in most of the teams. This was mainly due to the fact that the majority of practice nurses worked part time, were always fully booked for clinics and felt that they had little to contribute to the team or to the team discussions. Having different employers was also viewed as a problem by some of the practice nurses although they were always invited to training sessions and meetings and the nurse facilitator emphasised that she was there to help and support them as much as the nurses employed by the trust.

However, in the teams where there was practice nurse involvement it worked well. For several practices the GPs saw it as imperative that the practice nurses were fully integrated and encouraged them to attend team meetings and training. In these practices, joint protocols and policies were formulated, clerical assistants worked for the whole nursing team, not just for the community nurses, and communication increased dramatically.

From the initial meetings the nurse facilitator and the training and development advisor formulated a training programme which would begin with the basics of team development and build on the skills

Six Steps to **Effective Management**

and knowledge gained from this to enable the teams to function more effectively as a team rather than as a group.

TRAINING

The teamwork element of the training was seen to be key to the success of the project as was the interpersonal skills training. It had been noted that many of the nurses had excellent interpersonal skills when relating to patients/clients but that these were not so evident when relating to colleagues!

The initial training programme consisted of:

- financial management including budgets, legal requirements, payroll, statutory sickness and maternity pay
- teambuilding
- interpersonal skills
- managing meetings
- time management
- recruitment and selection of staff including legal requirements and interview skills.

Following further discussions with the nurses and to address problems that had arisen at various times, it was later expanded to include negotiating skills and managing relationships.

The training programme was written so that it could be delivered in a modular format, which would be team and practice based as far as possible. It was intended that this would prevent the nurses from being taken away from their practice for too long and to facilitate other members of the primary health care team to attend. This led to some interesting training sessions, including team building in a GP's consulting room!

Delivering the training in this manner was time-consuming for the trainers and as the philosophy of SMINTS was 'rolled out' within the trust, it was delivered more centrally and on an inter-team basis. This also allowed more flexibility for the nurses within the teams who were not all committed to training on the same day. It also gave them the opportunity to meet and mix with nurses from other SMINTS and to learn from each other's experiences.

During the teambuilding, along with fun games and puzzles, the process of effective team working was discussed and the teams were asked to evaluate themselves in relation to the recognised stages of team formation. Each member was also given a Belbin Team Type Inventory to complete and the team composition was then discussed. Following this, the strengths of the team members

Changing relationships in health care

and areas of development could be explored to enable them to use the strengths and weaknesses of the team types. For example, in all teams there was a majority of nurses who scored highly as team workers but in most there was no nurse who scored as a complete finisher.

For the team to monitor their progress and ensure that they were delivering effective and efficient care, it was necessary for them to set team norms and values that could be used as standards against which they could monitor performance. This has been a particularly useful starting point for team performance reviews, which the nurse facilitator established with several of the teams who felt that they were at a crossroads or had reached a plateau.

Training sessions that were pertinent to other departments in the trust were written and delivered by them. This ensured that all of the information given was factually accurate and enabled the nurses to meet members of the personnel and finance departments, which was an asset when they had queries or concerns as they could relate to a person and not just to a name on a piece of paper.

Handouts were provided at the end of every training session so that the nurses collected a comprehensive folder of information to which they could refer as necessary. In addition, the participants evaluated each training session and the trainers and changes were made to the programme as required.

Although the training was positively evaluated, there were concerns that there was 'too much crammed in too quickly' and some nurses commented that the training would have been more effective had it been carried out before the project started. However, the majority felt that a 'rolling programme' that could be accessed for refreshers and by new staff would be more beneficial. For this reason, the training programme has been included in the trust's in-house training manual.

NURSE FACILITATOR INVOLVEMENT

The nurse facilitator gained the support and confidence of the nurses by working with them and supporting them on issues that they felt strongly about. She was able to unblock some of the frustration that the nurses felt about not being heard by the senior management of the organisation, being on the periphery and not being involved within the trust by ensuring that communication channels remained open and by inviting directors and senior managers to training and study days.

Although this role was initially seen as being one which would enable the nurses to work independently and that it would no longer be needed, it became clear that the nurses valued the support that they were given. It has been perceived by some that the nurse facilitator would find it difficult to withdraw from teams who were working effectively but the converse was true. She found that by forming relationships with the nurses in the early days she could be assured that they would contact her if she was needed.

The input and contact that the nurse facilitator had with each of the teams therefore varied depending upon their particular needs at that time. She could, and often did, act as a 'go between' for the teams and other trust functions such as finance or personnel when the teams were experiencing difficulties. Although she encouraged the nurses to deal with challenging relationships within the practices, she would support them at meetings and facilitate meetings within the team if there were problems that could not be resolved.

The approach used was non-directive, non-threatening, gave support when it was asked for and did not interfere in the team dynamics unless asked to do so.

EVALUATION

The project was evaluated by an independent management consultant by means of questionnaires to the nurses involved and to those in eight similar sized control practices. These were administered at the beginning, middle and end of the pilot period. The first two followed the same format and used a Likert scale with room for comments to allow some freedom of expression. The final questionnaire contained more open-ended questions. The nurse facilitator also administered questionnaires to the GPs and practice managers at the practices involved with the pilot.

In addition, extra codes were added into the service activity monitoring system (SAMS) which the community nurses use to collate data on a daily basis to allow for time spent on project administration and project training. Some of the nurses and the nurse facilitator also kept reflective diaries that enabled them to recall critical incidents at the end of the pilot period.

The evaluation showed that the majority of nurses felt that there was more teamwork and integration although practice nurses did not demonstrate this as strongly as district nurses and health visitors.

It also demonstrated that there was more commitment to the organisation as well as to the nurses' practice. Senior managers and board members became visible to them: 'they have been interested, available and approachable and are no longer viewed as "the suits" in the board room/office', and nurses felt part of the trust. This can best be demonstrated by entries into reflective diaries, for example:

> If anyone had said that after 15–20 years working for the Trust I would work six times as hard on Trust related work they would have got a flat denial . . . it's been a lot of hard work and caused irritation at times but I have enjoyed this aspect and seeing things from a fresh angle.

> I feel that we can effect change rather than have it imposed upon us. We don't have a great deal of power but we have a lot more that we did have!

FULL IMPLEMENTATION

Lessons have been learned from the full implementation of SMINTS across the trust.

Following the successful evaluation, a programme to implement SMINTS across the trust was started. This was slow to begin with and the nursing teams were given the same level of training and support as those in the pilot. However, it soon became apparent that there were insufficient resources available to continue with a dedicated training programme for SMINTS and the modules were combined with the general trust in-house training programme.

This change to the training programme has resulted in the nursing teams being less confident in their abilities than those who had received the dedicated programme. In turn, this has resulted in more reliance on input from the nurse facilitators and, in some teams, the concept being lost. The problems engendered by this have been recognised by the nurses, nurse facilitators, senior managers and directors and steps are being taken to revisit the training needs of the community nursing teams.

ORGANISATIONAL CHANGE

The New NHS: Modern, Dependable (DoH 1997) has brought further changes and challenges to community nursing. WBPCS has disestablished and merged with local primary care groups (PCGs) to form primary care trusts (PCTs). The remit of PCTs is to bring community and primary care services closer together. There is an emphasis on health improvement and a greater focus on community and locality health rather than individual health.

The collaboration between general practices and the closer working within the PCT should see an end to the employment barriers between practice nurses and their community nursing colleagues. However, it is clear that GPs remain independent contractors and employ their own staff, so these barriers still remain. Locally, there has been no greater engagement of practice nursing than when the traditional trust structure was in place. It is of course early in the formation and development of the new organisation and every effort will be made for greater integration of practice nursing.

CONCLUSION

This project began as a 6-month pilot 5 years ago with seven nursing teams, who consisted of district nurses, health visitors and practice nurses. It was successfully evaluated by means of questionnaires and reflective diaries and has now been extended to all nursing teams. A management reorganisation has removed the traditional nurse manager and all nurses will be facilitated to enable them to make the change.

The success of the SMINTS in West Berkshire Priority Care Service NHS Trust appears to have been partly through the gradual introduction process and working with the nurses involved rather than forcing them into the changes. It was also due to the training programme that was delivered and tailored according to need. Nurses have commented how useful it was to have a comprehensive folder of handouts that they could refer to as necessary. It is also important to have a 'rolling' programme, which can be easily accessed by new staff joining the team. The lack of such a dedicated programme proved to be detrimental during the full implementation.

There is an acknowledgement that the full implementation was not as successful. This has been attributed to lack of attention to the training and support in the initial stages of team development.

If nurses are to really embrace the ethos of the modern and dependable NHS of the 21st century, they must first break down the barriers which have traditionally existed for so long and learn how to respect each other and work more closely together. PCTs should help this to happen to some extent.

In the initial phases of SMINTS, the nurse facilitator's (originally nurse consultant) motivation and commitment to the teams was helped by the energy, enthusiasm and commitment of the nurses.

The challenge is to replicate this energy and enthusiasm in the remaining nursing teams.

Reference

Department of Health 1997 The new NHS: modern, dependable. Department of Health, London

Self-managed integrated nursing teams

Section **Three**

DEVELOPING SKILLS IN INNOVATION

OVERVIEW

This third section picks up the reality of implementing change, but most importantly addresses the way in which a shift in culture must become embedded in health care. Three main areas are addressed in this section: the changes in nurse education that are helping to sustain lifelong learning, the complex issues associated with managing change and developing a learning organisation, and finally an example of imposing change in a large bureaucratic organisation that did not go according to plan.

Julie Hughes writes about the changes in nurse education that have encouraged nurses to develop the skills of critical analysis and embrace a problem-solving approach to health care. She shows how reflective learning is now part of all educational programmes, thus encouraging nurses to take a critical approach to their practice. Julie develops the importance of lifelong learning principles and how they have been adopted by health care to ensure that learning becomes implicit in the job and not, as in the past, associated only with academic courses. The various ways of sustaining and promoting lifelong learning are addressed in the chapter, but Julie argues that although the professional and regulatory bodies have a role to play, the most significant way of embedding lifelong learning in practice is by nurturing the learning environment. The associated application by Linda Chapman provides an example of practice-based learning. Linda uses the example of how a nurse was able to empower her patients by giving them a choice in their care. She also shows how practice-based learning can bridge the theory/practice gap through the use of learning contracts and the process of reflective learning. And above all else it shows how this process develops a learning culture which is part of day-to-day work.

The same theme of developing and sustaining a learning culture forms an important part of the next chapter by Jeanette Thompson and Sharon Pickering. The focus here is on the whole organisation in promoting creativity and growth. The concept of a learning organisation is introduced and described as one that values the individual, listens to their ideas and supports innovation and change. New ways of thinking are allowed and nurtured as people are encouraged to learn, and to learn collectively. In a learning organisation the lifelong learner is able to develop practice in innovative ways but also to ensure that the patient remains central.

Application 8.1 describes a project about shared governance that shows how an organisation has developed a system which optimises the contribution of every staff member in decision making. The example written by Linda Lilley shows how the implementation of the project went through the many stages of change management but that the key goal was ownership of the project by all staff through the system of shared governance. It illustrates how change theory and action research can be effectively implemented in practice to facilitate a major innovation and change programme. The introduction of shared governance required a major change within the organisational culture. The implementation and evaluation of the project was undertaken collaboratively by an acute hospital trust and an institute of higher education. The aims were in line with the government's modernisation programme and included the provision of best health care and increased collaboration between professionals, patients and the public to optimise the contribution of each member of staff and to develop multiprofessional team working. It is an inspiring example to those leaders who are prepared to accept the challenge of working collaboratively to create new ways of working in the provision of health care.

Developing skills in innovation

In Chapter 9 Colin Dale, James Gardner and Shirla Philogene cite the issue of staff ownership as one of the main reasons that change at Ashworth Hospital did not go according to plan. The theory of change management is discussed and then related to a case study of attempted change in a large hierarchical and bureaucratic organisation. One of the main weaknesses raised by the evaluation of the change process was the lack of communication. The managers' perception was that there was adequate communication whereas the staff and patients' perception was that they were 'left in the dark'. The authors make the point that in any process of change people must be involved at all levels and that they must have a sense of ownership. As this did not happen there was discontent felt by the staff and the change was viewed as an imposition. The authors support the view that the difficulties could have been overcome if a fully representative change group comprised of staff and patients had been set up.

Developing skills in innovation

Chapter **Seven**

Sustaining creativity and innovation through learning

Julie Hughes

Developing skills in innovation

- Continuous professional development
- The emergence of postregistration education and practice
- The personal professional portfolio

- Lifelong learning
- Innovative roles to support the lifelong learning culture

OVERVIEW

The purpose of this chapter is to explore and critically evaluate how as practitioners we might sustain creativity and innovation in the clinical setting. There have been significant changes over recent years in the educational preparation of nurses and there is a drive from within the nursing profession towards an all graduate status (Council of Deans 2000). Alongside this there is the government agenda to promote a lifelong learning society. The principles of lifelong learning should be evident in the health care profession with commitment from the profession to adopt a learning culture across educational settings and practice environments.

This chapter will endeavour to address the implications, for both the educational and practice settings, of creating a lifelong learning culture on the personal and professional development of health care workers.

DEVELOPMENTS IN NURSE EDUCATION

Over the past decade nursing education has undergone a transition from the traditional schools of nursing (generally based on or close to the hospital site where the students would undertake the practice component of the course) to a higher education institution (HEI). The drive for such a move was related to the curricular changes imposed by the introduction of Project 2000 promoting an academic advance to delivery of a diploma or degree level of education for nurses.

This transition has been subject to much balanced argument over recent years throughout HEIs, the NHS and through the media. The shift is supported by the professional bodies for nursing, midwifery and health visiting as they endeavour to secure a professional status for nursing.

Whilst health care education as a whole would be no stranger to the HEI (health visiting, district nursing and professions allied to medicine already having established links), for nursing this was a fundamental change. Quinn (1995) argues that for nurse teachers this created a need to ensure they would avoid becoming isolated from practice. This risk is enhanced by the demands on nurse teachers from the HEI to be research active.

Although research activity will greatly benefit the nursing profession, teachers would be expected to balance the demands of teaching, research, administration and clinical credibility – a daunting prospect.

Whilst recognising the climate of organisational change, Maslin-Prothero (1997) argues that this cannot be considered in isolation from significant professional changes influencing nurse education that have already taken place.

Examples of professional change are twofold:

1. From the clinical perspective there have been advances in research, technology and practice resulting in changing care patterns (DoH 1999, UKCC 1998). There has also been a reduction in the working hours of doctors and a subsequent exploration of the clinical roles of nurses and doctors which has led to the development of clinical nurse specialist and nurse consultant roles (Council of Deans 2000).

2. There have been substantial professional education changes with the emergence of Post Registration Education and Practice (PREP) from the governing body for nursing, midwifery and health visiting, the UKCC (1994). PREP embraces the principles

Creativity and innovation through learning

of lifelong learning as it will ensure that continuous professional development (CPD) is mandatory for nurses to maintain their professional registration. White (2000) suggests that initial qualification is merely the beginning of a long journey, thus supporting the argument for nursing to embrace a lifelong learning culture.

Whilst considering organisational and professional issues there must also be a commitment to the wider political agenda. *Making a Difference* (DoH 1999) links the adoption of a lifelong learning culture into health care to recent government initiatives to promote continuous quality improvement within the NHS:

- *Clinical governance* – it is widely recognised throughout the NHS that there is an element of 'blame culture' in the practice environment and 'whistle blowing' has had media recognition to support this argument. The introduction of clinical governance should address this through encouraging practitioners to discuss, in an open and supportive environment, issues related to patient care. It provides practitioners with the opportunity to explore patient care and identify areas for improvement.
- *Commission for Health Improvement (CHI)* – The CHI has an auditing remit whereby a team will be responsible for auditing and reporting to a designated trust. The team reports on how well the trust has adopted the culture for continuous improvement, and the significance placed on clinical governance as a tool to support this culture.
- *National Institute of Clinical Excellence (NICE)* – NICE is responsible for producing evidence-based guidelines for clinical practice. This is a government initiative to address the diversity of any given practice that may be noticeable across trusts. National guidelines will enhance clinical excellence on a national scale, thereby promoting equity for the patient.
- *National Service Frameworks (NSF)* – The Department of Health for England has been working with a multitude of professionals across health, social, education and the voluntary sector to compile National Service Frameworks, the purpose of which is to underpin practice with a set of standards/principles of care. The CHI will audit how well a trust integrates the NSF into practice and it therefore becomes a tool for continuous health improvement.

This drive for continuous improvement requires practitioners who are innovative and creative and who assimilate critical enquiry into their everyday practice. This has implications for health care as lifelong learning can no longer be a slogan to which lip service is paid, nor can education and training be an aspiration. Nurse teachers and nurse managers need to recognise and accept lifelong learning as a concept (Council of Deans 2000). They must therefore acknowledge the qualities of a lifelong learner and endeavour to facilitate their students to develop the qualities of:

- adaptability
- self-reliance
- responsiveness to change (Maslin-Prothero 1997).

If these skills are to be developed as students enter the profession, then creating an environment where such skills are recognised and valued is prerequisite to their continued development. If the commitment to lifelong learning is to be sustained, the philosophy must pervade the organisation and this is equally true of the HEI and the practice setting.

Sustaining creative learning environments across practice and HEI settings is challenging and requires innovation and collaboration to promote the integration of theory and practice.

IMPLICATIONS FOR THE HIGHER EDUCATION INSTITUTION

Perhaps one of the most significant arguments for the nursing profession in recent years relates to the relationship between theory and practice. Many theorists have argued that there is a 'divide' between theory and practice and that it is the remit of the educational establishment to attempt to build a bridge across the divide (Jordan 1998, Lathlean 1995, Wilkinson 1999).

As the nursing profession endeavours to embrace the principles of lifelong learning, and to apply these principles to the classroom setting and the clinical environment, it becomes apparent that creative and innovative leaders of health care must be aware of the significance of the concept. They must have the skills to recognise opportunities for development and identify appropriate teaching and learning strategies both for themselves and their colleagues.

Many theorists argue that the identification of appropriate teaching and learning strategies within the curriculum will support the development of leaders with these necessary skills (Conway 1994, Durgahee 1997, Jordan 1998, Wilkinson 1999). Thus the challenge to the HEI is to ensure that lifelong learning principles are implicit to the curriculum and appropriate teaching

Creativity and innovation through learning

and learning strategies (including theories of learning) are adopted.

Theories of learning

Whilst traditional nurse training was influenced by behavioural objectives to acquire specific skills, more recent education programmes have demonstrated a more holistic, humanistic approach embracing psychomotor and affective domains of learning. Strategies for teaching and learning that support the humanistic philosophy include reflection and experiential learning whereby the teacher/facilitator endeavours to marry the artistry and the science of nursing. Educational theories that have influenced current day curriculum planners are twofold: the adult and the experiential.

The adult learning perspective

Carl Rogers (1983) and Malcolm Knowles (1990) are among theorists who have explored the humanistic approach to learning to which they argue adult learners are more receptive. They suggest there is human inborn potential for growth and development and a subsequent willingness to learn. Where adult learning theories are utilised the consumer of education will be an active participant in the process and the teacher will undertake a facilitative role. This perspective marries well with the lifelong learning culture and the core principles as advocated by the ENB (1997) of lifelong learning being student centred and the responsibility of the individual to achieve (Box 7.1).

Box 7.1 The learning contract (adapted from UKCC 2001)

The emergence of the learning contract in nurse education is an example of how humanistic theory has been upheld. The contract requires the student to identify areas of learning need and work with the facilitator to identify how to meet those needs.

The UKCC PREP requirements are based on the principles of the learning contract recommending that the professional portfolio demonstrates the following:

- review of competence
- set learning objectives
- develop action plan
- implement plan
- evaluate and record.

The experiential learning perspective

Jordan (1998) argues that whilst adult learners may manifest an inherent willingness to learn, it will only apply where the theory delivered is relevant and applicable to the recipient. Theorists have addressed the issue of generating theory through reflecting on clinical practice in a cyclical manner (Fig. 7.1), thereby enhancing the relevance to the learner.

Recognising the value of experiential learning and reflective practice is paramount to the continuous professional development of nurses, midwives and health visitors and is the principle underpinning PREP. A further example of the value of such strategies is the emergence of the accreditation of prior experiential learning (APEL) (Box 7.2).

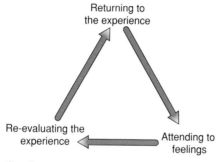

Figure 7.1 Reflection: turning experience into learning (adapted from Boud et al 1985)

Box 7.2 Accreditation of prior learning experience (APEL)

An example of APEL is the transitional arrangements that were put in place by the ENB to support practice nurses (GPNs) and community children's nurses (CCNs) following the development in 1994 of the specialist practitioner education programme.

At that time there were a number of GPNs and CCNs who were employed and very competent in their specialist role. The ENB produced outcomes and the practitioner could demonstrate, through the compilation of a portfolio of evidence, how they had achieved the outcomes in practice. The portfolios were assessed by a HEI and through prior experiential learning the practitioner would be awarded the specialist practitioner qualification.

This system is also apparent in the recent publication (ENB/DoH 2001a) relating to the preparation of mentors and teachers for health and social care. APEL may be utilised to illustrate how specific course outcomes have been met, thereby releasing the student from that component of the course and preventing repetitive learning.

Creativity and innovation through learning

Wilkinson (1999) argues that it is the responsibility of the academic establishment to ensure they recognise both adult and experiential learning theories in the curricula and that they utilise reflective learning to build a bridge across any theory/practice divide. This presupposes a fluent and effective working partnership between service and education and joint recognition of the implications of the practice setting as a learning environment.

Bridge building across the theory/practice divide

Since the move of nurse education into the higher education setting there has been growing concern that nurse teachers are more isolated from practice and at risk of jeopardising their credibility (Council of Deans 2000, Lathlean 1995). This lack of credibility would widen the theory/practice divide considerably as learners become aware that the theoretical underpinning negates the real world of practice. This scenario would not be conducive to sustaining innovation and creativity as a perceived theory/practice divide is likely to depress nurses' motivation to learn (Jordan 1998).

Bridging the divide is therefore fundamental to nurse education. The implications for the HEIs are that they must work in a collaborative fashion with the trusts that they serve and with the local education confederation. They must recognise teaching and learning for professional practice as a shared issue.

Innovative models for teaching

The emergence of the role of the lecturer practitioner (LP) is one example of collaborative working (the recent guidelines in relation to the preparation of teachers (ENB/DoH 2001a) suggest the title of practice lecturer).

The LP role has been subjected to an abundance of critical discussion over recent years. The role evolved from a model utilised in Oxford in the mid-1980s and the philosophy behind the evolution was to address the potential theory/practice divide that could result from the shift of nurse education into HE (Lathlean 1995).

Most LP roles are jointly funded by a university and a trust and postholders therefore require skills to integrate clinical and educational leadership. Gibbon & Kendrick (1996) argue that it is the minority who can demonstrate such skills and in line with other critics advocate that the serving of two masters can only be successful in supportive, creative environments across education and practice (Quinn 1995, Willis 1998).

Despite the demands of the LP role there is overwhelming evidence to support the strengths of the concept:

- LPs are considered by students/learners to be clinically credible due to still having roots in practice
- LPs promote reflective practice and problem-based learning thereby supporting the lifelong learning culture
- the appointment of LPs can serve to improve working relationships between service and education; this is essential to support the professional acceptance of PREP
- they contribute to curriculum planning and support the notion of a practice-led curriculum
- LPs are effective role models demonstrating expertise in practice
- on a personal level they have the opportunity to advance their career whilst still maintaining their clinical interest
- LPs can create and support a research culture in the clinical environment which is fundamental to enhancing the quality of patient care.

These arguments have been well supported by the literature and through anecdotal evidence offered by colleagues in the LP role (Lathlean 1995, Shepherd et al 1999, Tamlyn & Myrick 1995) (Box 7.3). Commitment and motivation are crucial to underpin the LP role and other necessary qualities have been suggested:

- flexibility
- resilience
- good time management
- ability to listen
- empathy (Willis 1998).

Box 7.3 The community practice lecturer

Over the past 4 years the University of Reading has had community practice lecturers (CPLs) in the Health Studies teaching team. The CPL is involved in planning and delivering the specialist component of the BA(Hons) Primary Care that comprises:

- general practice nursing
- community children's nursing
- mental health nursing
- health visiting
- district nursing
- learning disabilities nursing
- school nursing.

The CPL role has been well evaluated by the students and by colleagues as being an effective model in addressing the theory/practice divide.

Creativity and innovation through learning

Such a list reinforces the argument that the LP role is challenging and demanding and not for the faint hearted! To ensure that the LP can manage the role, both the service and the education side must provide a supportive environment and must recognise and respect the joint demands of the role.

There are now an increasing number of LP posts emerging, some with a very specialist focus and others more generic. The very early model that emerged from Oxford has been evaluated and critiqued and it is clear that the LP would benefit from not having any managerial responsibilities. Many of the initial posts were filled by senior clinical staff who had a management remit and as a consequence were attempting to juggle three balls. More recent posts have had a focus on those nurses, midwives and health visitors who have a commitment to teaching and assessing and to practice development and who have excellent clinical skills. This would seem to be a more acceptable model (Box 7.4) and this evolution is well supported by the literature (Lathlean 1995).

In the light of the challenges for the HEI to sustain creativity and innovation lecturer practitioners, with a 'foot in both camps', are well placed to support the development of the curriculum to include relevant strategic approaches to the teaching and learning needs of the profession. They are equally well placed to influence the creation of a suitable learning environment in the practice setting.

Box 7.4   The lecturer practitioner – a personal account

From a personal perspective I have practised as a lecturer practitioner for 5 years. For the first four of these I was a lead sister in my specialist field and consequently juggler of three balls. On reflection I became aware of the difficulties of shared loyalties both personally and professionally. I now practise and teach but have relinquished my managerial position.

My personal perspective is that my joint role is now more manageable, more enjoyable and I can provide a more qualitative service to my students and my clients.

IMPLICATIONS FOR THE PRACTICE SETTING

To sustain creativity and innovation in health care the practice setting must envelop a learning culture. Practice settings as learning

Developing skills in innovation

environments have been the focus of much discussion among nurse educators, increasingly so since the advent of P2K (ENB/DoH 2001b). The P2K programme aspires to equip nurses with the theoretical foundations on which to base their practice and to develop them as autonomous, enquiring practitioners. This preparation requires a commitment to teaching and learning across both the education and practice settings. Suitable practice placements are fundamental to nurse education and to continuous professional development.

The P2K cohorts have tended to be large and require an equivalent number of practice placements offering a diversity of learning opportunities. The educational establishment running the programme has an obligation to the national body and to quality assurance assessors to audit all the practice placements for suitability as a prerequisite to the validation of their education programme (ENB 1997).

Alongside the obligation to students undertaking programmes of study, the practice setting also has to recognise the government initiative *Making a Difference* (DoH 1999) to strive for continuous quality improvement in the delivery of health care. Creating an effective practice learning environment should be the collaborative responsibility of the managers, teachers and practitioners and will require effective leadership from a clinically credible role model (Kitson 1997). Assimilation of the philosophy of lifelong learning into the practice setting is fundamental to the professionalism of nursing and it is the responsibility of the leaders of the profession to equip nurses with the necessary skills for lifelong learning:

- ability to identify learning need
- access and retrieve information
- filter the information
- utilise it to enhance practice (Maslin-Prothero 1997).

In a practice setting where such skills are notably encouraged and nurtured, the characteristics of innovation, resourcefulness, adaptability and self-reliance should emerge, enabling nurses to meet the requirements of the profession and their clients and patients. Richardson (1998) suggests that a lifelong learning environment would increase motivation for learning through self-awareness, thereby facilitating continuous development. However, such an environment could have the opposite effect and appear threatening within the professional and organisational changing climate of health care (Box 7.5).

Promoting a practice environment that offers learning opportunities, supports learning and continuous development for all staff

Creativity and innovation through learning

Box 7.5   Threatening or supportive?

Whilst the philosophy that underpins clinical governance is that of continuous quality improvement, lack of understanding of the concept could mean it would be construed as a whistle-blowing exercise.

The Department of Health advocates that the Commission for Health Improvement (CHI) will visit a trust to compile a report of areas of good practice and make recommendations for improvements. This could be construed as a destructive force looking to name and shame!

Whilst the emergence of clinical governance and the CHI challenges the values and culture of the organisation it advocates a bottom-up approach to health care where the clients' and practitioners' experiences are explored as a quality improvement initiative. This must be seen as a positive challenge and an opportunity for health care professionals. Practice environments must enhance confidence and self-assurance to remove any element of threat perceived to be present.

---

and is non-threatening is a challenge to service and education. Over recent years collaboration between the HEI and the practice setting has resulted in the development of innovative professional clinical roles to support education in practice.

Nurse consultants

The nurse consultant is a recent innovation generated from a political agenda relating to the retention of expert clinical nurses. It has been recognised that the existing grading structure for nurses, midwives and health visitors is restricting for committed, expert practitioners. Once they reach the top of the clinical grading scale they can only progress through education or management. Recognising the need for the NHS to retain these clinical experts the government announced the development of the nurse consultant role. No formal evaluation of the role has yet been undertaken but the post must be seen as crucial to further development.

The Council of Deans (2000) supports the innovation and recognises the value of the nurse consultant in improving patient care through evidence-based practice. The academic underpinning for the role would be equivalent to Masters level education, which may be achieved through academic study and/or experiential learning. The concept of the nurse consultant is supported across education and service and the role modelling and educational capabilities of such a role must be nurtured as the post develops.

Practice development nurses

Many NHS trusts have begun to create practice development posts to promote and support the development of practice through change and innovation. Practice development nurses are required to be excellent clinicians and have an academic profile that supports a research culture, as well as the skills to initiate practice development and support practitioners with innovation and change in the clinical area, thereby enhancing a lifelong learning environment.

Practice educator

Recent guidelines jointly published by the ENB and DoH (2001a) announce the development of the practice educator role. Preparation for this role is to be through a postgraduate teacher training course with relevant outcomes (ENB/DoH 2001a, Appendix 1). The practice educator will be responsible for creating and sustaining a lifelong learning culture throughout the organisation in which they practise in order to support colleagues with continual professional development needs. Unlike other practice teacher models where teachers are responsible for meeting the learning needs of students, the practice educator will have a wider remit and commitment to professional development that will include multiprofessional education issues.

Like other emerging roles the evaluative process is crucial to future development. If practitioners are equipped with the skills for teaching and assessing and supporting professional development they will have the foundations for enhancing the teaching and learning culture throughout the organisation. Consequently the needs of the individual and the profession will be met and ultimately the patient will receive ever improving quality of care.

All the above posts support the government and professional agenda to promote the skills of leadership within the nursing profession. The ENB (1997) argues that leadership skills are enhanced through lifelong learning, that good leaders enhance a lifelong learning culture and that the concept thus becomes cyclical.

Creativity and innovation through learning

DEVELOPING INNOVATIVE, CREATIVE PRACTITIONERS THROUGH LIFELONG LEARNING

To sustain innovation and creativity throughout the profession the lifelong learning culture must become the norm. Although lifelong learning has been much discussed on the political agenda, nursing and midwifery have unique professional needs and blanket adoption of lifelong learning, without recognition of professional needs, could create a complex, unwieldy environment (Council of Deans 2000). The ENB explored the phenomenon in some detail and in the 1997 publication *Lifelong Learning in Europe* offered some core principles. Lifelong learning should be:

- practice based
- student/learner centred
- evidence based
- responsive to individual need
- upheld by the individual as well as the organisation.

The ENB also promotes lifelong learning as an active process underpinned by a multitude of personal characteristics:

- adaptability
- flexibility
- creativity
- confidence
- ability to challenge
- initiative
- enthusiasm.

The UKCC supports the ENB publication and argues that the introduction of PREP has enhanced the need for the profession to envelop the culture. Gopee (2000) argues that lifelong learning must become ingrained in health care to support initiatives such as PREP. It could be argued that the development of a personal professional portfolio supports the practitioner in developing self-assessment skills through reflection (Box 7.6).

Whilst lifelong learning within the profession has been implicit with the *Code of Professional Conduct* (UKCC 1992) it has now become explicit through PREP and 'keeping up to date' can no longer be for the motivated professional but must be adopted by all. Sayer (1998) argues that creating a supportive, nurturing lifelong learning culture will be more fruitful than trying to impose

Box 7.6 Reflection through clinical supervision

The art of reflecting on practice is slowly being integrated into the practice setting and initiatives such as clinical supervision support this. Clinical supervision allows the practitioner to share, in a confidential environment, issues about their practice. The supervisor will facilitate exploration of a critical incident, encouraging the practitioner to consider the what, why, how, what next elements of a reflective cycle and engage in the process of reflection.

such an environment by PREP alone. Where nurses have access to suitable facilitation they will recognise the value of PREP for its commitment to individual learning needs and to the need for the individual to reflect on issues that are pertinent and relevant to their own area of practice.

All the research and discussion that has taken place in relation to the concept of lifelong learning supports the notion that conducive and flexible learning environments across education and practice are fundamental. Extolling the values of education to a workforce that is for the most part underresourced, and where morale can as a consequence be low, would be ineffective. It requires the educationalist to be innovative and creative in designing teaching and learning that will be feasible and accessible for all.

REFERENCES

Boud D, Keogh R, Walker D 1985 Reflection: turning experience into learning. Kogan Page, London

Conway J 1994 Reflection, the art and science of nursing and the theory practice gap. British Journal of Nursing 3(3): 114–118

Council of Deans and Heads of UK University Faculties 2000 Breaking the boundaries: educating nurses, midwives and health visitors for the next millenium: a position paper. http://www.nursing.man.ac.uk

Department of Health 1999 Making a difference: strengthening the nursing, midwifery and health visiting contribution to health and healthcare. Stationery Office, London

Durgahee T 1997 Reflective practice: decoding ethical knowledge. Nursing Ethics 4(3): 211–217

English National Board 1991 Framework and higher award for continuing professional education for nurses, midwives and health visitors. ENB, London

English National Board 1997 Lifelong learning in Europe: developing a strategic approach. Executive Summary. ENB, London

English National Board/Department of Health 2001a Preparation of mentors and teachers. ENB, London

Creativity and innovation through learning

Six Steps to **Effective Management**

English National Board/Department of Health 2001b Placements in focus. ENB, London

Gibbon C, Kendrick K 1996 Practical conflicts. Nursing Times 92(1): 51–54

Gopee N 2000 Self-assessment and the concept of the lifelong learning nurse. British Journal of Nursing 9(11): 724–729

Jordan S 1998 From classroom theory to clinical practice: evaluating the impact of a post registration course. Nurse Education Today 18: 293–302

Kitson A 1997 Developing excellence in nursing practice and care. Nursing Standard 12(2): 33–37

Knowles M 1990 The adult learner: a neglected species, 4th edn. Gulf Publishing, Houston

Lathlean J 1995 The application and development of the lecturer practitioner roles in nursing. Ashdale Press, London

Maslin-Prothero S 1997 A perspective on lifelong learning and its implications for nurses. Nurse Education Today 17: 431–436

Quinn FM 1995 The principles and practice of nurse education, 3rd edn. Chapman & Hall, London

Richardson A 1998 Personal professional profiles. Nursing Standard 12(38): 35–40

Rogers C 1983 Freedom to learn for the 80's. Merrill, Ohio

Sayer J 1998 PREP and lifelong learning: whose responsibility? Nursing Times Learning Curve 2(6): 2–3

Shepherd B, Thomson AM, Davies S, Whittaker K 1999 Facilitating learning in the community with lecturer practitioner posts. Nurse Education Today 19: 373–385

Tamlyn D, Myrick F 1995 Joint nursing appointments: a vehicle for influencing health care change. Journal of Advanced Nursing 22: 490–493

United Kingdom Central Council 1992 Code of professional conduct for nurses, midwives and health visitors. UKCC, London

United Kingdom Central Council 1994 Standards for education and practice following registration. UKCC, London

United Kingdom Central Council 1998 A higher level of practice. Consultation document. UKCC, London

White C 2000 The three degrees. Nursing Times 96(7): 56–58

Wilkinson J 1999 Implementing reflective practice. Nursing Standard 13(21): 36–39

Willis J 1998 Lecture-practitioners: serving two masters for a common cause. Nursing Times Learning Curve 1(12): 6–7

Developing skills in innovation

Application **7:1**

Linda Chapman

Embracing creativity and innovation in the workplace

This application will demonstrate how practice-based education has facilitated a community nurse to learn and develop her practice to ensure that creativity and innovation are embraced in the clinical workplace using Case study 7.1.1.

Case study 7.1.1

Development in practice
- Empowering practice nurses to assess patients and their leg ulcers so that patients have a choice to be assessed either at home or in the surgery

Rationale for developing practice
- To give patients of all ages the choice of having their legs assessed either at home, often at the district nurse's convenience, or in the surgery at their own convenience
- A third of patients who had their legs assessed by district nurses in their homes in the practice area in 2000 would have preferred to be assessed in the surgery
- The development of a group of practice nurses' skills in the assessment of legs had previously been unsuccessful

Learning needs
- To develop leadership skills to assist a group of practice nurses in developing expertise in assessment of patients' legs
- To differentiate between teaching nurses new skills and empowering nurses to integrate new skills into practice

Evidence-based learning in practice
- Reflective accounts
- Learning contract   *(Cont. overleaf)*

179

Case study 7.1.1 (*Cont.*)

- Documentation from teaching sessions
- Critical analysis and self-evaluation
- Minutes of meetings
- Completed questionnaires by practice nurses
- Audit

Developing skills in innovation

PRACTICE-BASED EDUCATION

The value of experiential learning and reflective practice is paramount in lifelong learning. However, as with any learning, the concept of a theory/practice gap is recognised (i.e. the difficulty experienced by some nurses in transferring classroom theory to practical settings). Practice-based education is a way of addressing this balance successfully and achieving praxis so that individual nurses can improve their knowledge and translate that knowledge into clinical practice so that it has a positive impact on patients, staff and the health care system. Practice-based education provides learning opportunities for nurses whilst they remain in clinical practice, permitting the patients and the clinical environment to remain at the heart of learning. This integrated form of learning adopts the combination of face-to-face teaching and distance learning, promoting the linking of theory to the workplace.

Independent and self-directed learning is encouraged using educational strategies focusing on the learning process rather than the teaching process. This ensures that each nurse is at the centre of learning, prompting each to take responsibility for their own learning and enhancing their ability to develop skills to facilitate lifelong learning. Practice-based education takes into consideration the rich professional experiences a nurse has and uses the principles of adult learning to facilitate learning and practice developments. The approach incorporates collaboration between nurse education and nursing practice, seeking to maximise the relevance of education to the local working situation. The strategies for implementation include:

- reflection
- learning contract
- mentorship
- practice educator
- collaboration between managers, nurses and HEI.

180

Reflection

Experience in practice can be a rich source of learning; however, experience alone is not enough. Reflecting on practice helps a nurse to facilitate learning though practice and provides a mechanism to review clinical practice by examining and questioning day-to-day practice. It helps nurses to reconsider practices and identify areas of their work in need of improvement. In examining how nurses actually practise and the relevant theories, comparison can be made between actual practice and recent evidence-based practice.

In Case study 7.1.1 the community nurse was aware of current research that stressed the importance of correctly assessing patients' leg ulcers so that appropriate treatment could be provided. Although she had this knowledge and had previously shared this with practice nurses, the practice nurses had not used the knowledge to develop their skills or practice. Using reflection the nurse realised that although she had 'taught' practice nurses how to assess patients with leg ulcers, these skills had not been turned into practice. Instead of leading practice nurses to develop their own skills she had set herself up as 'an expert' and received all of the referrals for assessment of patients' legs. This impacted on her workload as well as reducing patients' choice of having their assessment in the surgery or at home. From the reflection on her practice and prior experience the community nurse therefore identified that her learning needs were to develop her skills in leadership to 'empower' practice nurses to develop their leg assessment skills, rather than just 'teach' the skills of assessment to them.

Learning contract

During the process of reflection a nurse considers the theory that arises out of the examination of practice and what is required for professional development. Negotiating a learning contract incorporates the required knowledge, skills and attitudes necessary for effective practice development by providing a tool for nurses to identify the required resources and strategies to achieve successful change. In Case study 7.1.1 the nurse had sound knowledge of how to teach the assessment of clients with leg ulcers; however, she had little knowledge of how to effectively 'empower' nurses in her area of work to put into practice the taught skills. In negotiating a learning contract with a mentor she was able to clarify her own learning needs and identify the resources and strategies to facilitate the implementation of a change in practice. Identified resources included distance learning materials which encouraged the nurse to discover theories of leadership.

Creativity and innovation in the workplace

Six Steps to **Effective Management**

Mentorship

Fostering reflective learning encourages individual nurses to explore their experiences and practice in depth. For reflection to make a difference to practice it is important that the outcome includes action, which improves clinical practice. A mentor facilitates this by helping each nurse to identify what the nurse has learned in practice and needs to learn to develop practice in the workplace. A mentor facilitates and supports the learning experience of the nurse by acting as a 'thinking partner', helping to identify strengths and learning needs in the context of the practice environment. The mentor is a trusted professional who helps the nurse work through difficulties associated with learning and developing practice and is someone with whom the nurse could talk, gain support from and receive honest and constructive feedback. The mentor's understanding of the practice area informs and enhances learning from both the wider service perspective and through the learning contract. In Case study 7.1.1, by the community nurse and mentor listening to each other and working together, the mentor helped the nurse to recognise learning needs and identify learning opportunities for development.

Practice educator

A practice educator facilitates the integration of theory and practice by helping the nurse to relate new knowledge to local circumstances and actively urging nurses to explore and lead initiatives in order to improve upon current practice. Often a nurse can provide good descriptions and comprehensive accounts of incidents from practice, but when deeply involved in a situation it can be difficult to identify key factors that are important in the way care is delivered. There may be feelings beneath the surface which, through questioning and exploration, a practice educator can help the nurse examine more carefully. The practice educator can facilitate a nurse to both challenge assumptions and scrutinise personal knowledge of changing practice. Within Case study 7.1.1, on a personal level the community nurse faced conflict between best practice and the custom and practices used in the workplace. Although best practice is for clients to be given a choice in their care, custom and practice dictated that district nurses assess all patients with leg ulcers in the patient's home, and patients were not given the option of being assessed in the surgery. The practice educator actively encouraged the nurse to explore new knowledge around styles of leadership and empowerment and to integrate relevant theories into local practice. The changes in practice the nurse made became real and visible for the practice educator.

Collaboration between managers, nurses and the higher education institution

Without opportunities for nurses to question practice, ways of working become stifled and ritualised. By contrast, work settings where learning is actively encouraged provide a supportive environment and the quality of patient care ultimately benefits. Creating an effective clinical learning environment should be the collaborative responsibility for the managers, teachers and nurses, which must be achieved in practice. In Case study 7.1.1 the manager recognised that if services are to be developed to meet rapidly changing needs, nurses are the key resource. By valuing the nurse's learning needs and providing a commitment to continuous professional development it allowed the nurse to be creative and innovative in the workplace.

Accredited learning is an ideal way of acknowledging learning and emphasises strongly the application of academic study to the practice area. A higher education institution (HEI) provides the necessary infrastructure that supports the delivery of accredited learning including assessment and quality assurance. Assessment of a portfolio, for example, provides a framework for acknowledging that a nurse has identified and reflected on experience and clearly clarified learning needs and what has already been learned. It encourages further development of nurses' skills of critical and reflective practice and assesses their contribution to professional development and improvements to client care. The nurse in Case study 7.1.1 compiled a portfolio containing a range of information providing a comprehensive picture of progress and performance, as outlined in Box 7.1.1.

Box 7.1.1 Portfolio of progress and performance

- Identification of learning needs and evidence of learning in a learning contract
- Mapping of progress and drawing together the eclectic experiences of practice with theoretical components of the programme in reflective accounts
- Evidence of activities undertaken including:
  —documentation for teaching sessions
  —self-assessment and reflective accounts
  —critical analysis and self-evaluation
  —minutes of meetings
  —completed questionnaires by practice nurses
- Evidence of how personal learning has benefited clinical practice using the audit

---

Creativity and innovation in the workplace

183

Six Steps to **Effective Management**

Following assessment the nurse was accredited with 20 credits that can be used as part of the modular degree programme.

The HEI makes a significant contribution to the development of specified, high quality programmes that meet the needs of individual nurses. It ensures that student learning meets the university's commitment to theoretical content, equality, delivery and accessibility of the programmes. The practice educator collaborates with colleagues in the HEI, managers, mentors and nurses to ensure that learning meets nurses' needs and in actively seeking to incorporate their evaluation as part of continuing improvement.

CONCLUSION

Practice-based education facilitates bridging the theory/practice gap by encouraging individual nurses to explore their knowledge and introduce new theories. By providing support and fostering reflective learning it helps nurses to identify what they have learned in practice as well as which skills they need to develop. Negotiating a learning contract allows each nurse to deal with their own feelings and thoughts, which very often have practical applications. The relationship between the nurse in practice and educationalist in a higher education institution becomes a partnership and allows learning based on personal needs for nurses at all grades and varying levels of academic study. Practice-based education adopts the view that providing nurses with the resources to develop their skills and knowledge will enable them to apply theory to practice which impacts on patients, staff and the local health care system. In achieving this it prepares nurses to work in environments that are changing rapidly. It actively encourages professional development and competence to practise by allowing nurses to use professional experiences in the learning process and envelops a learning culture whereby practitioners are given the opportunity to explore their daily work and reformulate their practice.

Developing skills in innovation

Chapter **Eight**

Developing a culture for change

Jeanette Thompson and Sharon Pickering

- Drivers for change and understanding the impact of personal, professional influences on organisational culture
- Organisational cultures
- Developing and sustaining a learning culture

- Leadership
- Using reflection to influence change
- Implementing change

OVERVIEW

This chapter will begin by acknowledging the complexity of the context in which the NHS functions and the drivers that are generating the need for change. The development of a learning culture and the role of the leaders within the organisation are presented as key factors in promoting creativity and growth. The chapter is presented in three parts: Part 1 defines the role of management and leadership and explores the concept of the learning organisation; Part 2 focuses on leadership approaches and the relevance of transformational leadership in the facilitation of innovation and change; Part 3 considers the impact of the culture of the organisation upon the implementation of the change process, with reflection being presented as a vital management tool and the value of an inclusive approach to change emphasised.

INTRODUCTION

Drivers for change

Recent years have seen a significant change in the ethos driving the NHS. Notably the Labour government has introduced accountability for the quality of health care delivery (DoH 1997, 1998, 2000, 2001), achieved in part by making chief executive officers not only responsible for the financial stability of their organisation but also for the quality of clinical care within their organisation. Changes such as those in public health and the increasing focus upon a primary-care-led NHS have resulted in fundamental changes in the ways in which the NHS workforce operates. Consequently managers and leaders within services now need to be more innovative and creative in their approach to supporting and developing both staff and the organisation.

The need for this creativity is further reinforced by the complexity of service delivery within the current welfare system. This complexity is influenced by the number of variables that affect care delivery and the number of structures and systems that underpin it. Contemporary organisations have to operate not just in the context created by political imperatives but also those that come from professional bodies and the belief systems of each individual. Figure 8.1 illustrates the interrelationship between each of these systems and it is within this context that both the management of change and the development of organisational cultures must be considered.

Developing and sustaining a learning culture

Schein (1986) identifies organisational culture as the way in which employees behave and also the values that are important to them.

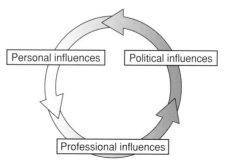

Figure 8.1   Influences on organisational culture

Carson (1999) translates this into the way that things are done in a particular organisation. Likert (1961) established a profile of organisational characteristics which when analysed can help in understanding the way an organisation carries out its functions and therefore the culture of that organisation. These characteristics are:

- leadership processes
- motivational forces
- communication processes
- decision making
- goal setting or ordering
- control processes.

Often the emphasis for developing the culture is invested within the managers of that organisation. This chapter will argue that it is not purely the role and responsibility of this group of people but is also that of the 'leaders' within that organisation, many of whom may not have the positional power of their managers. This is particularly relevant from the health care perspective where many of the leaders may be clinicians working directly with service users.

In many texts the terms 'manager' and 'leader' are used interchangeably; this appears to be based upon the perception that managers are often seen as having leadership functions. However, recent literature is beginning to further define these two concepts and some differences are beginning to emerge. These differences between management and leadership can be an important consideration in the context of encouraging both individual and organisational learning and development. It is not the intention to suggest that one approach should take precedence over the other but to demonstrate that both concepts have value and therefore are of equal importance. As such therefore they should not be viewed as mutually exclusive.

PART 1: MANAGEMENT, LEADERSHIP, LEARNING ORGANISATIONS

Defining management and leadership

Management is generally seen as a skill, technique or profession; however Autry (1991) suggests that it is a 'calling and a sacred trust' in which the well-being of staff (and clients/patients) is at the core of every decision made. Management and all the associated research and academic exposition clearly identify a series of tasks

Developing a culture for change

187

as being the role and responsibility of the manager. These frequently include activities such as planning, organising, managing staff, directing and coordinating activity, communication and budget management. Lindolm et al (1999) describe a manager as a member of an organisation who is granted the authority to direct the work-related activities of at least one other member of the same organisation by virtue of their position – a situation often described as positional power.

Mullins (1996) identifies leadership behaviours as mutual confidence and trust, an ability to understand work problems, having a genuine interest in personal problems, helping with personal and professional development, sharing information, seeking opinions about work problems, being friendly and approachable and finally, giving credit and recognition when due. Fagin (1990) defines leadership as the ability to bring about change whilst Tappen (1995) describes leadership as being about the process of influencing others. Naish (1995) suggests that although most leadership literature focuses upon the actions of the leader, the other side of the coin is about the way in which others respond to the actions of that person. Barnum & Kerfoot (1995) describe leadership based upon who the leader is, and how they motivate those around them. Maxwell (cited in King's Fund Project Paper 1985) stated that leadership is about power and charisma. He also emphasised the need for breadth, relevance, coherence of vision, the ability to communicate that vision, identifying good people to work with and helping individuals to develop.

Lindolm et al (1999) state that a leader is a person who does not necessarily have positional power in the same way as managers, but who has followers within an organisation irrespective of their hierarchical position. A further distinction between a leader and a manager is the focus of the leader upon managing learning.

Batten (1991) when discussing management and leadership draws the distinction between the 'simple hard' and the 'complicated easy'. The 'simple hard' can be represented by behaviours such as acting with integrity, transparency and managing the learning of others whilst the 'complicated easy' may be encapsulated in functions such as redesigning organisational structures. The risk that faces organisations is that managers or some leaders may focus upon the 'complicated easy' in order to achieve their defined tasks. This is not unusual in today's NHS when we consider the legacy, not only of competition within and between organisations, but also that of management and/or leadership within the sector. The challenge is therefore to develop strategies to move the culture of the organisation from one of competition, secrecy and a focus upon outcomes at the expense of process, to one that embraces the concepts of partnership, collaborative working, empowerment and transparency – in essence therefore, the development of an organisation that promotes innovation and creativity in its workforce. Implicit to the success of this is the need to consider how effective management approaches can be integrated with leadership styles that lead individuals to focus not only upon the 'complicated easy' but also upon the 'simple hard'.

The development of this or any other culture within an organisation can only be seen as a long-term effort. French & Bell (1995) identify it as a process that is led and supported by managers/leaders and aims to improve the organisation's capacity by using methods such as visioning, empowering, problem solving and learning which require managers/leaders to be collaborative and facilitative in the way they work with their employees.

Visioning

When implementing change and attempting to influence the culture of any organisation it is essential that the sense of purpose of the organisation is shared across all its constituent parts and by most, if not all, of its members. The common-sense approach to achieving this is for all members of the organisation to feel they have been represented and have had an opportunity to contribute to the process in which the vision of the organisation was established. This can be particularly important in an organisation where the culture is well embedded (Schein 1986). Essentially the most opportune part of any change process for developing the vision and the support for that vision is during the process of unfreezing, a term used by Lewin (1952) to describe the first stage in any change process. Visioning is equally important in situations where formal change is not on the agenda but where new members have joined the team. This situation may result in change of a different nature.

Empowering

Traditional cultures have not always operated on the premise of empowering those people who work within them, they have more characteristically focused upon traditional objectives and structured ways of achieving these. Current philosophies are, however, more focused upon valuing the employee and releasing the potential within each of us, as described in McGregor's 'theory Y' (1960). Essentially, therefore, empowering the workforce is an integral

Developing a culture for change

189

part of organisational and cultural change. Figure 8.2 illustrates the interrelationship between an empowered workforce and organisational and cultural change, with each of the component parts impacting directly upon the other in a positive way.

Problem solving

In traditional organisations we are often guilty of assuming that all things can be understood in relation to cause and effect. This can lead to failure to identify the actual problem as well as utilising a limited repertoire of solutions. This approach can be seen to have influenced the development of rigid and intransigent organisational cultures in which the values and experiences of those people who have organisational memory have the greatest power and influence. Within the current context of care there is now an acknowledgement that the problems that face us are complex and intractable. Consequently this traditional culture and its approach to problem solving can no longer be seen as the most effective strategy and that all staff need to be involved in problem-solving activities in order to effect cultural change.

Learning

Learning is an all-embracing term that encapsulates change of an enduring and persistent nature. Learning includes not only knowledge and skills but also attitudes and social behaviour. Learning links the individual to the social and organisational world and as such is both personal and professional. Consequently, developing the capacity of employees to learn is central to effective cultural change. Two of the most common approaches to developing an individual's learning in the context of the organisation are clinical supervision and action learning sets (Box 8.1).

It is through the principles of adult learning and reflective practice that clinical supervision and action learning can contribute to developing a learning culture and subsequently organisational change and development. The concept of reflection and how it can be used to inform change is discussed later in this chapter.

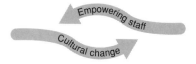

Figure 8.2 The correlation between staff empowerment and cultural change

> **Box 8.1** Methods to develop personal and team learning
>
> **Clinical supervision**
> Clinical supervision is defined as 'an exchange between practising professionals to enable the development of professional skills' (Butterworth & Faugier 1992). Barber & Norman (1987) suggest that clinical supervision is an interpersonal process by which a skilled practitioner helps a less experienced practitioner to develop skills and abilities appropriate to their role.
>
> There are some fundamental principles that underpin the concept of clinical supervision and which are crucial to the contribution of this approach in developing and sustaining the organisational culture. These include the practitioner focus, the reflective nature of the process, its relationship with continuous (professional) development and lifelong learning, as well as others such as empowerment and problem solving.
>
> **Action learning**
> Action learning is another way of facilitating the development of an organisation through the individuals working within it. Action learning aims to use the world of work to influence and inform the learning that takes place and therefore provides a powerful learning tool. The concept is based upon Revans' (1970) principle that there is no action without learning and there is no learning without action. This principle considers that experience is fundamental in any learning situation, as such work is the best place to learn when you are dealing with real issues. Revans' work is based upon the principles that are expounded within adult learning theories which value learning that is directly derived from experience. Such philosophies require that individuals are able to reflect upon their actions, but may yet not be able to see solutions to practice-based problems.
>
> The core of action learning is the establishment of action learning sets. These are groups of people who are willing to share problems, bring different perspectives and experiences and offer genuine solutions to other members' issues. Often individuals who belong to such sets are of a similar background and managerial level. Members of action learning sets need to have commitment not only to the idea of group problem solving, but also to the other group members. Such a group requires some organisation and structure; however, in true adult learning style, group processes must be negotiated and set within the group itself.

Learning organisations

The emphasis on learning within organisations demands a critical reappraisal of the traditional assumptions that underpin the NHS. Within this there is also a need to explore the wider historical,

Developing a culture for change

cultural and contextual imperatives that impact upon current management practice. For nurse managers within the NHS this is often a difficult task, not only as a result of the pace of change, but also because of the importance placed upon the role of the profession and the culture that comes with professional ideologies. The principles outlined above are fundamental to the capacity that any organisation has to change its culture and consequently improve the service it delivers. The concept of a learning organisation is one that is seen as a positive way forward in contemporary public services.

Pedler et al (1991) defines the learning organisation as an organisation that facilitates the learning of all its members and continuously transforms itself. Senge (1990) alternatively suggests that learning organisations are those organisations where people within them continually expand their capacity to create the results they really want and where new ways or patterns of thinking are allowed and nurtured. Senge (1990) also states that such organisations encourage people to continually learn and learn collectively. Learning organisations are essentially about building trust and confidence between employees and employers. It is this trust and confidence across the organisation that allows people to grow and develop and supports the interrelationship between the empowerment of individuals and the development of an organisation (see Fig. 8.2).

The realisation of this approach is predicated upon the optimistic philosophy of liberating human potential that is exemplified in McGregor's (1960) theory Y. This theory has an opposing view in theory X. In each case, fundamental assumptions about human nature are implicit within the theory. Theory X suggests that people are in the first instance inherently idle, will only work if coerced or threatened, only feel secure and comfortable in predictable situations, with set patterns of knowledge and hierarchies that control behaviour. The alternative view, or theory Y, supposes that people have a natural potential for learning and will expend physical and mental effort willingly in the service of objectives to which they feel some commitment. Those characteristics exemplified within theory Y can be seen as fundamental to the skills and approaches implicit within transformational leadership and related management styles. These concepts are described later in this chapter.

There are a number of major assumptions that underpin McGregor's theory, not least the belief that all individuals are either creative and imaginative (theory Y) or are unable to think 'out of the box' (theory X). The latter can be seen to underpin traditional management styles and theories, particularly those that present management as a controlling function. However, the development of organisations using learning as the prime focus relies heavily upon the belief that all human beings are able to learn and are willing or can be motivated to develop themselves and their organisation.

It also has to be recognised that within these ideas is the assumption that not only must individuals be willing but they also need to be able to participate in, and also take on the responsibility of, self-directed learning (Marsick 1987). The speed of learning and therefore change is heavily dependent upon organisational factors such as the culture and structures within it. Timpson (1998) argues workplace/organisational learning will always be governed by the need of the organisation to be productive or meet the aims of the service.

Essentially therefore, in order for an organisation to develop its culture in a way that acknowledges the inherent value of its key human resource (i.e. the staff team), the managers and leaders within that team have to be aware of the implications of the perception they hold of that workforce (theory X:theory Y). In addition, they have to consider the environment in which they ask staff to operate. This is particularly relevant as a converse relationship appears to exist between the speed and pace of change and the ability of people to respond positively to that change at all levels.

Until recently, the traditional view of management was predominantly seen as a scientific and rational process with only one way of achieving success. Within this the organisation is seen as a rigid mechanistic system which needed to be hierarchical in order to function well and be effective. Such processes breed 'top down' views and as such breed dependency by workers upon the hierarchy. Covey (1990) describes what he has named a 'maturity continuum' that at one end is a mode of behaviour which he labels 'dependency' and at the other 'interdependency' with the concept of 'independence' in the middle. In the dependent mode individuals believe that their feelings, behaviours and their fortunes are entirely caused by factors external to themselves and beyond their control. Within this context such individuals are essentially reactive and will not consider a situation to be their responsibility. These characteristics are essentially reflected within theory X and do not appear to be conducive with developing a learning organisation.

The independent mode is where individuals accept responsibility for themselves and generally their behaviour is proactive. Within an interdependency mode individuals recognise that they can achieve much more if they take responsibility not only for themselves but also for collaborating effectively with others. Covey (1990) contends that the position of individuals on this continuum strongly influences the degree to which they possess genuine self-confidence, with dependency typically coexisting with low self-esteem.

Self-confidence within members of any organisation is rarely established as a goal to be achieved, yet it is a crucial element. The potential power that exists within each individual when they are confident and self-aware ensures their contributions to the organisation are driven by the business of the organisation (in health care this is essentially client or patient focused). If self-confidence is manifested in all individuals within the organisation this creates a culture of mutual understanding, openness and positive regard. A service operating from this basis must surely have enormous potential both for users and for the overall development of the organisation. It would appear that self-confidence and all those associated traits identified as being part of a learning organisation's culture should become an acknowledged part of a service's education and training needs analysis and its supporting continuous professional development programmes. Conversely, an organisation that ignores such potential and reinforces hierarchical approaches to service management will not necessarily fail in service delivery, but may not maximise its potential.

Organisational culture is fundamental when exploring how an organisation works. In order to truly develop an organisation that engages in learning from its experiences there is a need to ensure that leadership and effective management exist at all levels. A well-led organisation is one that not only transacts its business effectively (i.e. within its financial resources) but also makes good use of the skills of the individuals who work within it. In addition, an effective organisation develops, evolves, improves and plans. Such an organisation is willing to take risks which are likely to pay off because the people who are taking the risks have a clear vision of what they are trying to achieve and are supported by those who will help them achieve it. The concept of leadership therefore has a great deal to offer the NHS in its current context.

PART 2: THE CONTRIBUTION OF LEADERSHIP IN ORGANISATIONAL CHANGE

As already noted organisational change occurs in a variety of ways – in some instances it is revolutionary and in others it may be much

Developing skills in innovation

more evolutionary – but one crucial factor in any approach to change is that of leadership. Leaders of any change need to have the ability to create the vision within an organisation, to empower the workers within it, create the followers that are needed for successful change and in so doing develop and change the culture within the organisation. This is also important as a consequence of contemporary health care environments, that is, environments characterised by turbulence and increasingly complex problems (Alimo Metcalfe 1996).

Types of leadership

Tannenbaum & Schmidt (1958) identified seven types of leadership. These operate on a continuum and include:

- making the decision and announcing it
- selling the decision
- presenting ideas and inviting questions
- presenting tentative decisions that are subject to change
- presenting the problem and seeking suggestions to inform the decision-making process
- defining the parameters in which the decision should be made and inviting the group to make the decision
- working with the 'subordinates' to make the decision.

Whilst continuing to acknowledge their importance and relevance, Tannenbaum & Schmidt have acknowledged the changing nature of organisations and the impact of this upon organisational development. Important contemporary influences outlined by Tannenbaum & Schmidt include the interdependency of the manager or leader with the workforce and the influence of the behaviour of each of these on the other. Within the health care context this is highly pertinent, for example, when considering the role and function of multiprofessional teams whose main focus is to meet the needs of service users. This is particularly important in circumstances where such teams do not have clear leadership, managerial or otherwise, and the organisation operates within a professional management hierarchy rather than a general management structure. Within this context the leader and their behaviour are fundamental to the success of the team in meeting its set goals.

In addition, Tannenbaum & Schmidt identify the crucial influence of external phenomena upon the work of any organisation. This includes both political and professional imperatives, as illustrated in

Figure 8.1. Of further relevance is the interrelationship between each organisation and their environment; data to inform this process are often collated in the form of approaches such as PEST (political, economic, social and technical) or SWOT (strengths, weaknesses, opportunities and threats) analysis. The influence of external elements and interfaces is particularly important when considering the changing nature of the environment in which health and social care is now delivered. Within this environment, the need for partnership is now crucial in order to maximise available resources and deliver a quality service to the consumer.

In addition, Tannenbaum & Schmidt's original work portrayed the manager as the principal actor who initiated and determined group function with little cognisance of other players. Such situations in contemporary health care services are becoming increasingly unlikely, particularly with the increasing specialism that often characterises contemporary health care. Clinical and managerial decisions need to be made on the basis of expert knowledge, not just hierarchical position. It is in this context that alternative approaches to management and leadership are gaining momentum.

Malby (1996) identifies the re-emergence of value-based leadership and the need to create a feeling of community within the service. The ideas of value-based leadership have relevance in the effort to create a public service ethic in a NHS that has experienced an internal market ethos. This concept is seen as important in the creation of an ethical base for decision making and priority setting within health care. Fundamental to this are effective communication structures and processes that enable any gaps that may exist between managers and workers to be satisfactorily resolved. The process of resolving differences assists in developing shared values that create a feeling of community and a clear sense of direction for everyone. This leads to a highly committed and energetic staff because they have shared values upon which their community is organised. Such a culture implicitly conveys feelings of value and worth. This is highlighted in work by Barnum & Kerfoot (1995) which states that people who do not feel cared for in today's health service will be unable to care for others. In such a context value-based leadership can be seen as synonymous with transformational leadership.

Transformational leadership

Burns (1978) suggests that there are two kinds of leadership: transactional and transformational. In transactional leadership one person takes the initiative for the activities, actions or exchanges. In doing so one person can be perceived as having greater control and power and each person having a different investment in that situation. In transformational leadership the leader and the followers have the same purpose, vision and similar philosophies about their area of work. Hein (1998) argues that transformational leadership is defined in terms of attitude rather than tasks. This means that the element of consistency required from a good leader is not necessarily found in the context of how the leader behaves, or performs tasks, but more in the leader's view of what is happening in the environment and how they translate those changes. As such, transformational leadership is holistic and is strongly underpinned by the individual's philosophy and value base about both people and life.

Within transformational leadership the most important focus of an interaction or function is the person. Such a leader mobilises others then grows and develops together with the followers. As this dynamic process continues, original needs and values are satisfied and new ones surface and contribute to the development of all involved. With this approach it is easier to see results than to actually plan the process. Leaders and followers make sense of the process of change by focusing upon goals and outcomes that can contribute to the overall vision. This process is supported, in the context of transformational leadership, by building a social architecture that provides meaning for the organisation's employees and will outlive the leader's employment within that service (Stevens Barnum 1998).

The role of the leader is to build and sustain trust, both in the organisation and themselves, and also to ensure that they are credible both professionally and personally. Other areas that the transformational leader needs to address are those of building self-esteem and self-confidence both personally and in the work that individuals do.

Transformational leadership interfaces very clearly with many of the changes currently being experienced within the health service. The move from transactional leadership styles towards a transformational leadership culture mirrors the changes from management to leadership and from a cost-effective, cost-conscious, competitive NHS to one that is more collaborative. It also mirrors the changes that are taking place within society as nurturing and caring become more respectable characteristics and are seen as more acceptable within the workplace.

As the health of individuals is reflected by what society looks like, reference can also be made to the changes in the world view. Barker & Young (1998) argue that most organisations and institutions will not survive in the 21st century unless they embrace the elements of transformational leadership that reflect the post-modern era. It is therefore crucially important both for the NHS and those that use health care services that we nurture and develop the skills implicit within transformational leadership.

Becoming a transformational leader

As already stated, transformational leadership is fundamentally about the individual, how they think and what they believe. Excellence in leadership and particularly transformational leadership is typified by both leader and followers acting, not on individual needs, but more in keeping with the visions and goals of the organisation. Charisma and personal power are important attributes in achieving this. Bennis & Nanus (1985) indicate that charismatic leaders foster inspiration, increase levels of personal confidence and communicate high expectations to team members. Transformational leaders also demonstrate a considerate approach to their followers based upon mutual trust and respect. Such consideration is often evidenced by individual attention, clinical supervision and mentoring experiences, all of which can stimulate the recipient to problem solve in a creative way.

Fundamental to developing approaches in keeping with the concept of transformational leadership is the issue of self- awareness. The concept of self is complex and has been of interest to philosophers, psychologists and theologians for centuries. One concept of transformational leadership is the idea of individuals who have a strong sense of 'real' self and are able to act authentically and honestly and have security of being. This security can enable the individual to make decisions, to feel able to act rather than be acted upon, and generally to be an autonomous being. The combination of self-awareness, self-confidence and reflective skills can be a powerful ingredient in developing transformational leadership styles (Box 8.2).

PART 3: IMPLEMENTING CHANGE AND ORGANISATIONAL CULTURES

Having considered the contribution of leadership to successful change and the impact of organisational cultures upon that process,

> **Box 8.2** Attributes of transformational leadership (adapted from Barker & Young 1998, Stevens Barnum 1998)
>
> - Works in networks not hierarchies
> - Considers the individual
> - Is value based
> - Develops relationships based upon mutual dependence and trust
> - Builds self-esteem in others
> - Develops others
> - Listens to intuition and balances this with analysis
> - Empowers others
> - Communicates well with others
> - Is self-aware
> - Has a strong sense of self
> - Has vision
> - Acts authentically and honestly
> - Is cooperative and collaborative

it is now important to consider the relationship between organisational culture, structure, strategy and the decision-making process that underpins these elements.

Machiavelli (1513) is often quoted on the issue of change and change management with particular reference to the difficulties of bringing about change and also the attitudes of different stakeholders affected by any proposed change:

> It must be considered that there is nothing more difficult to carry out, nor more doubtful of success, nor more dangerous to handle, than to initiate a new order of things. For the reformer has enemies in all those who profit by the old order, and only lukewarm defenders in all those who would profit by the new order . . . . (Machiavelli 1513, translation 1950, p. 21)

Schein (1986) further develops this concept by highlighting the implicit nature of the assumptions developed within any group or organisation and the way in which this informs the culture. Schein indicates that this culture exists to such a level that it informs the way in which all decisions are made within a team or organisation. As such, this influences every aspect of the team and subsequently the philosophy within which it operates. This is reinforced from the beginning of an individual's involvement with the team by the way in which they are inducted into the systems and value base of that group.

This ethos has direct transferability to the organisation as a whole, not least because individual teams make up the total organisation

199

but also because the organisation influences the team and the way in which people are introduced to the service. Within such a system any changes can be seen as a direct threat or challenge to both the team and the organisational status quo. Essentially therefore even the most unsatisfactory organisational culture or system can become one that is to be defended.

Challenges to change

In order to successfully implement change the concepts of partnership and collaborative working are essential and underpin many of the proposed changes within current welfare services. In a complex setting such as that of health and social care, uniprofessional, interprofessional and interpersonal networks and cultures can superimpose a myriad of motives upon this agenda. The successful implementation of such developments is therefore fraught with challenges. These particularly include:

- the seeking of status for the professions
- the encouragement of professional rivalry
- fear of failure and possible self-interest.

Nocon (1989) identified the concept of ignorance and its role within the joint planning process and consequently the process of collaborative working and the development of partnerships. Within this work, Nocon suggested that there were a number of forms of ignorance: personal, positional, structural, procedural, ideological and professional. Essentially, each of these forms of ignorance creates and sustains individual belief systems and professional ideologies, as well as team and organisational cultures. When focusing upon the management of change and the development of organisational cultures, it is therefore imperative to consider the implications of each of these forms of ignorance (Box 8.3).

Using reflection in management

Graham & Johns (1994) identify the interrelationship between effective management, optimum utilisation of resources and effective outputs from management actions. In addition they clearly acknowledge the role that reflection can have in helping to achieve this objective.

Reflection has been defined in many ways. Boud et al (1985) state that reflection is a generic term for those intellectual and affective activities by which individuals explore their experiences in

Box 8.3 Forms of ignorance (reproduced with permission from Nocon 1989)

Personal ignorance relates to ignorance with regard to knowledge and skills that are required for the effective execution of a specific role. In particular, when that knowledge is readily available.

Positional ignorance refers to decision makers' ignorance of available information in the context of their goals and the associated decisions. This may be due to genuine ignorance or simulated ignorance. Important within this is the personal decision made by the individual about whether or not to actively seek to reduce their level of ignorance. In some situations decision makers may choose not to reduce their level of positional ignorance as this makes the process of decision making easier.

Structural ignorance refers to the lack of understanding of the structures and procedures operating within the partner organisation. Examples include decision-making processes, planning systems, funding structures and financial cycles.

Procedural ignorance affects every aspect of partnership and collaborative working. This includes an understanding of the purpose and nature of the relationship through to the realities of making those relationships real and effective.

Ideological ignorance refers to ignorance about the political ideologies and drivers underpinning each of the partnership agencies. For example, health organisations do not always understand the concept of democratic accountability that is implicit in the work of local authorities. Conversely, local authorities are not always clear about the management structures and ideologies of the NHS.

Professional ignorance refers to ignorance about the value base, educational context and roles and functions of the many professional groups involved in service delivery, both within and across partner organisations.

order to lead to new understandings. Boyd & Fales (1983) defined reflection as being the process of creating and clarifying the meaning of past and present experience in terms of self. They perceive the outcome of the process as changed conceptual practice.

Reflection is perceived as being of crucial importance in many areas of professional activity. It has also been identified as a method of enabling professionals both to articulate more clearly the intuitive element of their practice and to learn from their own actions whilst based in practice (Schon 1991). Having identified the value of reflection within professional practice, and in particular nursing, it has to be noted that much of the literature refers to the role of reflection in individual learning whilst in practice and caring situations. When considering the value of reflection within a management context (Graham & Johns 1994) it is possible to identify this value from two different perspectives. First, in keeping with much of the literature, is its importance in developing the management/leadership practice of individuals. The second approach is that of utilising reflection to inform the overall efficiency and effectiveness of a service. As such, reflective skills within the leaders in an organisation are therefore vital in order to take forward the development of that organisation.

Managing personal reflection

Beckett (1969) suggests that only by fulfilling their own potential are individuals able to assist others in fulfilling their own. Becoming reflective is a process of empowerment and if managers/leaders are not themselves empowered then they will struggle to work in empowering ways with their employees. Within this context it is recognised that reflection is about a person's lived experiences and therefore 'who is the manager' is fundamental to the manager's appropriate and effective response within practice/management situations. This places the 'self' firmly at the centre of the learning agenda.

Humanistic approaches to managing can be clearly related to the individual's value and belief about learning, nursing and, more fundamentally, people. Managers operating from this end of the spectrum will invariably find reflection both before (Greenwood 1998), in and on action (Schon 1991) a useful tool in their personal and professional development.

When considering the value of reflection to inform management practice it is necessary to explore the varying methods and approaches to the concept. Within the literature there are a variety of models of reflection, all of which have different component parts (Box 8.4).

Greenwood (1998) introduces the concept of single and double loop learning within the context of reflection. She is critical of many of the UK models of reflection as being overly simplistic and only focusing upon single loop learning. Greenwood identifies that those professionals/teams/organisations who are serious about reflection will strive to engage in double loop learning. The former approach to reflection essentially focuses upon the effectiveness of the actions undertaken to achieve the identified end, whereas the latter will

---

Box 8.4 Models for reflection

Smith & Russell (1991) specify five key stages to reflection on action:

- background information such as time and place
- your account and the account of others as to what happened
- concerns and thoughts at the time of the incident
- what was demanding about the incident
- what aspects of the incident you need to reflect upon.

Burrows (1995) also uses a five-stage approach. These stages include:

- a description of the event(s)
- a description of your feelings
- what you have learnt
- how you would behave in a similar situation in the future
- how the theories of psychology, sociology, biology, philosophy and nursing research help to explain your experience.

Johns' (1995) framework considers five key stages, each of which has a number of questions within it. The first stage is aesthetics; within this Johns asks the following questions:

- What was I trying to achieve?
- Why did I respond as I did?
- What were the consequences of that for the patient? Others? Myself?
- How was this person (people) feeling?
- How did I know this?

The remaining perspectives within Johns' model are:

- personal
- ethical
- empirical
- reflexivity.

---

encourage the individual to consider whether the identified end-point is genuinely the most desirable outcome. This by its very nature involves the individual in reflection upon the norms, values and social interactions that inform human action. By reflecting in such a way it is anticipated that habitualisation will be avoided and the outcome of changed practice and culture will be made possible.

This avoidance of habitualisation is further developed through considering Munhall's (1993) pattern of knowing, paradoxically known as 'unknowing'. This 'unknowing' is an awareness by the individual that they cannot know or truly understand the service user/client upon first meeting. This meeting as strangers allows the nurse to remain alert to the client's experience and their

Developing a culture for change

perception of the situation in which they find themselves. This alertness will allow the individual to always remain cognisant of the issues facing the team in which they work from a client, team member or stakeholder perspective.

Managing team reflection

From the team perspective reflection can be an equally powerful tool. Two key areas for consideration are the skills required for developing reflection within other team members and subsequently within the team, and the skills that are required to implement any change that may result from the process.

Atkins & Murphy (1994) identified the skills of reflection as self-awareness, description, critical analysis, synthesis and evaluation. Whilst not exhaustive, this list can form a baseline from which a manager may need to operate when considering how to develop a reflective culture within the service.

Having established a positive culture and the appropriate skills it is essential to consider how to transfer these into team activity. A natural progression from this is to consider how to implement and evaluate any proposed change.

The transition from a team of individuals who are able to reflect, to a team that reflects in a collective manner is inevitably complex. This is compounded by the power imbalances and vulnerability of individual members as a result of perceived difference in status. It is therefore essential for the manager/leader to create a culture in which all team members feel valued for their contribution and able to challenge other team members irrespective of their professional background. This cultural change may well be achieved through inclusive approaches to change management.

Having created the appropriate culture it is essential to consider issues relating to management of change in the context of reflection. Ochieng (1999) considered the interface between these two approaches and proposed the following model:

- self-observation
- self-apperception
- self-analysis
- self-contemplation
- self-conceptualisation
- self-management of change
- self-implementation.

Fundamental within this approach is the focus upon self. This is perceived as creating psychological ownership of both the reflection and the resultant change process. The first four stages of this process essentially focus upon reflection. Whilst it is possible for this to take place in the context of an individual from the perspective of team change, it is more effective within group supervision or peer review approaches. Self-conceptualisation as a stage in the process requires the individual or team to conceptualise the outcome of the reflective process. Whilst focusing upon the self, later stages address the thorny issue of change management. For these approaches to be successful it is imperative that all members of the team are fully involved in the process and that any change management system uses an inclusive approach.

Inclusive approaches to change

When specific tasks need to be completed in order to ensure successful change it is important to engender a culture of volunteering. Such cultures encourage feelings of value and inclusion and create the feeling within people that they have some control over the whole change process so that it becomes one that is owned by the people who will potentially be most affected by it, including service users.

Whilst acknowledging that there is no right or wrong answer, the following areas should be considered in the context of any proposed change:

- gathering support
- communication
- openness and transparency
- acknowledgement of external drivers
- generosity in success
- effective teamwork (Thompson & Saunders 1999).

Gathering support

The challenge when implementing any change is to ensure all stakeholders involved in the change are able to contribute to the process and have that contribution valued. In addition, it is extremely important that all members of the team are seen to have equal status; this may include non-professionally qualified staff as well as service users. It is essential that the composition of any team be determined by who needs to be involved and who will be affected by the change, rather than just by the hierarchy of an organisation.

Developing a culture for change

Communication

Formal communication systems are often seen as the most appropriate method for communicating change to those involved. However, the use of existing structures can underestimate the value, or lack of value, placed upon these mechanisms by those working within the organisations. Managers often place great emphasis upon formal communication structures, whilst other workers often fail to see that they are effective. An example of this can be seen in organisations that use wage slips to attach written communications on the premise that all members of the organisation are paid and therefore they will all receive the communication. Receiving a communication, however, is not just about someone being able to say you have been given the information, it is also about understanding it and being given the opportunity to explore what the information means to you as a person. This is particularly relevant when considering the introduction of change within an organisation.

This approach fails to acknowledge the importance of informal communication processes during any change. It is therefore important to disseminate information both as widely and as often as possible, and through many channels, including structures designed specifically to communicate issues relating to the proposed change. When communicating any issue, the principle to be followed is to over-communicate. Other important principles include carefully selecting the time, place and content of the message as it is of little use establishing any communication strategy if it is inaccessible in terms of venue, medium chosen to deliver the message or the language used. For example, a message delivered to service users or their carers in technical and professional jargon may not have the desired impact and level of understanding that is useful.

Openness and transparency

Any change process will inevitably create advantage for some people more than others. This situation can occasionally lead to tension and to failure of the proposed change. However, if the change is desirable and worthwhile, it can be more helpful to be honest about how the change will affect all individuals and allow people the opportunity to discuss it.

Acknowledge external drivers for change

Changes to national and organisational policy inevitably impact upon the framework within which local services are delivered.

For some of the people affected by changes it can be quite difficult to see this and subsequently for these individuals the reason for some of the proposed changes is unclear. People are more likely to accept service changes if they can understand the reason behind them and can see what they need to contribute to the overall process.

Be generous in success

If changes are successfully put in place it is usually the result of the work of the team rather than one individual. As such it is important to explicitly acknowledge the work undertaken by all those involved. It is critical that positive feedback is given and people feel rewarded for their contribution. This can also be a successful strategy to use when a change is only partially achieved.

Effective teamwork

Bicknell (1988) suggests there are specific measures that can be used to support and encourage effective teamwork. For example, valuing the contribution of each individual as unique and important, identification of core and shared skills within the team and the utilisation of this information to create a positive feeling within the team as well as to manage workloads. Weinstein (1998) identifies the following as the key considerations in achieving an effective team:

- common understanding and common goals/objectives
- clear, jargon-free communication
- effective leadership
- regular interaction between members
- equal participation by and valuing of all members
- meaningful and challenging tasks for all members
- joint evaluation and action planning
- clear decision-making processes
- small enough number of people to facilitate thorough and regular communication
- open acknowledgement of power issues
- open acknowledgement and resolution of conflict
- recognition of the unique contribution of each member of the team.

Each of the above areas is important to consider in the context of teamwork, particularly when this crosses professional and organisational boundaries.

Developing a culture for change

CONCLUSION

This chapter has identified that to develop a culture for change it is essential for a manager/leader to create an environment which encourages and supports change. This will require structures and systems that facilitate the professional and personal development of individuals in order to encourage creativity and innovation. This type of organisation is called a learning organisation and is based upon a philosophy that values individuals, listens to their ideas and supports innovation and change. New ways of thinking are allowed and nurtured as people are encouraged to learn, and to learn collectively. Trust and confidence across the organisation are essential in order to allow people to grow and develop.

This new learning culture will be linked to service needs, ensure that the patient/client remains at the centre of care and that the professional becomes a lifelong learner who is able to change and respond to developing practice needs.

References

Alimo Metcalfe B 1996 Leaders or managers. Nursing Management 3(1): 22–24

Atkins S, Murphy K 1994 Reflection: a review of the literature. Journal of Advanced Nursing 18: 1188–1192

Autry J 1991 Love and profit: the art of caring leaderhip. William Morrow, New York

Barber E, Norman B 1987 Mental handicap – facilitating holistic care. Hodder & Stoughton, London

Barker AM, Young CE 1998 Transformational leadership: the feminist connection in post modern organisations. In: Hein EC (ed) Contemporary leadership behaviour: selected readings. Lippincott, New York

Barnum BS, Kerfoot K 1995 The nurse executive. Aspen, Gaithersburg, Maryland

Batten J 1991 Tough minded leadership. Annacom, New York

Beckett T 1969 A candidate's reflections on the supervisory process. Contemporary Psychoanalysis 5: 169–179

Bennis W, Nanus B 1985 Leaders: the strategies for taking charge. Harper & Row, New York

Bicknell J 1988 The mental handicap service – modern concepts of care. In: Sines D, Bicknell J (eds) Caring for mental handicapped people in the community. Harper & Row, London

Boud D, Keogh R, Walker D 1985 Reflection: turning experience into learning. Kogan Page, London

Boyd EM, Fales AW 1983 Reflective learning: key to learning from experience. Journal of Humanistic Psychology 23(2): 99–117

Developing skills in innovation

Burns JM 1978 Leadership. Harper & Row, New York

Burrows DE 1995 The nurse teacher's role in the promotion of reflective practice. Nurse Education Today 15(5): 346–350

Butterworth T, Faugier J 1992 Clinical supervision and mentorship in Nursing. Chapman & Hall, London

Carson S 1999 Organisational change. In: Hamer S, Collinson G (eds) Achieving evidence-based practice: a handbook for practitioners. Baillière Tindall, London

Covey S 1990 The seven habits of highly effective people. Simon & Schuster, London

Department of Health 1997 The new NHS: modern, dependable. Stationery Office, London

Department of Health 1998 A first class service: quality in the new NHS. Stationery Office, London

Department of Health 2000 The NHS plan. Stationery Office, London

Department of Health 2001 Guidance on implementing the NHS plan. Stationery Office, London

Fagin CM 1990 Nursing leadership global strategies. National League for Nursing, New York

French WL, Bell CH 1995 Organisational development: behavioural science interventions for organisation improvement. Prentice Hall, London

Graham J, Johns C 1994 The growth of management connoisseurship through reflective practice. Journal of Nursing Management 2: 253–260

Greenwood J 1998 The role of reflection in single and double loop learning. Journal of Advanced Nursing 27: 1048–1053

Hein EC 1998 'Sizing up' the system. In: Hein EC (ed) Contemporary leadership behaviour: selected readings. Lippincott, New York

Johns C 1995 Framing learning through reflection within Carper's fundamental ways of knowing in nursing. Journal of Advanced Nursing 22(2): 226–234

Lewin D 1952 Group decision and social change. In: Maccoby EE, Newcomb TM, Hartley EL (eds) Readings in social psychology. Holt Reinhart & Winston, New York

Likert R 1961 New patterns of management. McGraw-Hill, New York

Lindolm M, Uden G, Rastram L 1999 Management from different perspectives. Journal of Nursing Management 7: 101–111

Machiavelli 1513 The prince. Translated by Ricci L, published 1950. The Modern Library, New York

Malby B 1996 King's Fund ignites the leading lights. Nursing Management 2(8): 11–13

Marsick V 1987 Learning in the workplace. Croom Helm, London

Maxwell R 1985 cited in Johnson & Johnson/King's Fund 1995 Needs assessment study, unpublished. King's Fund, London

McGregor D 1960 The human side of enterprise. McGraw-Hill, New York

McGregor D 1987 The human side of enterprise (reprint with introduction by David Nickson). Penguin, London

Mullins LJ 1996 Management and organisational behaviour, 4th edn. Pitman, London

Developing a culture for change

Munhall P 1993 'Unknowing': towards another pattern of knowing in nursing. Nursing Outlook 41(3): 125–128

Naish J 1995 Clinical supervision – can you trust nurses' professional MOTs? Health Care Risk Report July/August: 16–17

Nocon A 1989 Forms of ignorance and its role in the joint planning process. Social Policy and Administration 23(1): 31–47

Ochieng BMN 1999 Use of reflective practice in introducing change on the management of pain in a paediatric setting. Journal of Nursing Management 7: 113–118

Pedler M, Burgoyne J, Boydell T 1991 The learning company: a strategy for sustainable development. McGraw-Hill, New York

Revans RW 1970 Action learning: new techniques. Blond & Briggs, London

Schein EH 1986 Organisational culture and leadership. Jossey-Bass, San Francisco

Schon D 1991 The reflective practitioner. How professionals think in action. Avebury, Aldershot

Senge PM 1990 The fifth discipline: the art and practice of the learning organisation. Doubleday, New York

Smith A, Russell J 1991 Using critical incidents in nurse education. Nurse Education Today 11(4): 284–291

Stevens Barnum B 1998 Leadership: can it be holistic? In: Hein EC (ed) Contemporary leadership behaviour: selected readings. Lippincott, New York

Tappen RM 1995 Nursing leadership and management: concepts and practice. Davies, Philadelphia

Tannenbaum R, Schmidt W 1958 How to choose a leadership pattern. Harvard Business Review March–April: 95–101

Thompson J, Saunders M 1999 Audit in teams. Association of Practitioners in Learning Disability, University of York

Timpson J 1998 The NHS as a learning organisation: aspirations beyond the rainbow? Journal of Nursing Management 6: 261–274

Weinstein J 1998 The professions and their interrelationships. In: Thompson T, Matthias P (eds) Standards and learning disability, 2nd edn. Baillière Tindall, London, pp 323–342

Developing skills in innovation

Application **8:1**

Linda Lilley

Shared governance: turning decisions over to staff

The introduction of a professional practice model of shared governance has resulted in a collaborative decision-making structure. This has optimised the contribution of each member of staff, encouraging empowerment, leadership and participative decision making. Recruitment and retention of staff are enhanced, harnessing the skills of staff and motivating them to give their best.

Objective measurements are available within the data collected through the 2-year action research project being undertaken by the Institute of Health Service Research, University of Luton. These data include surveys, interviews, focus groups and non-participant observations.

INTRODUCTION TO THE PROJECT

During 1997 changes within the nursing management structure within Kettering General Hospital involved a review of the clinical manager's role and led to the introduction of general managers. This provided an opportunity to reconsider the decision-making structures and processes for nursing and midwifery. The aim was to establish a flatter, broader model of governance which represented more than just a shift towards decentralisation or devolved management. Shared governance aims to develop a style of management where staff nurses and midwives have increased formal participation in the decision-making processes, functioning with a higher level of professional accountability and autonomy. The introduction of the shared governance model started initially with nurses and midwives in 1997 but quickly progressed to include all health care professionals and since July 2000 has also included a Patient and Public Council. Kettering General Hospital's human resources strategy identified the staff as the key resource in providing high quality service. Shared

> **Box 8.1.1** Summary of project aims
>
> - Provision of the best possible health care in a holistic, compassionate, cost- and clinically effective manner by empowering those who deliver care to have control over the decisions affecting their work.
> - Increased collaborative decision making, authority and accountability in a climate of innovation, harnessing the skills of staff, patients and public, and motivating them to give their best.
> - Optimising the contribution of each member of staff, aiming to encourage empowerment, leadership and participative decision making which would eventually replace the traditional authoritarian chain of command.
> - Provision of a base for developing a multiprofessional shared governance system enabling empowered multiprofessional teams to underpin and enhance the implementation of clinical governance within the trust.

governance was seen as a possible strategy to retain as well as recruit health care professionals by providing power and opportunity for innovation, intrinsic and extrinsic rewards and increased professional opportunities, thus improving job satisfaction. The shared governance system fosters professional development and a sense of ownership relating to standards of professional practice. By providing staff, patients and the public with an opportunity to articulate and define practice and to make decisions relating to practice the quality of patient care is enhanced.

In order to make the best use of resources and maximise value for money the trust must base decisions about patient care on the basis of evidence about clinical effectiveness. It was felt that this could be accomplished only by the introduction of a system where the decisions were made by the staff and the patients working closest to where they are implemented. The project aims are summarised in Box 8.1.1.

PROJECT PROGRESS AND TIMESCALE

Managing change

Shared governance was a relatively new concept in nursing and midwifery in 1997 and required a huge cultural change which could occur only through effective change management that considered the process of introduction, adoption, implementation and evaluation (Wright 1989). The significance of how the individuals involved came to understand the meaning of this change, and the effect it was to have on them, could not be underestimated. The process of preparing for the implementation of the concept of shared governance began with the appointment of an internal change agent, the Assistant Director of Nursing/Practice Development. The initial stages of the project involved a review of the literature and analysis of the ripeness of the environment within the trust to support a structure for change and empowerment of nursing and midwifery staff.

Getting people on board

To facilitate the ownership and involvement of staff and assess their individual perceptions of the value of shared governance a series of road shows took place within the trust. As well as receiving information relating to shared governance and possible models identified from the literature, attendees also had an opportunity to discuss their perceptions as to the benefits and the possible weaknesses of introducing this concept within Kettering General Hospital.

Beginning the implementation – the structure

The 'counsellor' model of shared governance, adapted from work by Tim Porter O'Grady (1994) and Rob Reeves (1996), was identified as the way forward for the organisation. This involved the development of four working councils with specific responsibility for:

- research
- clinical practice
- education and professional development
- quality.

In 1999 a Management Council was included in this model and in July 2000 a Patient and Public Council was added (Fig. 8.1.1).

Councils bring individuals together to consider, investigate, commence, make decisions and report on issues of interest and relevance. The result of the work generated in each of these six councils is forwarded to a Coordinating Council to assist in the coordination of activities and provide a direct line of accountability to the trust board. Each of the six working councils has a membership of approximately 12 people representing all the clinical areas, with the majority at staff nurse or equivalent junior level. Self-nomination was encouraged with the proviso that the nominee had the support of their directorate and line manager to enable them to undertake the role. Since the early days of development the councils have now expanded to include health care assistants and student nurses. A junior member of staff was elected as chairman for each council to demonstrate a clear shift from the traditional hierarchical decision-making committees. It also provided a valuable opportunity

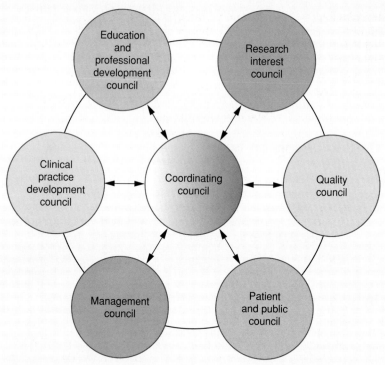

Figure 8.1.1 The counsellor model

for individual staff development. The Assistant Director of
Nursing/Practice Development attended the council meetings in the
first instance to provide support for the chairman and help facilitate
the group growth processes. The Coordinating Council comprises the
Medical Director, the Director of Nursing, Assistant Director of
Nursing/Practice Development, the chairmen of the six councils, a
Directorate General Manager and more recently the shared
governance coordinator who was appointed in 1999 from the
funding received by the trust from the NHS Department of Health
Beacon Awards for their work on shared governance.

Implementing the process

From the beginning it was recognised that all council members
nominated to represent their directorates, and in particular the
chairmen of the councils, would need education and training in
order to fulfil their roles. Through the Education and Professional
Development Council in conjunction with the Organisational
Development Department a series of training programmes were
facilitated and resulted in the council members being confident in
producing their terms of reference, roles and responsibilities,

agendas and a communication strategy for referral of issues to the councils. The council chairman, shared governance coordinator and the Assistant Director of Nursing/Practice Development have also continued to educate, train and inform all members of the health care team who are not members of the council on the purpose of shared governance, the form of shared governance being implemented and the achievements of the council. This is done through regular newsletters, articles in the hospital newspaper, information within recruitment packs and included in the trust induction programme, drop-in sessions, a shared governance bulletin board on the hospital email system and formal teaching sessions within the preregistration curriculum for all health care professionals.

The project plan

The project commenced in April 1996 with a three-stage plan covering the period from April 1996 to September 1999. Stage 4 of the development of shared governance commenced in 1999 and is currently being implemented.

Stage 1 (April 1996–June 1997)

The main aims of the project plan in this initial period were to define our vision for the development of an empowerment model of decision making for nurses and midwives within the trust and to review the literature for appropriate models:

- Assess the organisation climate, readiness, resources, barriers and opportunities, and our abilities to commit to an alternative model of decision making within the organisation.
- Explore the process of selecting a model of shared governance in conjunction with health care professionals and general managers within the trust.
- Identify the structures and processes to be established to enable the development of the model of shared governance.
- Consider the communication and reporting structures, the accountability lines, the education and training issues and changes required within individuals' current roles.
- Propose indicators for evaluating the process of the introduction of shared governance and the benefits to staff, patients and the organisation.

Stage 2 (June 1997–June 1998)

This involved:

- identifying the change agent (Assistant Director of Nursing/Practice Development) to lead the introduction of the model of shared governance

215

Six Steps to **Effective Management**

- developing and implementing the counsellor model structure for shared governance (Porter O'Grady 1994)
- continuing to develop and implement the processes involved within shared governance
- obtaining funding and entering into a joint collaborative action research project with a higher education institution to evaluate the process of introducing a model of shared governance within an acute hospital trust.

Stage 3 (October 1998–September 1999)

The main aims of the project plan at this time were:

- to link the shared governance model with the emerging model of clinical governance within the trust, developing directorate clinical and shared governance joint working
- to review and publish results of the evaluation study (Mitchell et al 1999) and implement the recommendations from this study
- to produce and implement plans for facilitation of the ongoing development of shared governance within the trust.

Stage 4 (September 1999–September 2001)

The main aims of the project plan at this current time include:

- development and implementation of the Management Council within the counsellor model: members of this council have a dual role – first as a Management Council member making decisions in relation to national and local management agenda items affecting staff and patients within the trust and, second, each Management Council member also sits on one of the other councils to provide managerial support
- the appointment of a shared governance coordinator for 2 days per week to work with the Assistant Director of Nursing/Practice Development in developing the framework, including supporting the chairs and vice chairs of all the councils
- the appointment of a dedicated secretary for 15 hours per week to support the development of shared governance within the organisation
- investigating the possibility of including patients and the public within the shared governance model to increase user involvement and patient and public participation in decisions affecting the trust
- obtaining funding for a joint collaborative research project with a higher education institution to evaluate:

   —the implementation of the Patient and Public Council and the effect on the culture of the organisation
   —the impact of the Patient and Public Council on health service users

—the value of the model of patient and public involvement in shared governance that has been implemented at Kettering General Hospital.

These elements of the plan are now well under way.

PROJECT OUTPUT

The project outputs can be determined at the individual level in terms of patients and public and staff involvement, feelings of empowerment and being part of the decision-making process. At operational level this is in terms of the development of clinically and cost-effective practices to improve the quality of patient care and at strategic level in terms of recruitment and retention. The initial evaluation included a baseline survey which at that time indicated staff were aware of shared governance but not fully aware of how the specific structures and systems worked. However, at the exit survey data in 1999 92% of staff surveyed had heard of shared governance and 90% knew that it operated at Kettering General Hospital. More staff knew of the shared governance councils and who their representatives were and for some staff shared governance had raised expectations about their involvement in decision making and was overwhelmingly associated with positive concepts rather than negative concepts.

Most staff surveyed stated that they had some degree of impact from shared governance within their personal work environment. Of these, 87% thought that the impact had been positive, 86% felt that shared governance had increased their opportunities for networking, sharing best practice and increased communication and collaboration between departments. The staff who have been council members reported that they developed their skills in mastering meetings and report writing and had increased confidence to approach trust board members and senior staff. Decision making and leadership skills are also identified as being more developed, all of which has enhanced their working lives, with 88% of staff saying they felt more empowered and more accountable for decision making within the hospital. There has been a series of practical outcomes from each of the councils which has resulted in developments of clinically and cost-effective practice:

- a review of the intravenous drug administration guidelines
- nurse referral of patients to physiotherapy and occupational therapy
- a training needs analysis and subsequent purchase of appropriate education and training
- a series of critical appraisal skills workshops
- a complete review of all the written patient information including a trust-wide audit of compliance with the standards
- the development, implementation and monitoring of the nursing and midwifery strategy

Shared governance: turning decisions over to staff

- the development, implementation and monitoring of the carers' policy.

BENEFITS TO THE ORGANISATION AND TO PATIENT CARE

Improvement in staff involvement, patient and public participation and decision making has led to an increased feeling of empowerment, increased confidence and a feeling that there is a mechanism in place for health care professionals and for patients and public to express their views and implement changes in practice. There have also been improvements in:

- the quality of patient care as a result of the development of evidence-based, clinically and cost-effective protocols for practice
- the multiprofessional working practices now that councils are fully multiprofessional in composition
- team working with a reduction of hierarchy and a feeling that all staff were learning about shared governance on equal terms
- the skills of council members (e.g. chairmanship skills, planning and organising, negotiating, project management, assertiveness, presentation skills, listening and debating)
- the reputation of the trust as an employer who respects the ability of first-line staff to shape new patterns of delivering, organising and managing health care.

LESSONS LEARNT FROM THE PROJECT

Commitment from the Chief Executive and the Director of Nursing is vital and an assessment of the ripeness of the environment to begin the adoption process of implementing this major cultural change is essential. A project leader should be appointed to maintain enthusiasm, get people on board and provide support for council chairmen as they develop their skills and their confidence. Communication regarding the purpose, process and achievement of shared governance with all non-council members is essential, particularly in terms of patient care and staff development. The communication mechanism needs to be wide-ranging and far-reaching. There need to be clear terms of reference, communication procedures between councils and identification of roles and responsibilities of council members. There should be a continuous process of selection of new council members, each of whom should remain on the council for a maximum of 18 months. When implementing a major change there should be a formal evaluation of the process and the outcomes of introducing shared governance to enable credible dissemination of the information and shared learning with a wider audience.

CONCLUSION

The introduction of a model of shared governance has resulted in a collaborative decision-making structure within Kettering General Hospital. Through this, staff, patients and the public are involved in decisions affecting their working lives and the quality of patient care. The introduction of this model has optimised the contribution of each member of staff and the patient and public council members, encouraged empowerment, leadership and participative decision making. Recruitment and retention of staff are enhanced, harnessing the skills of staff and motivating them to give their best, and involving the public has enabled us to provide the best possible health care to our patients. This has been achieved by empowering those who deliver care and those who have experienced care to have control over decisions affecting the working lives of staff and the quality of care for patients in the hospital.

References

Mitchell M, Brooks F, Pugh J 1999 Shared governance – a collaborative project with Kettering General Hospital NHS Trust. Report No 55 IHSR, University of Luton

Porter O'Grady T 1994 Whole systems shared governance – a model for the integrated health system. Journal of Nursing Administration 25(5): 18–27

Reeves R 1996 Shared governance: does it make a difference? Professional Update 4.7: 51–52

Wright S 1989 Changing nursing practice. Edward Arnold, London

Shared governance: turning decisions over to staff

Chapter **Nine**

Overcoming barriers to change: case of Ashworth Hospital

Colin Dale, James Gardner and Shirla Philogene

Developing skills in innovation

OVERVIEW

In writing this chapter, the authors aim to address the importance of creativity when change does not go according to plan in the NHS. Literature on the theory of organisation development and change will be reviewed and its relevance to the wider NHS as a human activity system will be identified. A case study on the management of change in Ashworth Hospital Authority, a specialist health authority dealing with high security forensic psychiatric patients, will be presented. Conclusions will be drawn from the use of creativity as an approach to the management of change in what was a bureaucratic and hierarchical subsystem.

INTRODUCTION

Peters (1990, p. 9) stated 'Organisations simply must poise themselves to innovate, to change, or they risk decline and death'. Whilst this comment is obviously aimed at the commercial sector, the modern NHS with its internal markets and mergers has long recognised the need to embrace change as a constant force to be dealt with. As is often stated the only certainty is that change will continue. Peters & Waterman (1982) show that the most successful companies are those that respond rapidly and are willing to change. However, although the management of change is essential to the survival of any organisation it is also the most complex and demanding of managerial tasks.

Change can have a very unsettling effect on the whole of an organisation as shown by research into the phenomenon of why one company is successful at change management when another is not (Peters & Waterman 1982; Woodward 1958).

Republished management texts are increasingly in vogue among publishers of management books, even though the genre is barely 50 years old and most of the best-known gurus are still alive and writing. Russell Ackoff (1999) has revived his collected works and is best known for his systems theory and its effect on business. In 1981 he warned that independently designed management information systems foisted on an entire organisation from the top do not work: 'It is better to start with the way managers work and build a system based on their experience' (Ackoff 1999, p. 36). It sounds sensible, but the proliferation of off-the-shelf solutions peddled by management practitioners today suggests that his ideas have not caught on.

Intelligent managers do not read management books to find out how to do their jobs. The better books may contain insights into human behaviour, interesting case studies, salutary lessons and even the rare joke, but not practical solutions to the issues facing managers each day, and honest management thinkers know this. John W Hunt, professor of organisational behaviour at London Business School, admitted that academics had limited knowledge of what made organisations work. 'What we cannot give you is a right answer, simply because there is no right answer. And believe me, this is as infuriating for us as it is for you.' Managers must therefore learn how to adapt and apply theory to their own specific situations (Hunt 1999).

THE IMPACT OF CHANGE AND THE RESISTANCE TO IT

Developing skills in innovation

Kubler-Ross (1969) argued that impending and actual loss is dealt with by moving through a series of stages, each characterised by a particular emotional response. This response cycle (Box 9.1) has been used to understand resistance and other responses to organisational change, which some individuals can find particularly traumatic and stressful.

Change can be studied from the perspective of the individual, group or organisation. Organisational change influences conditions of work, occupational identities and divisions, the training and experience of employees, and hierarchical relationships. Change is complex to research as the different levels on which change can be studied are intimately related and this makes it difficult to disentangle cause and effect. It is particularly difficult to stand back from a process in which one is closely involved and examine it objectively.

Some authors (Ahituv & Neumann 1986, Buchanan & Huczynski 1997) recommend a problem-solving process for any change implementation including the steps:

1. Identify problem
2. Gather data
3. Analyse data
4. Generate solutions

Box 9.1 Stages of the emotional response to change

Stage	Response
Denial	Unwillingness to confront the reality: 'This is not happening.' 'There is still hope that this will all go away.'
Anger	Turn accusations on those apparently responsible: 'Why is this happening to me?' 'Why are you doing this to me?'
Bargaining	Attempts to negotiate, to mitigate loss: 'What if I do it this way?'
Depression	The reality of loss or transition is appreciated: 'It's hopeless, there's nothing I can do now.' 'I don't know which way to turn.'
Acceptance	Coming to terms with and accepting the situation and its full implications: 'What are we going to do about this?' 'How am I going to move forward?'

---

5. Select the solution
6. Plan for implementation
7. Implement and test
8. Continue to improve.

There are many such models in the project management literature. Successful change in this approach depends on the clarity with which project objectives are stated, and on the effectiveness of monitoring and control to ensure that the project stays on target with respect to time and money. Ineffective change in this model is usually blamed on the failure to specify goals, tasks, milestones and budgets clearly, and to poor project control.

Project management models of change have one striking feature in common – they rely on the assumption that planned organisational change unfolds in a logical sequence:

● Solutions are not identified until the problem has been clearly defined.
● The 'best' solution is not chosen until the options have been compared and evaluated.
● Implementation does not begin until there is agreement on the solution.
● Each key actor in the implementation process has clearly defined roles and responsibilities.
● Implementation is closely monitored and deviations from a plan are detected and corrected.
● The implementation process is bounded in terms of resources (people, money, space) and time, with a clear project completion date.

It is sometimes possible to anticipate responses to organisational change and to use that knowledge to build on support and address potential resistance to change at an early stage. Resistance to change can be defined as an inability, or an unwillingness, to discuss or to accept organisational changes that are perceived in some way to be damaging or threatening to the individual.

One cannot expect everyone in an organisation to respond in an identical manner to specific change proposals. Different individuals and groups are likely to be affected in different ways and are also likely to perceive the implications differently from those proposing to implement the change. Anticipating responses becomes possible when one knows and understands the stakeholders (anyone likely to be affected directly or indirectly) concerned with a particular organisational change.

Resistance to organisational change includes parochial self-interest (seeking to protect a status quo with which people are content) and misunderstanding and lack of trust (when people do not understand the reasoning behind the change, its nature and possible consequences) (Bedeian 1980). In some instances the way in which change is introduced can be resisted, rather than the change itself.

Eccles (1994) lists 13 sources of resistance to change and identifies a hierarchy of five antiresistance techniques (Box 9.2).

ORGANISATIONAL DEVELOPMENT THEORY AND THE MANAGEMENT OF CHANGE

General reflections on organisations

At the most simplistic level, 'organisation' is a matter of dividing work amongst people whose efforts have to be coordinated. Every organisation is a system of work activities and a system of social

---

Box 9.2 Organisational change: resistance to change and antiresistance techniques

Resistance to change

1. Ignorance (failure to understand the problem)
2. Comparison (the solution is disliked as an alternative is preferred)
3. Disbelief (feeling that the proposed solution will not work)
4. Loss (change has unacceptable personal costs)
5. Inadequacy (the rewards from change are not sufficient)
6. Anxiety (fear of being unable to cope in the new situation)
7. Demolition (change threatens destruction of existing social networks)
8. Power cut (sources of influence and control will be eroded)
9. Contamination (new values and practices are repellent)
10. Inhibition (willingness to change is low)
11. Mistrust (motives for change are considered suspicious)
12. Alienation (alternative interests valued more highly than new proposals)
13. Frustration (change will reduce power and career opportunities)

Antiresistance techniques

1. Convince your critics of the validity of your chosen strategy
2. Demonstrate that the change may mean promotion in the long term and that it is in their interests to support the change
3. Buy their support, or flatter them
4. Marginalise critics and use their skills for the benefit of the rest of the organisation
5. Neutralise or 'exit' critics by termination if necessary

relations. It is concerned with specifying objectives for the business as a whole, as well as determining the activities and decisions necessary to accomplish these objectives. In addition, the activities of each individual and/or subsystem must be controlled and coordinated in order to ensure that the objective of the organisation as a whole is served. Where the above is permitted to lapse, systemic problems that require interventions arise, as in the case of 'The Ashworth Hospital Inquiry' (DoH 1992).

Traditionally, the management and coordination of an organisation has been achieved by setting up a hierarchy of authority and a system of superior/subordinate relationships. Authority is seen as stemming from the apex of the organisational pyramid and it is exercised through successive levels of management and supervision, with each level responsible for controlling and coordinating the activities of those at the inferior level. In the case of Ashworth, the hierarchy of authority was also reflected in the staff/patient relationship and interaction.

The system of work activities and the organisational structure described above are based on the requirement of the task rather than the needs of members of the organisation. The organisational structure in this sense exists independently of the people who happen to belong/work within it at any given point in time. They are regarded as replaceable components, in that an individual can leave his job and be replaced by another without necessitating the change in the organisational structure that is concerned not so much with people as with jobs, roles and office.

Human beings however do not normally confine their behaviour at work to the performance of their roles: they interact as whole people and establish relationships with one another. They develop their own attitudes to work, to the organisation and to management; they have their own aspirations and their hopes and fears for the future are all part of the organisation's life. These factors cannot be ignored because they have a very considerable impact on the ability of the organisation to achieve its goals effectively.

Ashworth Hospital Authority is established to provide a mental health service for high security forensic psychiatric patients. The management structure is a hierarchical one, the staff respond positively to the environment and the culture reflects a custodial rather than a therapeutic approach to care. The custodial approach has an influence on the culture of the organisation. Using Roger Harrison's definition of culture (Harrison & Stokes 1992), it is possible to identify a mixture of power and task elements. This mix is complementary as it fits the values of the employees and the contingencies with which they have to work. This custodial accord

Overcoming barriers to change: Ashworth Hospital

does not exist within the NHS main system where the culture is therapeutic in nature.

Human relations approach

The human relations approach starts with the study of human motives and behaviour from which criteria are derived which help in designing an organisation that stimulates people to cooperate in order to achieve the aims of the organisation. Effective coordination of activities relies on the willingness of people to cooperate. More specifically this approach is concerned with individual and group productivity, individual development and job satisfaction. Unlike the hierarchical structure associated with the classical approach, the human relations approach favours a flat structure which can be brought about by the delegation and simplification of decision making, decentralisation and the forming of subunits with different managers.

One major criticism of this approach/arrangement has come from McGregor (1960) whose XY theory represents a different view of human nature – X representing the negative aspects of humans, whilst Y promotes the positive. McGregor implied that people's conduct is either the cause or effect of classical management policies.

The classical and human relations approaches to the study of organisations have been succeeded by the approach concerned with the study of organisations as systems. This approach stresses the interdependency and interrelatedness of the parts to the whole, and is based on the principle of natural sciences (e.g. Ashworth Hospital Authority is a subsystem of the NHS).

Classical approach

'Influencing' in order to change and to develop a service will not be possible unless there is a basic understanding of the theory relating to organisation development. The classical approach focuses on the study of activities that need to be undertaken in order to achieve the organisation's objectives. Once defined, these activities are grouped to form individual jobs, sections and higher administrative units. The rationale for this arrangement is to maximise specialisation and coordination, whilst at the same time maintaining the equilibrium of supervisors and managers. Coordination is also further facilitated by linking people together in a chain of command and by ensuring that each person knows where their responsibilities end and those of others begin.

The classical approach also attempts to establish rules to act as criteria for developing an organisation. The linking of people together in a chain of command follows the view that there are an optimum number of subordinates within a span of control. This approach fits those organisations that are bureaucratic in nature and hierarchical in structure. Some common factors that influence behaviour in organisations are concerned with the organisation as a whole, the organisation in relation to its environment, the dynamics of organisation life and the process of growth, adjustment to change and organisational development. Adverse elements of these common factors were present at Ashworth and contributed to the need for an inquiry.

Contingency approach

The contingency approach, sometimes called the structural approach, recognises the complexity involved in managing modern organisations. This approach uses patterns of relationship and/or configurations of subsystems in order to facilitate improvement in practice and starts with the premise that no single design is best for all situations. It takes into account technology, economics, social factors and human resources as well as other variables; it therefore adopts a design that is conditional in nature.

Woodward's study of British companies (1968) reinforces the situational view. She showed that organisational structure and human relations were largely a function of the existing technological situation. Woodward's findings are applicable to the Ashworth situation where the structure and human relations can be said to be largely a function and reflection of the custodial nature of the organisation.

Process approach

In the early 1960s the process approach to management of organisations was seen as the approach that would lead managers out of the jungle of management theory. This has proved not to be the case and, instead, two separate paths have emerged, each veering in opposite directions. These new paths have become known as the quantitative and the behavioural approaches to management.

Quantitative and behavioural approaches

The quantitative approach incorporates quantitative decision techniques and model building, as well as operational management and research and computerised information systems; the behavioural approach relies on behavioural sciences and sees organisational behaviour as a result of interaction between human beings and the formal organisation.

Neither of these two approaches has been able to lead managers out of the jungle. However, both appear to veer towards the path of the systems approach which, although it has some appeal, will not of itself be a unifying factor, and as such was not deemed to be an effective approach to apply to the resolution of the problems of Ashworth.

Systems approach

In the 1980s the systems approach was seen as leading to what was defined as the 'contingency approach' and this was suggested as the path out of the jungle that managers were so keen to discover. The new direction that this was expected to take is illustrated in Figure 9.1.

Applying an organisation development approach in a clinical setting – Ashworth Hospital

Revans states: 'In any epoch of rapid change those organisations unable to adapt are soon in trouble, and adaption is achieved by

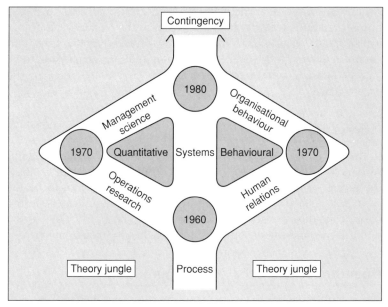

Figure 9.1 New directions in management theory

Developing skills in innovation

learning, namely – by being able to do tomorrow what might have been unnecessary today. Or, to be able to do today what was unnecessary last week' (Revans 1998, p. 11).

Organisation development (OD) is one of the many approaches to change. It is an approach that seeks to maximise human as well as organisational resources through the use of applied behavioural science knowledge. Organisation development has been defined as:

> a long-range effort to improve an organisation's problem solving and renewal processes, particularly a more effective collaborative management of organisational culture . . . with the assistance of a change agent as catalyst, and the use of the theory and technology of applied behavioural science including action research. (French & Bell 1973)

> the creation of a culture which supports institutionalisation and use of social technologies to facilitate diagnosis and change of inter-personal, group and intergroup behaviour, especially those behaviour-related to organisational decision-making, planning and communication. (Horstein et al 1971)

> a planned change effort, evolving the total system, managed from the top to increase organisational effectiveness through planned interventions using behavioural science knowledge. (Berkhard 1966)

> a process of planned organisational change which centres around a change agent who, in collaboration with the client's system, attempts to apply valued knowledge from the behavioural sciences to client problems. (Bennis 1965)

It is clear from the above definitions that the principal element is change. OD is involved in looking at the organisation and helping it to change in the direction it desires to go. It examines change in terms of a planned and systematic approach, its main objective being to increase the organisation's ability to perform its tasks and to meet its goals.

McGregor's XY theory has an influence in the behavioural approach. He made the point that assumptions about human nature colour and influence every managerial decision and action; the leader acts and behaves according to personal assumptions. Today's greater educational opportunities and higher expectations call for a reassessment of the outdated theory X, as it is felt generally that any attempt to motivate individuals with methods based on outdated assumptions will result in a negative response.

The following are some of the basic assumptions outlined by French (1969), as he perceived them to affect people in groups and people in organisations, from the individual's perspective. French stated that western people have needs for personal growth and development. These needs are most likely to be satisfied in a supportive and challenging environment. Most workers are under-utilised and are capable of taking on more responsibility for their own actions and/or making a greater contribution to organisational goals than is permitted in most organisation environments. Therefore the job design, managerial assumptions and other factors frequently 'demotivate' individuals in formal organisations.

From the perspective of people in groups, French held the view that groups are highly important to people and most people satisfy their needs within groups, especially the work group. The work group includes both peers and the supervisor and is highly influential on the individual within the group. Work groups as such are essentially neutral. However, depending on its nature, the group can be either helpful or harmful to the organisation and the case study demonstrates how the Ashworth staff group had become harmful to the organisation in the time leading up to the 1992 public inquiry.

Work groups can greatly increase their effectiveness in attaining individual needs and organisational requirements by working collaboratively. In order for a group to increase its effectiveness, the formal leader cannot exercise all of the leadership functions at all times and in all circumstances. Group members can become more effective in assisting one another. In Ashworth Hospital it was clear that groups became confrontational rather than cooperative and that a leadership vacuum emerged which was filled by militant trade unionists.

From the perspective of people in organisations, French contends that, since the organisation is a system, changes in one subsystem (social, technological or managerial/custodial) will affect other subsystems. Most people have feelings and attitudes that affect their behaviour, but the culture of the organisation tends to suppress the expression of these feelings and attitudes. When feelings are suppressed, problem solving, job satisfaction and personal growth are adversely affected. Evidence provided at the public inquiry into Ashworth Hospital demonstrated this problem with staff feeling that there was no legitimate outlet for pent-up anger and frustrations and that they were in effect repressed.

In most organisations, the level of interpersonal support, trust and cooperation is much lower than is desirable and necessary. Although 'win–lose' strategies can be appropriate in some situations, many win–lose situations are dysfunctional to both employees and organisations and also between organisation, staff and the patients they care for in the long-term care situation such as

Developing skills in innovation

Ashworth Hospital. Many 'personality clashes' between individuals or groups are functions of organisational design rather than of the individuals involved. When feelings are seen as important data, additional avenues for improved leadership, communications, goal-setting, intergroup collaboration and job satisfaction are opened up.

Shifting the emphasis of conflict resolution from smoothing to open discussion of ideas facilitates both personal growth and the accomplishment of organisational goals. Organisational structure and the design of jobs can be modified to more effectively meet the needs of the individual, the group and the organisation. A group of staff emerged from the Ashworth Inquiry who became known as the 'Ashworth four' who championed patients' rights and were seen to be whistleblowers on the organisation. These staff spoke of conflicts between staff groups, how brutality and ill-treatment of patients became commonplace and institutionalised and staff development was non-existent.

Creating change successfully

Eccles (1994) identifies eight preconditions for successful change:

- pressure for the change
- a clear and shared vision of the goal and the direction
- effective liaison and trust between those concerned
- the will and the power to act
- capable people with sufficient resources
- suitable rewards and accountabilities
- actionable first steps
- a capacity to learn and to adapt.

Assuming that the need for change is broadly accepted, Taylor (1994) identified eight successful strategies, based on the experiences of a number of organisations:

- *goals* – managers must define goals in terms of specific, measurable objectives
- *vision* – employees must be shown a 'promised land' where they will find a prosperous future
- *organisation* – line managers must be given a structure in which they can take charge and be held accountable
- *culture* – a more open style of leadership, communicating values, and working through teams
- *quality* – to succeed, organisations must measure themselves against the best

- *performance management* – every employee is involved in delivering high quality services
- *innovation* – the challenge is to harness workforce creativity, to do new things and to do things differently
- *partnerships and networks* – managers must learn to trust and to cooperate; partnerships must be formed with external agencies.

The recurrent themes from these suggestions are that organisations should have: a clear sense of purpose and direction; people should know what is expected of them; change implementation steps should be planned with care; goals should be interesting and challenging; and above all communicate, communicate . . . and keep communicating.

The single main problem with these change recipes is the extent to which they seem to oversimplify a complex issue. In particular, the 'rational–linear' model, which presents change unfolding in a logical sequence, seems to misrepresent organisational realities.

A popular method for considering the introduction of organisational change involves a technique known as 'force field analysis' (Torrington & Weightman 1994). This technique has been utilised for examining a broad range of issues within the human sciences and considers the dynamics of 'driving' forces (which help or facilitate a situation) and 'restraining' forces (which hinder or prevent progress). This technique is helpful in allowing for an analysis of the forces for and against change, and also allows for the position of each stakeholder to be considered (Fig. 9.2).

In the Ashworth case study the key forces were seen to be those outlined in Box 9.3. Once an organisation has been able to identify factors such as these the challenge is to consider how the restraining forces might be weakened to inhibit their negative effects and conversely how the driving forces can be strengthened to increase the likelihood of a successful project.

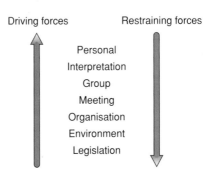

Figure 9.2 Force field analysis

Box 9.3 Forces for and against change

Driving forces	**Restraining forces**
Commitment to change	Poor industrial relations
Additional funds	Negative staff and patient culture
Stated values of organisation	Resistance to change
Desire for demonstrable	Poor leadership
improvements	Inadequate funding
	Poor record of previous successful
	change

The 'change agent'

In many instances the delivery of change is dependent upon the drive and energy of a 'change agent'. This can be any member of an organisation seeking to promote, further, support, sponsor, initiate, implement or deliver change. Change agents are not necessarily senior managers and do not necessarily hold formal change management job titles and positions.

Kanter (1989) identifies seven skills which the change agent requires to perform effectively:

● the ability to work independently, without the power, sanction and support of the management hierarchy
● the skills of an effective collaborator, able to compete in ways that enhance rather than destroy cooperation
● the ability to develop high trust relationships, based on high ethical standards
● self-confidence, tempered with humility
● respect for the process of change, as well as the content
● the ability to work across business functions and units, to be 'multifaceted and ambidextrous'
● the willingness to base reward on results and gain satisfaction from success.

Hutton (1994) claims that the change agent should be patient, persistent, honest, trustworthy, reliable, positive, enthusiastic, cooperative, confident (but not arrogant), a good listener, observant (of the feelings and behaviours of others), flexible, resourceful, difficult to intimidate, willing to take risks and accept challenge, and able to handle organisational politics. They should have a sense of humour, a sense of perspective and be able to admit ignorance and ask for help when appropriate.

Overcoming barriers to change: Ashworth Hospital

Applying theory to practice

One of the ways in which the OD approach accomplishes the balance between the maintenance of the main stem of the organisation whilst changes within its subsystem are occurring, is through the mechanism of survey research and feedback which has been a guiding principle in the OD approach ever since it was established.

This guiding principle was applied to the solution of the problem at Ashworth and the case study that follows describes how this principle was applied, what problems were encountered and how the guiding principle, coupled with creativity, became the final solution.

CASE STUDY: ASHWORTH HOSPITAL

The National Health Service Act (DHSS 1977) places a duty on the secretary of state 'to provide and maintain services for persons subject to detention under the Mental Health Act (DHSS 1983), who in his opinion require treatment and conditions of special security on account of their dangerous, violent or other criminal propensities'. Ashworth Hospital is one of three high security hospitals in England providing such conditions, caring for approximately 520 patients, who have diverse needs, and employing more than 1600 staff. The hospital became a separate health authority with effect from 1 April 1996. Whilst not a trust in its own right, the hospital does have a structure similar to that found in NHS trusts. The relationship between care, therapy and security is of fundamental importance and is a continuing theme that managers constantly need to address.

Change at Ashworth Hospital Authority – in context

One of the major barriers and factors to be considered when one examines change within any organisation, is the organisation's history and culture. Ward (1994, p. 98) gives the following advice: 'To help people to change, to create a new future, you must first understand the present. To understand the present, you must understand their past. This can only be achieved by considering the historical influences which have been at work'.

Ashworth Hospital was the subject of a major inquiry in 1992 where one of its key findings was the presence of a negative and damaging culture within the hospital. A selection of statements from the report underlining this fact would include:

- 'A vivid picture emerged . . . of life in a brutalising, stagnant, closed institution.' (p. 143)
- 'The all-pervading nature of an oppressive sub-culture at Ashworth Hospital, which persistently undermines the therapeutic approach and places constraints on those who do not conform to it, was made clear.' (p. 144)
- 'The changes that the hospital aspires to cannot be delivered in the current climate at the hospital.' (p. 148)
- 'Patients at Ashworth must be valued as individual people with specific and challenging needs who have a right to expect respect, warmth and empathy from staff.' (p. 205).

Historically, Ashworth Hospital was what Goffman (1961) would refer to as 'total institution', which he felt was symbolised by a barrier to social intercourse with the outside world. The hospital had become isolated and trapped into a time-warp with most of the changes occurring elsewhere in the health service passing it by. Between 1992 and 1997 tremendous efforts were made to change Ashworth from a total institution into one that was more open and less hierarchical.

Lewin (1948) first expanded his theories of 'unfreezing–movement–refreezing' in the late 1940s. In terms of a driver for change or an agent for 'unfreezing' an organisation, there can be few which will ever be as effective as a public inquiry. There can also be little doubt that many of the well-recognised barriers to change and virtually all resistance to change were overcome by the public criticism that the report contained. Consequently, following on from the publication of the Ashworth Inquiry Report, the pace of change picked up considerably at the hospital and any resistance from an organised perspective from trade unions virtually disappeared.

In November 1994, the Special Hospitals Services Authority, who had the responsibility for the management of all three high security hospitals covering England and Wales, requested the Health Advisory Service to undertake a review of the services provided by Ashworth Hospital. In their report entitled *With Care in Mind, Secure* (HAS 1995), they noted that 'patients and staff at Ashworth Hospital have tackled a programme of change since 1992, which elsewhere in the National Health Service has been managed through a period in excess of six years' (p. 101).

The range of changes that were achieved during that short period of time were the result of pressures from many different sources, both internal and external to the organisation. Whilst the hospital was concentrating on introducing the changes that occurred as a result of the inquiry, they were also not exempt from other changes that were taking place within the NHS.

Ashworth Hospital presented its own unique difficulties when considering change. In a closed institution with staff and patients in almost continual contact it is paradoxical that the organisation's 'customers' were the very people who were major contributors and reinforcers of the very aspects of the culture that was seen to need changing. Many of the patients had been transferred in from the prison service and continued to perceive the hospital and staff as extensions of that service and behaved accordingly.

This unique set of circumstances was analysed in depth by Dale et al (1995). In this article it is observed that because of the very close relationship between staff and patients, it is almost inevitable that they will share values and beliefs and that to some degree both the staff and the patients become 'victims' of the prison culture. The article concludes that a paradigm shift of the magnitude required to change the culture at Ashworth required intense activity which would focus on both patients and staff. This activity needed to target not only people's beliefs and values but also target many of the symbols, artefacts and routines that existed in the hospital.

Research into one aspect of change

Focusing on one specific example it was decided to research a major and controversial aspect of change and attempt to describe how the various groups perceived this and were affected by it. Care at Ashworth Hospital, as with all of the high security hospitals at that time, involved patients being locked in their rooms from 9.00 p.m. through until 7.00 a.m. the next day. For many of the patients, which included all of the women patients, this also meant no access to sanitary facilities and led to the prison system of 'slopping-out' each morning as receptacles filled with the nighttime waste were emptied. As well as this degrading practice, during nighttime hours patients had limited contact with the one nurse on duty, often unqualified, and could only converse through a narrow 'pill-window'. If a patient's room needed to be opened for any reason during the night, this entailed a major logistical exercise. Staff had to be brought over from other ward areas so that three staff could be present when a door was opened; as a consequence this was regarded as an emergency procedure and was a rare occurrence.

It was generally felt by the newly appointed Special Hospitals Services Authority and staff coming in from the wider NHS that this was a draconian and dehumanising practice and should be eradicated as soon as practicable. This did however present a major logistical and managerial challenge as it required significant additional resources (staff for an additional shift for each ward needed to be recruited), as well as the major policy and procedural changes involved.

The proposals were also not universally welcomed by all at the hospital as many existing staff predicted major disturbances and disruption from patients who would recognise the hospital's vulnerability at these times. In addition, many staff and patients felt that the money could be put to better uses. Undeterred, the eradication of slopping out and the introduction of what became known as 24-hour therapeutic care became a key objective for the hospital and was achieved in four main phases between 1993 and 1995.

It was anticipated that people's perception and opinions on this issue would vary quite noticeably, depending on their position within the hospital. It was also further anticipated that the views expressed by the strategic managers would be broadly in line with the views expressed by patients, and that these would be noticeably different to the views expressed by ward-based staff. It was decided to test this hypothesis to evaluate the change process.

Sample group

A random stratified sample group was selected and consisted of patients and staff from five wards, combined with ward and senior managers, to give a representative sample reflecting the population of the hospital.

Methodology

A Likert scale questionnaire was produced which focused on the areas of investigation. The questions were phrased as statements which the respondents were asked to comment on in the range of 'strongly disagree' to 'strongly agree'. The questionnaire also allowed for any comments to be made at the end. In order to provide more breadth to the information gathering and also to validate the information collected from the questionnaire, it was decided to undertake some semi-structured interviews with an equal number of patients, staff, ward managers and senior managers.

Overcoming barriers to change: Ashworth Hospital

Information analysis

Barnard (1980) suggests that 'thematic content analysis' is probably the most valid approach. This involves identifying a series of themes, headings and categories which can be refined into manageable sections of information, thus allowing conclusions to be drawn in a systematic (if not scientific) manner. Hard data concerning patient seclusion (the involuntary confinement of a patient in a room to protect themselves or other people) and incidents were also analysed to examine any impact following the introduction of the changes.

Findings

In total 270 questionnaires were sent out and an overall response rate of 43% was achieved. This relatively high response rate indicated that both patients and staff within Ashworth Hospital were interested in putting forward their views on the value of 24-hour therapeutic care.

The findings from the questionnaire fell naturally into two main areas: change implementation and culture change. The section on cultural change also examined the feedback relating to what respondents thought should exist in terms of values and what they thought actually existed.

Change implementation

Of the 26 questions, 18 were designed to explore various areas of change implementation but for the purpose of analysis these were grouped into five common themes: communication, ownership, consultation and evaluation, financial resources and culture and values.

Communication

The five questions targeted in this area showed some quite different responses. Both patients and staff felt that the objectives of 24-hour therapeutic care had not been clearly communicated to patients, yet both the ward managers and senior managers felt this had occurred.

A similar picture emerged in relation to communication with staff. Patients, ward managers and senior managers agreed that staff communication had occurred to a satisfactory degree, yet the staff themselves quite markedly disagreed, with 44% of staff either disagreeing or strongly disagreeing with this statement.

Given that excellent communication is seen as a prerequisite for success it is clear that the respondents to this questionnaire felt that this had not been adequately covered in the change process.

Ownership

All four groups clearly saw 24-hour therapeutic care as being imposed by senior managers and that it was 'owned' by them. There is of course a distinction between ownership and support and the evidence gathered shows that patients and staff did not feel ownership of the project. This in itself is not surprising, as ownership is often something akin to trust in that it can take time to evolve and is unlikely to occur at the start of the change process.

Consultation and evaluation

Most of the responses in this area were of a positive nature where all groups felt that they had been afforded the opportunity to be part of the consultation and evaluation process. It is quite interesting to compare the responses in this area to that of ownership. One of the methods which is suggested as effective in creating a feeling of ownership is to ensure that interested parties are involved in the consultation and evaluation process. The evidence here seems to suggest that consultation and evaluation occurred but this did not lead on to any feeling of ownership. Perhaps this can be explained by the strong response to the exercise being perceived as an imposition.

Financial resources

All groups were clearly of the view that insufficient financial resources had been made available and this was an expected outcome. There is no doubt that strenuous efforts were made to introduce this change as efficiently as possible and heated debates between managers at ward level and senior managers were not uncommon. A significant number of ward-based staff and managers felt that the resources could have been better used in other areas.

Culture and values

A very strong positive response from all groups was that Ashworth should be more like a hospital than a prison. There can be little doubt that this is an aim and a value that is commonly shared and is further reflected by an almost equally strong response regarding the notion of Ashworth being a prison. Whilst this ideal is shared by all groups, there are a small but significant number of staff who feel

Overcoming barriers to change: Ashworth Hospital

239

that Ashworth is still like a prison. Out of 58 staff, 11 did not feel that Ashworth had moved away from the prison culture.

Semi-structured interviews

Twenty interviews were conducted and consisted of five people from the four groups of patients, ward-based staff, ward managers and senior managers.

- *Communication* – the views expressed in this area were markedly different. All managers felt strongly that there had been considerable good communication with staff and patients, but the views of patients and staff did not reflect this. Patients in particular, and to some degree staff, felt that at best they were informed of what was happening but that was the extent of the communication. Managers and staff had been aware of 24-hour therapeutic care for a long time and nearly all recalled discussing the subject at meetings. Patients and ward staff knew of it in advance but felt they were not involved in ward-based discussions.
- *Ownership* – most managers accepted that the concept of 24-hour therapeutic care was a major strategic decision which high security hospitals were expected to implement. Ward managers appeared to have a degree of ownership as to 'how' 24-hour therapeutic care was introduced but patients and ward staff did not feel any great degree of ownership. Nearly all interviewees commented that this is something they would change in the future.
- *Consultation and evaluation* – it is known that four major reviews of 24-hour therapeutic care were undertaken as part of the contract monitoring requirements, all of which involved the use of major surveys to sample wards. Senior and ward managers appeared to be aware of these and felt that evaluation was of a high standard. Strangely, none of the patients and only two of the five staff interviewed could recall these quite major reviews taking place and felt that the consultation and evaluation had been very poor. Most respondents had been aware of the ward developing a policy, but most patients felt they had been excluded from the process and had been presented with a *fait accompli*.
- *Financial resources* – most people agreed that resources had been very limited and that this was problematic. However, everyone interviewed agreed that in terms of value for money, 24-hour therapeutic care was the most important and beneficial change that had happened at Ashworth for some considerable time. Everyone felt that this was the right area to pursue in principle,

Developing skills in innovation

but several managers felt that some alternative options as to how it was implemented should have been considered more closely.

● *Culture and values* – this was the area in which the most diverse opinions were expressed, ranging from the very negative to the very positive. The patients were very positive about the effect 24-hour therapeutic care had on the organisation and stated that it had greatly improved the culture. They now felt like patients, not prisoners, and this had improved their 'self-esteem'. The senior manager group broadly supported this view. However, both groups accepted that some of the prison culture still remained and that there were problems with some patients abusing the new system. Ward managers were less positive than the patients and senior managers and tended to highlight the problems of abuse of the system although they did accept that this was a problem of managing the ward rather than of the 24-hour therapeutic care itself.

The group mostly at variance were the staff at ward level. Only two of the five felt there had been a positive change and, even then, this was not very noticeable. The remaining three felt that 24-hour therapeutic care had not changed the culture positively, that the outcome had been quite negative in that staff had no control over patients and that the problems of managing 24-hour therapeutic care far outweighed any benefits. Reference was made to 'poor value for money', 'staff are no longer in control' and 'the hospital is now a doss house'.

Of the 20 interviewees, 3 thought 24-hour therapeutic care should be withdrawn and the other 17 were very keen for it to be retained. The patients especially regarded it as being highly valued.

Change implementation

In the theoretical section of this chapter there emerged some common themes which can be referred to as 'best practice' and are generally considered as key elements required for success. These inturn were the areas explored via the questionnaire and semi-structured interviews. This process allowed for the following conclusions to be drawn.

Top management support

This is a feature in some of the recommended frameworks and appears in the model suggested by Daft (1992). There appears to

Overcoming barriers to change: Ashworth Hospital

have been a great deal of confusion as to whether or not this was the case with 24-hour therapeutic care. There can be no doubt that virtually everyone perceived this as an imposition from top management yet some ambiguity was detected amongst some members of the senior management team. If top management support is to be given to any change project then that commitment should be clear and unambiguous.

Communication

This is probably the most important element in any change project and is noticeable in every model considered. The information obtained in the Ashworth project clearly shows that communication was a definite problem area. The managers expressed the view that communication with staff and patients was of a good standard yet this was not reflected by the patients and most especially not by the ward-based staff.

Consultation and evaluation

This is seen as a key element in the process and is recommended in the suggestions from Beer et al (1990), Daft (1992) and Loucke-Horsley & Herger (1985). Obtaining the commitment for change is aided by those who are affected by the change being involved in the process, ideally leading to a sense of ownership whereby they will own and protect the change as they view it as 'theirs'. The responses in this project indicate that efforts were made to consult and evaluate which was acknowledged by patients but rejected by staff, leading to the conclusion that consultation and evaluation was not as effective as it might have been.

Shared vision

Developing a vision of the change, which is understood by all, is again one of the features that is apparent in the conceptual frameworks on change management. Beer et al (1990) view this as being of particular relevance. The evidence gathered indicates that this was achieved, with the majority of patients and staff clearly understanding the concept.

Financial resources

This is acknowledged to be one of the major barriers to change which Daft (1992) refers to as 'excessive focus on costs'. There is no doubt that almost everyone felt that the 24-hour therapeutic care initiative was badly underresourced and some of the respondents were also unsure if this was the best use of resources. Underresourcing provides the opportunity for people to say 'it cannot be done', 'we don't have enough people', etc., etc., all of which can undermine the whole process. It can therefore be concluded, based on the information given, that lack of resources was a major inhibitor of this change process.

Culture and values

A significant number of areas relating to culture and values were explored and there are a variety of conclusions that can be reached. Based on the information received, 24-hour therapeutic care does appear to have had a significant, positive effect on the culture at Ashworth. There is little doubt that the hospital moved away from the prison culture but it may have gone too far in that a significant number of patients and staff refer to abuse of the system and the hospital being a 'doss house'. It can also be concluded that the hospital still has a lot of work to do in this area.

CONCLUSION

All organisations need to be able to cope with change and it is almost certain that they will need to cope with imposition, adaptation, growth and innovation. External agencies such as the government and purchasers may require imposition; changes in technology or practice may cause adaptation. Changes in service may cause both reduction and growth, and innovation must be encouraged and nurtured. The case study demonstrated that the key elements for successful change management were not in place. One of the causes for this may have been the lack of an accepted methodology or framework adopted by the hospital with sufficient flexibility and adaptability.

It is rare that any study of services does not highlight communication as a problem. The difficulty appears to be that managers perceive they have communicated well with patients and staff, but this is not reflected by them. This is indicative of a lack of monitoring and, to correct this, the manager responsible for the implementation of any change project should accept personal responsibility for communication. An auditable communication plan could usefully be included as part of any project, including methods of monitoring.

Overcoming barriers to change: Ashworth Hospital

Lack of resources is a major barrier to change and the strongly held view in the case study was that this project was seriously underresourced. Any project of change will be thoroughly scrutinised to keep expenditure to the minimum. To overcome this potential barrier to change, the costing for any change project should be widely communicated in order to demonstrate that funding is adequate.

In the case study it was evident that there was confusion about what style of management was being adopted in relation to the change process. Style can be very important and to adopt a very consultative or democratic approach during a change process of imposition will inevitably lead to confusion. Daft (1992) refers to force and coercion and the Copeland et al (2000) framework emphasises the need for the right style. For change management to occur successfully, it is essential that those responsible for its management receive the appropriate training. Services should consider organising training activities prior to change implementation.

It is important for people to be involved in the process of change to facilitate a sense of ownership. In the case study discontent was muted as some staff felt that they had little involvement. Consultation and evaluation was through ward meetings and surveys which did not prove very effective from a staff perspective. An alternative might have been the formation of a 'change group' with representation of all key stakeholders, including patients, as a matter of routine.

The evident progress in the case study to change the organisational culture has been relatively slow, but it would be naive to suggest that a culture which takes in excess of 20 years to develop can be changed quickly. This project provided powerful 'symbolism' for change with patients no longer suffering the ritual of being treated like prisoners by being locked in their rooms. More importantly, patients who come to Ashworth Hospital from prison clearly see the hospital as different, which helps to dissuade them from bringing the 'prison culture' to Ashworth Hospital. Any organisation, however, must be concerned when some of the responses from staff are at odds with the hospital's stated values.

References

Ackoff R 1999 Ackoff's best: his classic writings on management. Wiley, London

Ahituv N, Neumann S 1986 Principles of information systems for management. WC Brown, Dubuque, Iowa

Barnard K 1980 Tracing decisions in the NHS. King's Fund, London

Bedeian AG 1980 Organisational theory and analysis. Dryden Press, Chicago

Beer M, Spector BA, Eisanstat RA 1990 The critical path to corporate renewal. Harvard Business School Press, Harvard

Bennis W 1965 Theory and method in applying behavioural science to planned organisational change. Journal of Applied Behavioural Science 1: 337–360

Berkhard R 1966 An organisational improvement programme in a decentralised organisation. Journal of Applied Behavioural Science 2(1): 2–25

Buchanan D, Huczynski A 1997 Organizational behaviour: an introductory text. Prentice Hall, London

Copeland T, Koller T, Murin J 2000 Valuation: measuring and managing the value of companies, 3rd edn. Wiley, New York

Daft RL 1992 Organizational theory and design. West Publishing, St Paul, Minnesota

Dale C, Rae M, Tarbuck P 1995 Changing the nursing culture in a special hospital. Nursing Times 91(30): 31–35

Department of Health 1992 Report of the Committee of Inquiry into complaints about Ashworth Hospital. HMSO, London

Department of Health and Social Security 1977 National Health Services Act, Ch. 49. DHSS, London

Department of Health and Social Security 1983 The Mental Health Act. DHSS, London

Eccles T 1994 Succeeding with change: implementing action-driven strategies. McGraw-Hill, London

French W 1969 Organisation development: objectives, assumptions and strategies. California Management Review XII: 2

French W, Bell C Jr 1973 Organisation development: behavioural science interventions for organisation improvement. Prentice Hall, Englewood Cliffs, New Jersey

Goffman E 1961 Asylums. Penguin, London

Harrison R, Stokes H 1992 Diagnosing organizational culture. Jossey-Bass, New York

Horstein H, Bunder B, Horstein M 1971 Some conceptual issues in individual and group oriented strategies of intervention into organisation. Journal of Applied Behavioural Science 7(8): 57–67

Health Advisory Service 1995 With care in mind, secure. Department of Health, London

Hunt JW 1999 A case of guru fatigue. Financial Times March 24: 17

Hutton DW 1994 The change agents handbook: a survival guide for quality improvement champions. ASQC Quality Press, Milwaukee, Wisconsin

Kanter RM 1989 When giants learn to dance. Unwin, London

Kubler-Ross E 1969 On death and dying. Macmillan, Toronto

Lewin K 1948 Resolving social conflicts. Harper & Row, New York

Loucke-Horsley S, Herger LF 1985 Association for Supervision and Curriculum Development, Andover, Massachusetts

McGregor D 1960 The human side of enterprise. McGraw-Hill, New York

Overcoming barriers to change: Ashworth Hospital

Peters T 1990 Get innovative or get dead. California Management Review
  Fall: 9–26

Peters TJ, Waterman RH 1982 In search of excellence: lessons from America's
  best run companies. Harper & Row, London

Revans R 1998 ABC of action learning. Lemos & Crane, London

Taylor B (ed) 1994 Successful change strategies: chief executives in action.
  Director Books/Fitzwilliam Publishing, Hemel Hempstead

Torrington D, Weightman J 1994 Effective management. Prentice Hall,
  London

Ward M 1994 Why your corporate culture change isn't working and what to
  do about it. Gower, Aldershot

Woodward J 1958 Industrial organisations, theory and practice. Oxford
  University Press, London

Woodward J 1968 Industrial organisations. Oxford University Press, London

Developing skills in innovation

Section **Four**

MANAGING KNOWLEDGE IN HEALTH CARE

OVERVIEW

The amount of knowledge that is available to support health care is considerable and to the busy practitioner can be overwhelming. Successful implementation of any innovation and change is dependent upon a sound knowledge base that develops with the project and is owned and understood by all participants. The following three chapters will focus upon issues that are central to accessing, managing, producing and evaluating knowledge.

In Chapter Ten Thoreya Swage first considers the need for evidence-based practice, the impact of the related policies and their implications for the development of evidence-based health care. Clinical governance, National Service Frameworks, the National Institute for Clinical Excellence, the Commission for Health Improvement and the Modernisation Agency are all addressed. The second half of the chapter becomes practitioner focused and is informative in relation to both the sources of information that are available to support evidence-based practice and accessing and evaluating the information. Finally, the challenge of applying the evidence to practice is addressed.

Brendan Docherty enlarges upon this theme in Application 10.1. He suggests that evidence-based health care is part and parcel of the everyday work of nurses and that evidence-based practice is central to their role of patient advocate. The application demonstrates how evidence-based nursing practice can be measured and evaluates a measuring tool designed for use in the clinical area.

Information technology (IT) is acknowledged to be an essential element in the accessing, storage and management of knowledge. The value of the computer systems and their contribution to the effective delivery of health care services is not at issue but the skills gap that exists for many nurses must be addressed. Chapter 11 by Laurence Alpay, Gill Needham and Peter Murray provides a widely researched review of the literature written in order to discern the issues and trends that are relevant to nurses within primary care. Recent IT policies are highlighted, problems identified and possible solutions considered. The selection of the literature is not restricted to national publications and therefore provides a useful perspective in that the barriers identified represent an international experience.

Applications 11.1 and 11.2 are relevant to the IT theory chapter; the former is a practical implementation of IT in primary care and the latter is about the use of IT in school health. Judith James is a GP working in a fully computerised practice and in Application 11.1 she evaluates the system and recognises the benefits for patients, to health care professionals and improvements for communication between primary and secondary care. In Application 11.2 Mary Hollins presents an IT project which is both informative about health care for young children but presented to them in an amusing format using technology.

In Chapter 12 Cynthia Thornton takes a critical view of research and development and considers the implications for nurse leaders and managers. Nursing research is examined from a historical perspective prior to the acknowledgement of recent developments and illumination of the opportunities and challenges that are likely to face nurse leaders. A consideration of paradigms and their associated philosophical influences on research activity leads to a recommendation of action research as a tool to facilitate practice-based research and development.

The final application in this section is an account of an action research project led by Pam Denicolo which aims to improve services for people with severe or enduring mental health problems. Action research is recommended as a creative means of introducing practice-based research to facilitate the innovation and change that is needed to meet the needs of the NHS modernisation programme. The aim of this action research project is to improve the quality of health care provision and provides a useful contrast to the study in Application 8.1 which relates to a systemic change within the organisation. The emphasis upon the process is intentional in order to provide insight into the some of the practical issues that should be considered when planning a similar project.

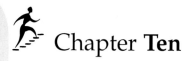

Chapter **Ten**

Evidence-based practice

Thoreya Swage

- ● The need for evidence-based practice
- ● The impact of recent policy changes on evidence-based health care
- ● National bodies to support evidence-based care
- ● Sources of information to support evidence-based practice
- ● The challenge of applying the evidence to practice

OVERVIEW

The purpose of this chapter is to introduce the reader to the importance of evidence-based practice within the National Health Service and how this is enshrined in much of recent health care policy. National bodies supporting and monitoring NHS organisations and clinicians applying evidence-based practice and related quality initiatives are discussed together with the practical aspect of implementing research into routine clinical care.

THE NEED FOR EVIDENCE-BASED PRACTICE

Although in the late 1990s the NHS celebrated half a century of working as one organisation with the simple aim of providing comprehensive health care free at the point of delivery, it was not until about 40 years after its inception that much thought was directed towards critically analysing effective methods of clinical practice in a consistent and systematic manner. Furthermore, it was only in 1991 that a cohesive strategy for research and development was launched for the NHS, the aim of which was to provide robust evidence to support the needs of the service. At around the same time the concept of clinical effectiveness and evidence-based care was introduced as a means of improving and measuring the quality of health care provided by clinicians.

The stimulus for examining health care in this way is due to an interaction of a number of factors which have increased the demand for services. They are an ageing population, new technologies and knowledge, and an increase in patient and professional expectations (Box 10.1).

Against this background, there has been a gathering of momentum in the promotion of clinical effectiveness initiatives within the NHS led by the NHS research and development strategy, the aim of which is:

> To create a knowledge-based health service in which clinical, managerial and policy decisions are based on sound information about research findings and scientific developments. The programme focuses on the needs of the service. It balances a centrally developed

---

Box 10.1 Factors stimulating closer examination of evidence-based health care

Ageing population	Larger numbers of older people requiring health care
	Greater expectations of health care and therefore more assertive in their demands
	Greater use of high technology medicine
New technology and knowledge	Developmental costs of new technology
	High introductory costs to the NHS
	Can identify unmet need
Patient expectations	Better access to services
	High quality services
	Service failures may result in complaints or litigation
	Better information on new technologies and treatment options
Professional expectations	New technologies may stimulate expectations
	Fear of litigation may increase the use of 'defensive medicine'

---

strategic framework and priority setting, with regional implementation. (DoH 1998a, front sheet)

Six key functions were identified to achieve the aim:

- To establish the requirements of the NHS for knowledge that is based on research and science
- To ensure that the evidence based on the identified requirements is made available to the NHS
- To disseminate the appropriate research evidence to decision makers (purchasers and providers of health care)
- To make the evidence easily available through the use of information
- To encourage a culture within the NHS that critically analyses and evaluates practice
- To continue to develop, monitor and evaluate the research and development strategy.

The importance of the research and development strategy was reflected by the NHS Executive in a number of Executive Letters to the service, highlighting the need to consider and implement clinical effectiveness in practice as part of the priorities and planning guidance for at least two separate planning cycles (EL(93)115 in 1993 and EL(94)55 in 1994). Other initiatives, including the founding of the UK Cochrane Centre and the Effective Health Care bulletin series in 1992, the Centre for Evidence-Based Medicine established in Oxford in 1993 and the NHS Centre for Reviews and Dissemination in 1994 reinforced the message of implementing evidence-based practice.

However, Walshe & Ham's (1997) survey of health authorities and trusts in England and Wales found that despite the direction from the centre, the implementation of evidence-based care by the various NHS bodies was poor. For example, the responses to three specific Effective Health Care bulletins were analysed according to the level of action subsequently taken by the relevant organisation. The main recommendation for the treatment of benign prostatic hyperplasia was to use a different operation (NHS Centre for Reviews and Dissemination 1995a); for the prevention and treatment of pressure sores to use low pressure foam mattresses (NHS Centre for Reviews and Dissemination 1995b) and for the management of cataracts to increase the day surgery rate (NHS Centre for Reviews and Dissemination 1996). Walshe & Ham found that trusts and health authorities implemented the recommendations in a differential manner. For example, many organisations were unable to say whether anyone had taken heed of the recommendations, and nearly four out of five health authorities did not know what action their trusts had taken for the management of benign prostatic hyperplasia and the prevention and treatment of pressure sores.

One of the possible reasons for the findings was a lack of commitment by the management of NHS organisations to clinical effectiveness as demonstrated by only 56% of health authorities and 32% of trusts having an agreed formal strategy (Walshe & Ham 1997). A key problem for clinicians was access to appropriate information. Often trust libraries were not open outside of office hours or were available only for medical staff; worse still were some situations where there was no library or information services at all.

Eldridge & South (1998) recorded similar findings among staff in community trusts; in particular many professionals (doctors, nurses, managers, etc.) felt that they lacked basic research skills – so much so that they did not know where to start.

Another factor stimulating the need for evidence-based practice was the increasing cost of claims for medical negligence and the greater onus on clinicians to demonstrate that care has been of the highest quality. Apart from asking questions on clinical risk management systems, the effect has been to examine the requirements of clinicians to maintain their professional knowledge and expertise (continuous professional development).

A major influence was that the only statutory function NHS organisations had to comply with was to ensure budgetary balance at the end of each financial year. As demand on services increased, the pressure not to overspend became greater and other issues including clinical matters were given less attention. This situation was recognised by the Labour government when it came to power in 1997 and, in its vision for the NHS, clinical and quality issues were firmly pushed further up the agenda.

THE IMPACT AND IMPLICATIONS OF THE RECENT POLICY CHANGES ON EVIDENCE-BASED HEALTH CARE

The White Paper, *The New NHS* (DoH 1997), announced two major changes to the workings of the NHS: the delegation of the commissioning of health care to primary care groups (PCGs) in England, local health groups in Wales and local health care cooperatives in Scotland; and the introduction of clinical governance, a statutory duty of assuring the quality of clinical care.

Evidence-based practice

What is clinical governance?

The White Paper, *A First Class Service* (DoH 1998b), defines clinical governance as:

> A framework through which NHS organisations are accountable for continuously improving the quality of their services and safeguarding high standards of care by creating an environment in which clinical care will flourish. (p. 33)

It is a structure on which to hang and interconnect a number of quality processes under one roof and comprises four main components:

- clear lines of responsibility and accountability for the overall quality of clinical care
- a comprehensive programme of quality improvement activities, e.g. audit, evidence-based practice and professional development
- clear policies aimed at managing risk, including clinical risk
- procedures for all professional groups to identify and remedy poor performance.

This has subsequently been developed into the seven pillars of clinical governance by the NHS Clinical Governance Support Team:

- clinical effectiveness
- risk management effectiveness
- patient experience
- communication effectiveness
- resources effectiveness
- strategic effectiveness
- learning effectiveness.

The cornerstone of clinical governance, essentially, is the application of the research evidence into practice and the accountability of the whole organisation right up to the chief executive for the quality of clinical care. Each NHS organisation is required to produce an annual plan for the improvement of clinical services which will have the scrutiny of the general public. Clinical governance plans do not sit in isolation of other strategic plans. They are a central feature of the Health Improvement Programme (DoH 1997), the strategic plan for the development of health services in a health authority area drawn up in consultation with social services and other partners. The delegation of commissioning to bodies such as PCGs which have general practitioners and nurses on the board means that there is now greater examination of clinical matters than in the past.

The establishment of primary care trusts (PCTs) (NHS Executive 1999) marks a progression in the development of PCGs. However, the composition of the trust board and executive team is different from that of PCGs and it appears that the clinical input and influence has been diluted. The challenge for PCTs is to ensure that the clinical input that has been harnessed by the predecessor PCGs continues.

The same issue applies to the development of care trusts (DoH 2000a) when PCTs join with their social services colleagues to provide health and social care services for their populations.

National Service Frameworks

It is with the introduction of National Service Frameworks (NSFs) that the concept of national standards of care were incorporated into the health services provided by the NHS. Essentially NSFs indicate a set of minimum standards of care that can be expected across the whole of England for particular conditions or client groups. At the time of writing NSFs have been published for mental health (DoH 1999), coronary heart disease (DoH 2000b), and older people (DoH 2001) with a framework for diabetes due imminently. Other NSFs in the pipeline include long-term conditions (e.g. neurological diseases such as epilepsy, multiple sclerosis and Parkinson's disease and brain and spinal injury). The NSFs set targets for the improvement in aspects of care which have been based on the latest research evidence at the time of publication over a period of 10 years, the endpoint being the targets highlighted in the national strategy for health, *Our Healthier Nation* (DoH 1998c). The implementation of the NSFs relies on a number of agencies (both statutory and voluntary) coming together as local implementation teams to oversee and monitor the process.

The National Institute for Clinical Excellence

In addition to the internal systems and structures set up by individual organisations, there are two statutory bodies which stand outside of the NHS but are associated closely with it, whose functions are to ensure that the process of clinical governance runs smoothly.

The National Institute for Clinical Excellence (NICE) is a special health authority which provides national evidence-based clinical guidelines for local adaptation, clinical audit methodologies and information on good practice. It covers the English and Welsh NHS. The Health Technology Board for Scotland and Scottish Intercollegiate Guidelines Network carry out a similar function in Scotland and, at the time of writing, Northern Ireland is still consulting about its structures.

To carry out these functions, NICE systematically appraises medical interventions before they are introduced to the NHS. It operates by working at the local level with NHS organisations, for example trusts, health authorities, PCTs and patient groups to facilitate dissemination of the guidance and, nationally, with the Department of Health, Royal Colleges, academic units and other health care industries to ensure that the appropriate information is fed into further clinical reviews or audit methodologies. Each NHS organisation must appoint a clinical lead to ensure the implementation of every guideline as it is produced by NICE.

The Commission for Health Improvement

The Commission for Health Improvement (CHI) is the second new statutory body whose function is to support the development of high quality clinical practice consistently across the NHS. CHI covers the NHS in England and Wales; in Scotland the Clinical Standards Board for Scotland carries out the same function and Northern Ireland currently is considering CHI's input into the province. The role of the CHI is to provide national leadership on the principles of clinical governance and to support those organisations that are having difficulty setting up clinical governance arrangements locally when all other usual channels have failed. The Commission has a programme of rolling reviews, in which every NHS trust, including primary care trusts, will be visited over a period of 3–4 years. In each review, evidence will be sought that clinical governance arrangements are working and that the national standards produced by NICE are being adhered to. Although CHI has a 'troubleshooting' function (i.e. investigate a local problem) if there is an issue that requires particular attention, it is the responsibility of the local NHS organisations to ensure that the recommended action plans are followed up. If there are problems with the performance of individual clinicians, the Commission will refer these to the appropriate regulatory body (e.g. the General Medical Council, the Nursing and Midwifery Council and the Health Professions Council) for further action.

The Modernisation Agency

It is a common situation within the NHS to have pockets of good practice and service redesign surrounded by areas which do not appear to have taken on board the experiences of others. To rectify this a national Modernisation Agency, part of the Department of

Managing knowledge in health care

Health, has been established to help local clinicians and managers spread good practice and stimulate change. The Agency encompasses a number of initiatives including (DoH 2000a):

- *The National Patients' Action Team* – this encourages service redesign around waiting lists and waiting times for outpatient and inpatient care.
- *The 'Action On' initiatives* on cataracts, dermatology, orthopaedics and ear, nose and throat services – these are initiatives specifically for streamlining waiting times and care for patients receiving treatments in these areas.
- *The primary care development team* – developing good practice in primary care.
- *The 'Collaborative Programmes'* in which local clinical networks are developed – e.g. the orthopaedic, coronary heart disease, cancer services and primary care collaboratives.
- *The Clinical Governance Support Unit* – provides training and support on clinical governance to the NHS.
- *The NHS Leadership Centre* – to develop and promote leaders at all levels of the organisation.
- *The NHS Beacon Programme* – sites of good practice.

So what are clinical effectiveness and evidence-based practice?

The Department of Health defines clinical effectiveness as:

> The extent to which specific clinical interventions, when deployed in the field for a particular patient or population, do what they are intended to do – i.e. maintain and improve health and secure the greatest possible health gain from available resources. To be reasonably certain that an intervention has produced health benefits, it needs to be shown to be capable of producing worthwhile benefit (efficacy and cost effectiveness) and has produced that benefit in practice. (DoH 1996, p. 45)

The Royal College of Nursing strategy document on the clinical effectiveness initiative (1996) provides a shorter definition:

> The application of the best available knowledge, derived from research, clinical expertise and patient preferences, to achieve optimum processes and outcomes of care for patients. (Royal College of Nursing 1996, p. 11)

Clinical effectiveness is a multifaceted process with a number of components (Royal College of Nursing 1996). For ease of understanding these can be summarised as:

Evidence-based practice

- the production of robust evidence through research and scientific review
- the production and dissemination of clinical guidelines that are based on the evidence
- the implementation of evidence-based, cost-effective practice through education and change management
- the evaluation of compliance to agreed practice guidance and evaluation of patient outcomes including clinical audit.

The application of clinical effectiveness is essentially a dynamic process that depends on a number of factors and involves a range of players. Clinical effectiveness is of concern to the purchasers of health care (e.g. PCTs) so that they can ensure that health priorities are addressed and the best outcomes are secured for the populations they serve. It is of importance to providers of health care in demonstrating accountability to the patients they treat in that they provide the best quality care.

Evidence-based practice is contained within the processes outlined above and is summarised succinctly by Martin (1998) as the 'ability to appraise and incorporate a body of evidence into one's clinical practice'.

Much of the work in this area has been developed by David Sackett (1997) who states that evidence-based practice can be divided into five stages:

1. The information need is converted into an answerable and focused question.
2. The evidence which answers the question is tracked down, e.g. by a literature search.
3. The critical appraisal of the research evidence needs to be done for its validity and application to practice.
4. The application of the evidence into clinical practice.
5. The evaluation of performance through audit and self-reflection.

From the above, it is clear that looking up the appropriate information in order to frame the right question, together with some skills to assess the available research, are essential in starting the process of evidence-based practice.

SOURCES OF INFORMATION

Although NICE has recommended national guidance to facilitate the application of evidence-based practice, there will still be occasions when local clinical teams will need to look up research papers and reviews in order to answer their specific questions and problems. For this, clinicians will need to know where to investigate sources of information and to acquire skills to assess the research critically.

It is at this point that issues around information, knowledge and evidence need to be established. The Collins Dictionary defines information as 'knowledge acquired through experience or study' and this can take many forms, such as written or verbal. Information, therefore, implies an active process of gathering facts obtained from various sources. There is an element of critical analysis in that the individual filters out the facts which are useful using a systematic process and applies this to their particular situation.

Knowledge is 'the facts or experiences known by a person or a group of people' or 'consciousness or familiarity gained by experience or learning'. There is always a danger that knowledge can easily become out of date if it is not maintained on a regular basis. This could be a problem, particularly if it is not recognised by the health professional concerned, and could lead to less effective clinical care. Another problem is the use of knowledge which does not have robust evidence to support a specific course of action and this therefore makes the rationale for its use rather weak.

Evidence augments and strengthens knowledge. It can be defined as 'the data on which to base proof or to establish truth or falsehood' (Collins Dictionary). Evidence can vary in its strength and reliability. The skill here is how to assess the evidence and to ascertain its relevance to the specific clinical situation.

The acquisition of knowledge, particularly of facts, is dependent on the dissemination of information which must provide the appropriate evidence in an easily accessible form to those who need to use it. It is also dependent on the skills of the recipients to relate the information to the local setting. The former is determined by access to appropriate information from various sources and the latter on upgrading the research and critical appraisal skills of clinicians.

Evidence arises from the results of research which can be found in two main forms: primary research and systematic reviews.

Primary research

This consists of original pieces of work focusing on patients or populations and are usually published in scientific journals. The quality of the research can be variable although most reputable journals do not publish papers that are not 'peer reviewed' (i.e. assessed by others who have an expertise in the field in question). As the primary research base is vast and expanding rapidly, the trend is now to look up the evidence in systematic reviews.

Evidence-based practice

Systematic reviews

Systematic reviews assess primary research papers. A systematic review is a piece of work in which evidence on a topic has been systematically identified from the literature, critically appraised and summarised according to predetermined criteria.

Accessing the information

Until recently health care professionals have had to use a number of sources in order to obtain the research information to support their clinical care, such as original journals, looking up medical databases and using local medical and nursing libraries. This has been simplified through the development of a National electronic Library for Health (NeLH) which was announced as part of the Information Strategy for Health (NHS Executive 1998). The aim of the NeLH is to provide health care professionals with the knowledge and knowhow to support health care-related decisions. This virtual library also provides information to the general public via NHS Direct On-line and the New Library Network. Access to the NeLH is via the NHSnet (the internal secure intranet for the NHS) and the wider Internet.

The library is organised on three levels:

● *Knowhow* – this contains NICE guidance and guidelines, NSFs and NeLH guidelines database
● *Knowledge* – e.g. the Cochrane Library, MEDLINE (biomedical research literature) and Effective Health Care bulletins
● *Knowledge management* – e.g. NHS Economic Evaluation Database and the British National Formulary.

Users can also go to the atrium where there is a help desk for their special interest and for an opportunity to share ideas with other members of their profession.

A similar initiative has been developed for professionals working in social work and social care called the electronic Library for Social Care (eLSC). This has a similar architecture to the NeLH in that there are four levels:

● *Knowledge* – containing key research evidence and guidance and standards across social care
● *Knowledge bases* – e.g. databases and journals
● *Knowledge skills* – this provides users with the skills to make use of the material held on the eLSC and to change practice
● *Service users and carers* – containing information about social care for users and carers and to collate and disseminate the knowledge and expertise of users and carers.

There are links between the two virtual libraries which are useful for health care professionals who work across health and social care such as mental health and learning disabilities.

A major factor in the effective use of these virtual libraries is the ease (or otherwise) of access of health care professionals to the Internet and NHSnet. Not all NHS organisations are currently able to provide this. In addition, health care staff do not necessarily have the IT skills to search the Internet. Investment in training staff in this area is therefore an issue.

Hierarchy of evidence

The quality of evidence can be variable. However, the generally accepted method of assessing the strength of the evidence is to follow the criteria outlined in Box 10.2 (Muir Gray 1997).

It is worthy of note that, although type V evidence is considered lowest on the hierarchy scale, there may be situations when this is the only source of evidence for interventions. It is in these circumstances that health care professionals need to stimulate and develop research where gaps have been identified.

Applying the evidence

Once the information has been identified, an appraisal of the research papers needs to made to assess the impact and importance of the findings to the clinician's own practice.

There are three broad issues to be considered when appraising a research paper:

Box 10.2	Hierarchy of evidence
Type	**Strength of evidence**
I	Systematic review in which many well-designed randomised controlled trials feature
II	Randomised controlled trials which are well designed and of appropriate size
III	Trials without randomisation or non-experimental study, e.g. cohort or case control studies
IV	Qualitative studies
V	Opinions of respected authorities, based on clinical evidence, descriptive studies or reports of expert committees

Six Steps to **Effective Management**

- Are the results valid?
- What are the results?
- Will the results help locally?

The Critical Appraisal Skills Programme at Oxford has developed an assessment tool that consists of about ten questions (a different set for each level of evidence I–IV) which are designed to take the assessor systematically through papers. Although the skill requires practice, it enables the assessor to make appropriate decisions about the relevance of the research findings to day-to-day clinical care. There are many courses available to help health care professionals develop critical appraisal skills and the reader is referred there for further details, for example the Critical Appraisal Skills Programme in Oxford (see Useful websites at the end of the chapter). A worked example is illustrated in *Clinical Governance in Health Care Practice* (Swage 2000, Ch. 4).

THE CHALLENGE OF APPLYING THE EVIDENCE

A major criticism of the concept of evidence-based care by clinicians is that it threatens to impose a more 'rational' approach to clinical practice, mainly fuelled by the need to make savings within a health care system. This is the perception, particularly if managers are seen to be the driving force for change rather than practitioners. It is also seen to be suppressing innovation and creativity in that clinical practice is 'restricted' by inflexible guidelines or protocols that do not relate to the needs of patients.

This picture is not helped by the apparently haphazard way in which the evidence from research is disseminated to clinicians, the messages on priorities from purchasers seeming to conflict with each other or are too many to deal with, and clinical effectiveness initiatives and service strategies bearing no relationship to the financial and contractual obligations required of providers.

When clinicians are asked about evidence-based practice and what it means to them, a wide range of reactions are elicited – from not understanding what the term means to 'I provide good quality care anyway, what is the point of it?'. Some of the usual responses are summarised below (Loach, personal communication):

- Lack of skills (e.g. how to do literature searches, critical appraisal, etc.)
- Lack of information on the process of evidence-based practice/unaware of the relevant information

- Not enough time to read research papers
- Do not understand research papers
- Cannot get to library/library not open at convenient hours/no library facilities available
- Do not see relevance of evidence-based practice
- The process is too complex, daunting and not appropriate for busy clinicians
- Too busy to do evidence-based practice
- A threat – if one has done something that is not evidence based
- Dangerous innovation – restricts clinical freedom
- Don't know where to start, i.e. what are the priority areas?
- What will be the action following the results?
- Nobody uses guidelines/guidelines restrict clinical freedom.

When first applying the evidence it can be overwhelming, particularly if it has not been usual practice within a clinical environment or team to do so. A common method for encouraging a change in practice is the simple distribution of printed educational materials to target health professionals as a means of modifying behaviour. For example, Mason et al (1998) assessed the effect of the Effective Health Care bulletin on the treatment of depression in primary care (NHS Centre for Reviews and Dissemination 1993) as measured by the levels of prescribing of selective serotonin reuptake inhibitors (SSRI) antidepressants by general practitioners. They found that there was a temporary halt of the otherwise constant increase in prescribing of SSRI antidepressants over the 6-year period of the study. Although the result was to save an estimated £40 m (representing the cost of the SSRIs had they continued to be prescribed at the pace at which they were increasing) this did not have a lasting effect in clinical practice.

A systematic, multifaceted approach is therefore required in order to change behaviour. In the Effective Health Care bulletin on getting evidence into practice (NHS Centre for Reviews and Dissemination 1999) it is suggested that before any change is implemented there needs to be a period of 'information and diagnostic analysis' to inform the development of an appropriate dissemination and implementation strategy for that change. The steps are outlined below.

1. The identification of all the relevant groups involved in, affected by or influencing the proposed change(s) in practice
2. An assessment of the characteristics of the proposed change that might influence its adoption, e.g. it is a recognised priority area or there is a specific problem connected with the topic
3. An assessment of the preparedness of the health professionals to change and an analysis of other potentially relevant internal factors within the target group

Evidence-based practice

4. The identification of potential external barriers to change
5. The identification of likely enabling factors, including resources and skills.

Once this analysis has been done then the implementation strategy can be designed.

As with many new areas which require introduction, the greatest chances of success are most likely with small projects. In this situation the task is manageable and can be tried initially with those who are interested in the innovative idea. The challenge of setting up an evidence-based culture within a team or organisation provides an opportunity for clinicians to lead on a clinical idea by explaining the process to others, playing the 'champion' for the cause as they are perceived to have an expertise in this subject, being a driving force for change and demonstrating the positive outcomes. This process can best be illustrated by an example.

Setting up an evidence-based culture – an example

The chief dietician in Bradford (Loach, personal communication), had studied the application of evidence-based practice. She decided to implement a similar process for her colleagues in the dietetics departments in the local area. When the idea was first aired with the local dieticians, the reactions resembled those identified above; in particular, there was a concern that there was no time for individuals to pursue the idea. The solution was to encourage the process of evidence-based practice in a group format so that the burden of work was shared amongst a number of dieticians. This was kick-started by a workshop for all dieticians in the locality on the principles and rationale of evidence-based practice. From that session, a smaller group was convened which addressed the following questions:

- What questions should be asked to which answers were required?
- Where is the evidence to be found?
- Who will do what task, by when?
- Which topics could be used for an initial study?

A large number of topics were identified initially for study which were then whittled down to a manageable size. The main criterion for selection was those areas which had been agreed as local priorities. Box 10.3 illustrates the different points in the process of evidence-based practice and the role of the group in implementing the key tasks (Swage 2000, p. 106).

(side text, vertical) Managing knowledge in health care

Box 10.3 Process of implementing evidence-based practice

Process	Group work
1. Decide on the question	Evolving, defining, refining, prioritising
2. Find the evidence	Ideas on search strategy, sharing materials and contacts
3. Appraise the evidence	Spot new angles and roles (i.e. who has the skill)
4. Agree on best practice	Adding clinical expertise, practical issues on application
5. Compare with current practice	
6. Identify any change needed	Agreed amongst group members
7. Action plan	Who is doing what, how and when. Share the workload
8. Set review date	Accountability (report to next meeting)
9. Keep notes of the action agreed	
10. Evaluate the progress, e.g. journal club, standard documentation, etc.	

The benefit of working as a group meant that no one was operating in isolation and ideas were generated and support provided from different members. It also provided an opportunity for discussion of the available evidence and comparison of different methods of disseminating clinically relevant research.

One of the main challenges faced by the group was that there was very little research evidence relevant to dieticians. This made the selection of evidence difficult, particularly as any evidence found was mostly for doctors and nurses. Interpretation of the evidence was therefore prone to be subjective or biased and often more questions were raised than answers given. Above all, this was found to be a time-consuming activity. However, the project stimulated much activity including:

● an assessment of current practice through baseline audits
● processes for maintaining current knowledge, e.g. journal clubs
● an increase in the dissemination of information to the public, referrers and other health professionals
● stimulation of further questions
● the development of guidelines and standard documentation

Evidence-based practice

265

- input to multiprofessional/multiagency guidelines, e.g. hypertension and wound care
- informing the training and education programme for dieticians.

For the participants themselves, the process boosted their credibility amongst their colleagues, new skills had been acquired and the group method of working saved time in an activity they were required to perform. Future plans included continuing the momentum of the process by revisiting the need for various skills, informing others of progress and feeding back the relevant questions to those who were carrying out the research.

HOW CAN MANAGERS SUPPORT EVIDENCE-BASED PRACTICE?

Managers in health organisations can provide much support to clinicians in their endeavours to apply evidence-based practice in a number of ways.

- Conduct a proper assessment of the main personnel and issues relating to the area to be examined and work up a robust strategy for achieving change in behaviour.
- Allow protected time for clinicians to look up the evidence and have discussions on critical appraisal of the evidence.
- Provide funds for specific evidence-based projects.
- Ensure that areas to be examined for evidence-based practice are consistent with other obligations of the organisation including internal and external priorities, e.g. health improvement programme.
- Ensure that clinicians have access to the evidence, e.g. libraries are open at appropriate times, information from NICE and other relevant organisations are disseminated to clinicians.
- Ensure that clinical information systems are appropriate and accessible for use in evidence-based practice.
- Ensure access to training on assessing and applying the research.
- Encourage clinicians to develop their own personal development plans which reflect their own training needs and which are also consistent with the needs of the organisation.
- Use the information gleaned from applying the evidence to develop better services.
- Ensure that other systems and structures, e.g. clinical audit, clinical risk management and complaints, are interconnected with the process of evidence-based practice.

Managing knowledge in health care

The application of evidence-based practice requires the efforts of both clinicians and managers for it to succeed. By focusing in the same direction, greater yields are more likely in terms of better patient outcomes, effective use of resources and stimulating clinicians' interests in creating innovative practice.

CONCLUSIONS

Evidence-based practice is very much here to stay. It has been enshrined in central NHS policy through the National Service Frameworks, the various support mechanisms to spread good practice such as the Modernisation Agency and NICE (and equivalent) guidance. It has been a statutory responsibility for all NHS organisations since 1999 so that quality issues have equal importance to financial obligations when delivering effective health care.

The challenge for all clinicians is to develop critical and analytical skills when faced with new research and to incorporate new ways of working into routine day-to-day practice. This involves not only a change in attitudes but also ready access to appropriate information and the development of IT skills as the National electronic Library for Health becomes the first port of call for health care professionals when seeking the evidence.

Health care managers also have an important role to play in facilitating access to the research evidence, by ensuring appropriate training of clinical professionals and ensuring the implementation of good practice to improve patient outcomes.

References

Department of Health 1996 Promoting clinical effectiveness. A framework for action in and through the NHS. Department of Health, London

Department of Health 1997 The new NHS: modern, dependable. Department of Health, London

Department of Health 1998a Research and development. Towards an evidence-base for health services, public health and social care. Information pack, issue 5, introductory sheet. Department of Health, London

Department of Health 1998b A first class service: quality in the new NHS. Department of Health, London

Department of Health 1998c Our healthier nation, a contract for health. A consultation paper. Department of Health, London

Department of Health 1999 National Service Framework for mental health. Modern standards and service models. Department of Health, London

Department of Health 2000a The NHS plan. A plan for investment, a plan for reform. Department of Health, London

Evidence-based practice

Managing knowledge in health care

Department of Health 2000b National Service Framework for coronary heart disease. Modern standards and service models. Department of Health, London

Department of Health 2001 National Service Framework for older people. Modern standards and service models. Department of Health, London

Eldridge K, South N 1998 Slow acting remedy. Health Service Journal May 21: 24–25

Martin J 1998 Evidence based practice. Primary Health Care 8(10): 18–20

Mason J, Freemantle N, Young P 1998 The effect of the distribution of Effective Health Care Bulletins on prescribing selective serotonin reuptake inhibitiors in primary care. Health Trends 30(4): 120–122

Muir Gray JA 1997 Evidence-based healthcare. How to make health policy and management decisions. Churchill Livingstone, Edinburgh

NHS Centre for Reviews and Dissemination 1993 Effective health care: the treatment of depression in primary care. NHS Centre for Reviews and Dissemination, University of York

NHS Centre for Reviews and Dissemination 1995a Effective health care: benign prostatic hyperplasia. NHS Centre for Reviews and Dissemination, University of York

NHS Centre for Reviews and Dissemination 1995b Effective health care: the prevention and treatment of pressure sores. NHS Centre for Reviews and Dissemination, University of York

NHS Centre for Reviews and Dissemination 1996 Effective health care: management of cataract. NHS Centre for Reviews and Dissemination, University of York

NHS Centre for Reviews and Dissemination 1999 Effective health care: getting evidence into practice. NHS Centre for Reviews and Dissemination, University of York

NHS Executive 1998 Information for Health. An information strategy for the modern NHS 1998–2005: a national strategy for local implementation. NHS Executive, London

NHS Executive 1999 Primary care trusts: establishing better services. NHS Executive, London

Royal College of Nursing 1996 The Royal College of Nursing clinical effectiveness initiative. A strategic framework. The Royal College of Nursing Institute, London

Sackett DL, Richardson WS, Rosenberg W, Haynes RB 1997 Evidence-based medicine. Churchill Livingstone, New York

Swage T 2000 Clinical governance in health care practice. Butterworth-Heinemann, Oxford

Walshe K, Ham C 1997 Who's acting on the evidence? Health Service Journal April 3: 22–25

Useful websites

Clinical Standards Board for Scotland – www.clinicalstandards.org
Commission for Health Improvement – www.chi.nhs.uk

Critical Appraisal Skills Programme – www.phru.org/casp
Department of Health – www.doh.gov.uk
Electronic Library for Social Care – www.elsc.org.uk
Modernisation Agency – www.nhs.uk/modernnhs
National Institute for Clinical Excellence – www.nice.org.uk
National Electronic Library for Health – www.nelh.nhs.uk
Primary Care National Electronic Library for Health –
www.nelh-pc.nhs.uk

Application **10:1**

Brendan Docherty

Brendan Docherty

Evidence for effective care

This chapter aims to give the reader some practical applications of how to measure nursing evidence-based practice, thereby promoting effective health care delivery where the patient is the central focus. A measuring tool is provided for use in the clinical area.

INTRODUCTION

Measuring the evidence that we use in practice will give us and our patients information on what we do well and where there is room for improvement. For example, where we find no evidence exists for practice, then a research proposal should be drawn up and conducted; where there is evidence then it should be critiqued and assessed for suitability and, if appropriate, translated into clinical effectiveness tools such as guidelines and integrated care pathways. These should then be audited for effectiveness and clinical endpoints measured that demonstrate favourable and quality-driven patient care. This will lead to a nursing and health care culture that values evidence for patient care, thereby optimising the patient experience.

DEVELOPING AND MONITORING PRACTICE

Health care delivery is complex. Practitioners must ensure that they use the best available evidence to guide clinical care and ensure that feedback mechanisms are in place to support continuous quality improvement. Evidence may come from one of three main areas (NHS Executive 1998; see also Fig. 10.1.1):

● research and development (R&D) – including theory and laboratory work

Managing knowledge in health care

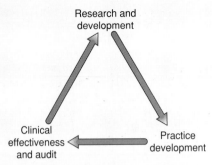

Figure 10.1.1 Continuous quality-driven practice

- clinical effectiveness and audit (CEA) – involving patients and populations
- practice development initiatives (PD) – how nurses and other health care professionals interface with the patient and their environment to develop care and practice.

In the clinical environment, there are many variations of what evidence for practice and patient care is – and it is multifaceted. Evidence from patients about care delivery is important and should be embraced, for example in the form of feedback about interventions or their views on planning or improving services (DoH 2000). This may include focus groups, patient advocacy and satisfaction surveys. However, caution should be exercised when acting on views from individual patients – views of larger groups and populations will make the issues and way forward clearer and more robust.

Theoretical evidence is also important, as is laboratory evidence. For example, in the early days of resuscitation guidance it was unethical to randomise patients in ventricular fibrillation to either the control group (no defibrillation) or treatment group (defibrillation administered). Controlled animal studies that were applied to human physiology were therefore seen as important methods to protect patients. Theoretical or high level research evidence (e.g. the randomised controlled trial) are also important guides for practice as they often indicate what the majority of cases will clinically respond to but are limited by the nature of their methods and the complex nature of individual patients (Docherty 2001).

The evidence hierarchy suggests, by the very nature of a hierarchy, that there are more favourable types of research or evidence depending on the rigors of the data collection method (Chambers & Boath 2001). This is a tension in the evidence-based practice movement as it implies that the health care professionals' and patients' experience may not be as reliable, when sometimes it is often the only evidence source available.

Evidence for effective care

There are also some historical debates about the use of quantitative and qualitative methods of research, with qualitative methods being seen as less powerful and therefore less useful (Cormack 2000). However, with appropriate application of qualitative methods or consideration given to triangulation of both research approaches, then qualitative and quantitative methods can be equally useful at solving clinical problems (Docherty 2000). Nursing can be viewed as an art and a science, and therefore mixed modes of research or enquiry approaches may be more appropriate and should be considered. Also, due to the uniqueness of the patient–nurse/health care team interaction, some research approaches may not be appropriate because of the inability to replicate a health care experience.

MEASURING HEALTH

A paper from the last decade sought to provide a historical perspective on patient outcomes, identifying that nurses and nursing philosophy were aligned to effective care, and attempted to classify outcome measurement that might reflect care being delivered (Lang & Marek 1990, see Box 10.1.1). These outcomes have been used as benchmarks for future work on measuring effective nursing care. The authors conclude that there is frequently a fear that certain measures are dynamic and may then not truly reflect the quality of care accurately. By using the measures outlined in Box 10.1.1 with identified clinical outcome indicators and robust care evaluation, nurses can ensure that their evidence for care and their measures of effective care delivery are unambiguous and patient centred. These measures can be used selectively depending on the care being measured and are not mutually exclusive.

Once evidence for best practice has been implemented however, clinical audit is the most common method of a systematic and critical analysis of the quality of care, and offers the following benefits:

- improves the effectiveness of patient care
- promotes efficiency of health care

Box 10.1.1 Categories of patient outcomes (Lang & Marek 1990)

- Physiological
- Psychosocial
- Functional
- Behavioural
- Knowledge
- Symptom control
- Home maintenance
- Well-being

- Goal attainment
- Patient satisfaction
- Safety
- Nursing diagnosis resolution
- Frequency of service
- Cost
- Rehospitalisation

- assists in updating clinical care documents (e.g. integrated care pathways and guidelines)
- influences and validates decision making
- encourages professionals to work together
- encourages innovation and creativity
- empowers staff.

Clinical audit embraces the notion of identifying what we are doing whilst seeing if we can do it better (Chambers & Boath 2001). For example, high volume, high risk, high cost, high variance and concerns about quality of care may all initiate an audit programme of care.

There is also evidence to suggest that by increasing the level, competence and amount of nursing care, patient outcomes are positively affected and that the role modelling of expert practice by specialists nurses will influence care given by junior nurses and lower overall patient mortality (Brooten & Naylor 1995).

MEASURING THE EVIDENCE BASE

Sackett et al's (1997) definition of evidence-based medicine is one of the most commonly cited and is 'the conscientious, explicit and judicious use of current best evidence in making decisions about the care of individual patients'.

Evidence-based practice (EBP) stemmed from evidence-based medicine in the late 1990s and occurred in tandem with the clinical governance agenda (DoH 1998a). EBP represents the health care agenda of delivering best care to patients utilising a team approach – moving from uniprofessional models that may have in the past duplicated effort and not acknowledged the impact that a health care team may have on the patient's experience (DoH 2001).

The development of EBP created a vehicle to lower the theory/practice gap through critical appraisal of clinically relevant information. However, it has come under criticism as it has also been perceived as lowering professional autonomy and focusing on utilitarian principles, thereby rationing possible health care options (Trinder & Reynolds 2000).

As health care teams become busier and patients' health care needs become more complex, there has to be a system by which parts of the health care team can assess evidence for practice and their specific patient groups so that the team can benefit from their review and decision. However, the decision about whether evidence is appropriate has to be transparent and consensus managed to maintain confidence in the process. A possible process flow is demonstrated in Figure 10.1.2, focusing on the three Ds of evidence for practice – demystify, deconstruct, disseminate.

A questionnaire interview was developed to measure nursing EBP (Cole et al 2000) and this tool was used to benchmark EBP across

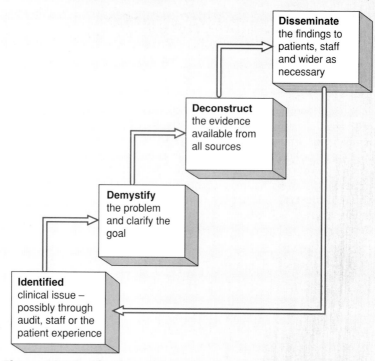

Figure 10.1.2 The three 'D'imensional elements of evidence-based practice

clinical geographically different areas so a forum for sharing of expertise could be facilitated. From this interview schedule it is possible to apply the critical elements to help nurses and ward teams assess, understand, strategise and remeasure the levels of evidence base that are used in nursing and health care practice. The crucial element, however, is the process undertaken to ascertain/investigate the level of EBP using audit.

When auditing EBP, the methods must be robust and should ideally be measured using a local member of staff and an external verifier. Information on conducting, analysing and utilising audit is available (NHS Executive 1998). From this a realistic and truthful level of EBP can be assessed and a more realistic and manageable action plan derived and executed.

An evidence assessment tool (Box 10.1.2) should be used to assess/audit the level of evidence that is used in nursing or health care practice. Ideally, views from the team should be taken, themes identified and concurrent views constructed. The process can then be repeated after any intervention or action plan aimed at improving EBP utilisation.

Managing knowledge in health care

Box 10.1.2 Evidence assessment tool (Cole et al 2000 adapted with permission from Emap publishers)

This tool is designed to give the assessor(s) a guide to how well evidence for practice is accessible, interpreted and shared. The cues should be used to elicit responses that can be collated, grouped and used to identify areas for improvement or to share as best practice. The cues can then be repeated regularly at intervals for improvement (after action planning) or to benchmark against other clinical areas.

Demystifying evidence

Q1. Do you think that a clear philosophy exists for EBP in your organisation and is this evident from your workplace strategic plan/mission statement?

Q2. What organisational support mechanisms are in place to support the implementation of EBP? For example your R&D directorate, practice development team, training and development team.

Q3. Do you know where to access research evidence relevant to your needs? For example, how might you undertake a database search and a hand search for evidence?

Deconstructing evidence

Q4. Is time allocated weekly/monthly for research or evidence-based practice discussions? For example a journal club or reflective practice clinical group.

Q5. Have you received any education regarding how to critically review research/evidence for practice? This may be a research module at an academic institution or in-service training.

Q6. Have you any experience in critically appraising evidence? How did you gain this experience and how is it utilised in your care delivery?

Disseminating evidence

Q7. Does your workplace subscribe to and make accessible nursing research or EBP journals that are peer reviewed (e.g. Journal of Advanced Nursing, Professional Nurse, Clinical Effectiveness in Nursing)?

Q8. When nurses in your area go on study days/courses, is there opportunity for them to share any findings of best practice and care? Is this formal or informal and in what format does it take place (lecture, communication book, ward meeting)?

Q9. Does your workplace make use of clinical guidelines or protocols that are evidence based? If so, give examples and describe why they are evidence based.

Q10. Are you encouraged to consider the multiprofessional dimensions of care? If so, what is in place to help facilitate this? For example multidisciplinary team patient care meetings, shared research meetings.

Evidence for effective care

Demystifying evidence

Understanding the importance of evidence for practice is crucial but this must also be contained within a social and political context, i.e. within the modernisation plan and applied to your local patient group or population (DoH 2000). Organisations that focus on developing services and staff should have a strategy for EBP and research that endorses and provides support (possibly in terms of facilitation, training, funding or specialised personnel) for underpinning EBP and patient-focused philosophy. It is also essential that national evidence is disseminated within organisations and that health care staff can access that information, thereby promoting EBP and health care equality. For example, this could be easily managed on intranet/internet sites or through other forms of communication (bulletins, magazines, journal clubs).

Deconstructing evidence

Critiquing evidence in small groups is essential to ensure that interpretation is more robust and rigorous. Qualitative and quantitative evidence has to be critiqued differently by the nature of the enquiry methods, but there are some core generic principles that assist in determining whether the evidence is the best available:

- Did any of the evidence come from a reliable and validated source (e.g. Cochrane, National Institute for Clinical Excellence)?
- Is it clear how the evidence was retrieved? For example when searching journal databases, which particular databases were searched using which years and which keywords? If someone were to repeat the search can the strategy employed be replicated yielding the same results? Searching the CINAHL database alone may not retrieve all the relevant work for a particular clinical question and therefore Cochrane and MEDLINE should also be considered as well as specific databases for certain specialties (e.g. psychology, cancer care).
- Is there a reference list available with the evidence being critiqued and does it include the appropriate evidence? Are the writers of the evidence credible and appropriate 'champions' of that particular area?
- Can the results of research/evidence be applied locally? For example, when critiquing and then applying evidence, ensure that cultural differences are accounted for if it applies to your local population. If a research study investigated only middle-class white men, then the results would not easily transpose into an Asian female population.

Managing knowledge in health care

Disseminating evidence

Duplication of effort and lack of sharing had been highlighted as an issue within the NHS (DoH 1998b, 2000, 2001). When solving clinical questions using research, audit or practice development the findings should be disseminated according to the scope and purpose of the work undertaken: locally, regionally, nationally or internationally.

There is a bias that exists when you try to publish work. When was the last time you read a clinical article which demonstrated that a method of health care delivery did not work? The nature of publishing is that it is a commercial market and therefore the cutting edge; novel information and findings will get published easily as opposed to a lengthy enquiry process that did not find the answer. However, by disseminating information about what is not the answer, we would help to reduce duplication of effort and the valuable time that other clinical practitioners use investigating something that we know will not work.

There is also scope to improve dissemination skills when presenting results to our patients – something that many health care practitioners will have little experience of, but which will in the near future become more common (DoH 2000). Nurses should also look towards disseminating findings at conferences (either as poster or oral presentations) and should seek training and experience of public speaking if they are unfamiliar with it.

ORGANISATIONAL PERSPECTIVE

We know that there is a slow uptake of research evidence being used and translated into clinical practice for patients (Trinder & Reynolds 2000) across both primary and secondary care. There may be many factors that are barriers to EBP including not having a comparative data collection culture, power and influence issues and individual responses to influence as well as the organisational culture (Lipman 2000). It is also recognised that research and EBP that contributes to clinical guideline development and implementation are also dependent upon robust audit methods for their success. This is a clear indication that audit – and the audit process – is essential to the clinical governance and modernisation agenda (Keaney & Lorimer 1999).

An unpublished systematic review of the effectiveness of organisations to support EBP was undertaken in 1999 (Foxcroft & Cole 1999). This review did not uncover any high quality studies on organisational interventions that may help support the development of EBP. Some of the studies – although they contained positive outcomes of effectiveness – could not be conclusive due to methodological weakness. What is clear is that organisations have to

Evidence for effective care

277

adequately resource interventions that support EBP development including both the individuals with skills and knowledge as well as the appropriate cultural and behavioural intent (NHS Centre for Reviews and Dissemination 1999). This may include the use of specialist nurses and health care professionals with theory and practice in EBP, as well as structures and processes that are interlocked to the organisational culture and everyday ways of working. Examples of structures that may support the development of EBP include shared governance and practice development initiatives (Docherty 2001).

CONCLUSION

Measuring evidence that is used in practice is not as difficult as it may sound. The important elements should already be in place if clinical governance arrangements are evident (e.g. patient feedback, clinical audit and research and evidence-based development strategy).

The critique (deconstruction) of evidence remains one of the pillars of EBP (Trinder & Reynolds 2000) and staff should ensure that they have the appropriate training and experience to evaluate evidence (from whichever source/level) and be able to apply the findings into their care after discussion and consensus with their teams, including the patient in partnership. Utilising the tool in Box 10.1.2 will help in the critique of published materials where the assessment of the written word can be validated and reliability checked.

Evidence-based health care is part and parcel of our everyday work as nurses, and we should embrace EBP as the patients' advocate. EBP is patient focused, is driven by a culture that responds to best practice and also allows health care professionals to optimise their contribution towards the patients' quality of care and overall experience of care delivery.

References

Brooten D, Naylor MD 1995 Nurses' effect on changing patient outcomes. IMAGE – The Journal of Nursing Scholarship 27(2): 95–99

Chambers R, Boath E 2001 Clinical effectiveness and clinical governance made easy, 2nd edn. Radcliffe Medical Press, Oxford

Cole N, Tucker LJ, Foxcroft DR 2000 Benchmarking evidence-based nursing. Nursing Times Research 5(5): 336–344

Cormack D (ed) 2000 The research process in nursing, 4th edn. Blackwell, Oxford

Department of Health 1998a A first class service: quality in the new NHS. Stationery Office, London

Department of Health 1998b Information for health. Stationery Office, London

Department of Health 2000 The NHS plan: a plan for investment, a plan for reform. Stationery Office, London

Department of Health 2001 Research governance framework for health and social care. Stationery Office, London

Docherty B 2000 Using triangulation in health-care research. Professional Nurse 16(2): 926–927

Docherty B 2001 An evidence base for nursing practice. Professional Nurse 16(9): 1355–1358

Foxcroft D, Cole N 1999 A systematic review of the effectiveness of organisational structure interventions to (1) promote nursing research; and (2) promote nursing research utilization. Unpublished investigation. (Email David Foxcroft *hcp@brookes.ac.uk* if you are interested in discussing this research)

Keaney M, Lorimer AR 1999 Auditing the implementation of SIGN (Scottish Intercollegiate Guidelines Network) clinical guidelines. International Journal of Health Care Quality Assurance Incorporating Leadership in Health Services 12: 6–7, 314–317

Lang NM, Marek KD 1990 The classification of patient outcomes. Journal of Professional Nursing 6(3): 158–163

Lipman T 2000 Power and influence in clinical effectiveness and evidence-based medicine. Family Practice 17(6): 557–563

National Health Service Centre for Reviews and Dissemination 1999 Getting evidence into practice. Effective Health Care Bulletin 5: 1

National Health Service Executive 1998 Achieving effective practice. Stationery Office, London

Sackett DL, Richardson WS, Rosenberg W, Haynes RB 1997 Evidence-based medicine: how to practice and teach EBM. Churchill Livingstone, New York

Trinder L, Reynolds S 2000 Evidence-based practice: a critical appraisal. Blackwell, Oxford

Evidence for effective care

Chapter **Eleven**

The potential of information technology for nurses in primary care: a review of issues and trends

Laurence Alpay, Gill Needham and Peter Murray

OVERVIEW

This chapter (which is reproduced from *Primary Health Care Research and Development* 2000; 1: 5–13, with permission from Arnold Publishers, London) presents a review of current issues and trends in the use of information technology (IT) by nurses in primary care. Its aim is to raise awareness of the particular problems faced by nurses, and so it is not aimed at the IT expert but at the primary care nurse, researcher or educator who seeks a wider perspective on the issues involved. The first section highlights recent policy changes in the area of information technology that are already affecting nurses in primary care. The second section addresses some of the barriers to progress in this

Managing knowledge in health care

area, which should be taken into account if the government's vision of an IT-rich health service is to be achieved. To draw attention to the fact that nurses in other countries face similar issues to those in the UK, a wide selection of international as well as national literature is included. Finally, the third section suggests how these barriers might be overcome, and identifies emerging trends.

BACKGROUND: INFORMATION TECHNOLOGY IN HEALTH CARE AND PRIMARY CARE

The launch of the recent information strategy for the health services, *Information for Health* (DoH 1998a), seems to promise a bright new dawn for the use of information technology (IT) within health care in the UK.

Coupled with the government's overall vision for the future development of the NHS as set out in the White Paper (DoH 1997) and other subsequent documents dealing with the delivery of quality services, such as *A First Class Service* (DoH 1998b), there certainly seems to be top-level commitment to widespread change in the nature of health services and the forms of delivery. However, there is still an important contrast between the current reality of nurses' computer use in primary care and the future vision as made explicit within this recent information strategy. If current reality is to be transformed into the future vision, a serious skills gap will need to be urgently addressed.

The use of IT is seen to be integral to the development and delivery of health services, with *Information for Health* setting out a 7-year timetable for the development of widespread electronic information storage and exchange across all parts of the health service. Such an implementation has profound implications for the way in which all nurses and other health professionals work and has equally vast implications for their education and training needs, to enable them to use the new technologies that the strategy promises.

The emphasis on the need for clinical benefit from computer systems has been widely welcomed within the health professions and is generally seen as a much-needed contrast to the previous finance- and management-driven information management and technology (IM&T) strategy. However, many of the factors that will determine the success or otherwise of these developments as we move into the 21st century are human factors. Furthermore, there

Information technology for nurses in primary care

is increasingly a shift from focusing on the intricacies of the technology to considering how best to manage information using it. These factors, rather than any detail of the technological issues, will be explored.

If we are to believe what has been said and written about the development of computer systems within the health service, primary care would already seem to be well served by the technology and well placed to take advantage of the benefits to patient and client care promised by the new direction and focus. There has been substantial financial investment in computer systems for general practices in recent years and it is now estimated that well in excess of 90% of practices in England are computerised. However, there is concern that although such systems may be in place, they have been – and will continue to be – used primarily by general practitioners (GPs) (e.g. for repeat prescribing and for financial and administrative purposes), and have generally not been used by or provided any direct benefit to nurses.

OBSTACLES TO ACCESS TO AND USE OF INFORMATION TECHNOLOGY

Although in the past few years most general practices in the UK have invested in computer technologies (Brown 1998), a number of problems associated with computerisation in primary care still remain. Some of the difficulties encountered in making information technology work for nurses in primary care include attitudes to computerisation, changes in work practices and education and training needs in IT.

Attitudes towards computer technology

For computerisation in health care to be successful, the attitudes and concerns of health care professionals, and particularly of nurses, need to be considered. Recent literature has reported on nurses' mixed and ambiguous attitudes towards the use of computers and information technology (Lacey 1993, Scarpa et al 1992). Such negative attitudes towards computer technology affect both the use of and access to IT. Negative attitudes have developed when, for example, nurses have had unsuccessful experiences with computer systems. In conjunction with nurses' own past experiences of computers, their perception of what computer technology can or cannot provide is very important. There is still a gap between the nature of nursing as provision of care and nurses' understanding of the benefits of IT to support patient care (Simpson & Kenrick 1997). Furthermore, there is also the perception that computers take away nurses' responsibilities. For example, some nurses view computers as a threat that challenges their traditional codes of ethics and confidentiality (Miller & Jeffcote 1997).

Another factor which influences nurses' attitudes towards computerisation concerns cultural differences. For example, Marin et al (1998) have investigated nurses' requirements for information technology in the USA and in Brazil. Nurses in the USA were found to be more comfortable with computers than nurses in Brazil, and in each country they had a different view of the role of computers within their work practices: nurses in Brazil tended to agree that computers should be mostly used in the administrative nursing area, whereas nurses in the USA believed that computers could help in other nursing areas as well. Mixed feelings about how IT can support nurses in different countries were also reported by Simpson & Kenrick (1997). They compared attitudes towards computerisation in the UK with a similar study in the USA. Although their results show that the UK situation was not too dissimilar to that in the USA, they found that other underlying factors were affecting attitudes towards computer technology, including age, gender and experience as a nurse. For example, it was found that older nurses who had not been trained in IT during their nursing studies were more likely to display negative attitudes towards computer technology. With regard to the gender factor, Simpson et al (1998) reported that in general practice it was more likely that male partners than female partners had responsibility for computer development.

Closely related to negative and ambiguous attitudes, anxiety about and resistance to computers contribute to the difficulties in accepting and using computer technologies. Negron (1995) reports on the impact of computer anxiety on nurses using IT. Resistance to computer technologies includes both resistance to learning and lack of information. Another type of resistance is that to change generally, including using computers. These are serious problems that need to be addressed or they will continue to hinder progress in the use of IT to support and deliver patient care.

Changes in work practices

The mode of health care delivery is undergoing major changes. Nowadays the style of patient care delivery is moving towards

Information technology for nurses in primary care

integrated care. Primary care centres are organised around multiprofessional teams and within the primary care team the role of the nurse is changing rapidly. Nurses in the UK now play an active role in disease management and health promotion, while primary care groups (PCG) can give nurses a clear role as part of PCG boards involved in commissioning health services for their local population.

Changes in work practices may be strongly influenced by technological changes and technological innovations may drive the change to progress. Many of the studies (Fogarty 1997, Hall 1996, Shepherd 1999) investigating current and projected use of information technology in general practice have identified areas where IT could be added to the existing activities of the general practice (e.g. links to digital medical libraries). However, although most GP practices in the UK are computerised, nurses tend to have little access to the system, especially for uses other than updating patient records (Miller & Jeffcote 1997).

Changes in work practices can also be hindered by technological and human factors. In some cases, the technology in place (e.g. electronic mail and connection to the world-wide Web or WWW) may not work efficiently, or the systems used may not fit the general practice's wider needs and requirements (Shepherd 1999). Furthermore, national and institutional guidelines for technological changes can be difficult to implement because health care professionals, including nurses, cannot always grasp the benefits and potential of IT. For example, there is some evidence that when nurses in primary care are not involved in the introduction of IT into the workplace, they will miss the opportunity to enhance their practice and status (Miller & Jeffcote 1997).

Changes in work practices also mean that health care professionals, including nurses, are faced with new challenges of communication and collaboration (Alpay & Heathfield 1997). However, health care professionals may be reluctant to alter their current modes of communicating and collaborating with colleagues – for example, in using electronic patient records in the practice (Swanson et al 1999). In addition, as Herbert (1998) has pointed out, socioeconomic and organisational factors impact on collaboration and communication. More and more health care institutions (such as primary care centres) need to contain their expenditure and aim to achieve increased quality of care and staff development while at the same time minimising costs. Thus members of the PCG must collaborate in order to maximise resources (Lock 1995, Whitecross 1999).

The introduction of information technology in the workplace impacts not only on changes in work practices but also on other related aspects such as changes in roles and responsibilities and changes in 'culture'. For example, the roles and responsibilities of health care professionals, including nurses, have been reported to change in relation to electronic access to and data entry of patient information (Herbert 1998).

It is recognised that a culture change in nursing is taking place and information technology is viewed by some nurses and nurse leaders as supporting rather than conflicting with activities (Procter 1998). However, such a change would seem difficult to achieve in the short term when computer resistance and computer anxiety still affect a large number of nurses (Negron 1995).

Are the changes in work practices brought about by IT always beneficial and desirable? This question merits consideration for, as Herbert (1998) points out, technological changes do not always result in better work practices. The need to spend more time using computers, and the necessary training for this, may result (at least temporarily) in less frequent interactions with patients.

Training needs and requirements in information technology

Information technology training for professional nurses

It has been recognised for some time that health care professionals, including nurses, have an inadequate knowledge of the principles of health informatics (Barnett 1995, Hasman 1994). One of the main problems is that there is still little empirical research reported in the literature which has assessed the current situation of IT training needs and requirements for nurses (see, for example, in Murray 1996, Simpson & Kenrick 1997, Wright 1994). Examples of studies investigating IT training for general practice have usually focused on GPs rather than on other members of the primary care team, such as nurses (Ahmed & Berlin 1997).

Unfortunately, computer training for nurses is often either non-existent or inadequate and targeted at audiences other than nurses, as was found for 80% of practice nurses interviewed in the study by Miller & Jeffcote (1997). It is also important to point out that GPs may not always give a high priority to the professional development of their colleagues, including nurses. Furthermore, in the UK the absence of any agreed accredited IT training for nurses, which has been highlighted in recent surveys (e.g. Miller & Jeffcote 1997), has certainly contributed to the low level of IT literacy within this health care group.

Information technology for nurses in primary care

Where IT training programmes do exist, nurses are not always provided with IT educators who can appreciate their educational and learning needs. Thus these instructors often fail to facilitate the teaching–learning process without provoking anxiety and discomfort (Nagelkerk et al 1998, Negron 1995).

Other problems associated with IT training arise from the nurses themselves, in that they may lack interest and concerns in IT and may not have aspirations to develop their expertise in this area. Nurses in need of training in IT will have received their formal education before this technology was integrated into the curriculum, and some of them will not have been inclined to find out about developing computer technologies (Roberts & Peel 1997). Furthermore, for some, training in IT is only seen as relevant when the information content is deemed to be directly helpful (e.g. if it is linked with training in the use of specific information management systems).

In addition, some nurses experience difficulties in prioritising their learning needs due to the magnitude of these needs, including computerisation and information technology (Lindner 1998). Moreover, some nurses are being increasingly challenged by new educational demands. Continuing education through open and distance learning is an attractive way to acquire informatics skills. However, recent courses for newcomers to computers (e.g. some of the courses developed at the Open University in the UK) expect their learners to be able to adapt to novel study modes of communication and collaboration.

Information technology within the nursing curricula

There are various problems associated with nursing curricula. First, the number of nursing curricula which include informatics is limited (Mantas 1998). This situation results in utilising existing materials developed for health or medical informatics courses, or using materials from outside the health care sector. Neither approach is desirable for nursing education. A related difficulty is the fragmentation of the nursing curriculum. That is, IT teaching modules are not always developed as an integral part of the curriculum itself (Carlile & Sefton 1998).

The curriculum content for teaching IT to nurses is still far from achieving its goal (Travis et al 1992). Although nurses are trained in the use of information technology, there are still areas of study that require attention. Frequently practical skills are limited (e.g. to word-processing software) and nurses lack knowledge of health information systems (Saranto 1998). Furthermore, not enough emphasis is placed on support for nursing practice and nursing research (Moritz 1990) and on bridging theory and practice in the use of IT (Crudele et al 1996).

The learning environment in which nursing students acquire their knowledge and skills is also a crucial factor. One recent study showed that nursing students were dissatisfied with the current learning environment, and that they wanted more depth and breadth to the teaching of information technology (Saranto et al 1997). The importance of learning in a peaceful environment when studying IT in nursing education has been stressed previously (Vanderbeek et al 1994). Nurses need to be away from work pressure and delivery of nursing care. Thus an inadequate learning environment will not reduce initial computer anxiety and enhance computer literacy.

Another set of difficulties in incorporating IT in nursing curricula arises from the teachers themselves. The selection of those who teach nursing students is important and needs to be done carefully. For example, in a study by Saranto et al (1997) it was found that nursing students felt that the best choice for a nursing informatics teacher was an IT teacher, rather than a nursing teacher. While some nursing academics feel comfortable teaching nursing students in informatics, others display negative attitudes towards computerisation and thus hinder the implementation of technological advances in their academic settings (Lewis 1997). Furthermore, with the advent of computer and telematics technologies, nursing educators need to rethink nursing education altogether. However, the need to re-examine and re-conceptualise the field of nursing in the light of IT still remains a problem for some (Ronald 1991). Many of the issues discussed above were identified and discussed by Nelson (1997) in the early 1990s, but there is little evidence of substantial progress towards addressing them.

OVERCOMING OBSTACLES VIA EMERGING TRENDS

Nurses' proactivity

Nurses need to work within a computer environment that can deal with the complexities of the care that they plan and deliver, rather than working with computer technologies that require them to adapt their practices to the computer environment. One way to achieve this is for nurses to be more proactive in finding out how IT coupled with adequate information management will improve

Information technology for nurses in primary care

their practice (Glen 1998, Marin et al 1998). The view that nurses ought to be involved in the IT revolution is also echoed by Keen & Malby (1992) and Negron (1995). It is through models like that proposed by Nagelkerk et al (1998) that nurses can prepare themselves for computerisation and change their negative attitudes. Those authors identified six factors that will successfully help nurses in nursing informatics, including strong leadership, effective communication and organised training sessions.

Furthermore, in order to be more proactive nurses need to be reflective. For example, they should assess and aim to raise their levels of concern in their use of and access to IT. Stages of concern as proposed by Hall & Hord (1987) range from no concern or awareness, through interest and information seeking to personal concern about how the computer innovation will affect the individual. These levels of concern can be applied to the nursing context (Barnett 1995). For example, a nurse may have reached the personal level of concern about the technical aspect (e.g. being uncertain about the personal demands and her competence in using the technology) and at the same time be at a different level for the policy aspect (e.g. having only a general interest in the new NHS information strategy).

Capitalising on 'nursing intelligence'

As work practices in primary care change, the role and responsibility of its nurses also change. Consideration is now given to 'nursing intelligence' (i.e. information gathered from nurses in their nursing work) and the nurse's role in utilising such intelligence (Ballard 1997). This view reinforces the idea of knowledge transfer as an evolving paradigm that will provide full and effective use of the technology by nurses (Ball et al 1997). Furthermore, it is through methods such as focus groups that nurses can capitalise on nursing intelligence, explore their role in depth, and identify their information needs and requirements (Torn & McNichol 1998). Strong leadership coupled with the capitalisation of nursing intelligence will put nurses in a favourable position to lead IT innovations in their practices.

Assessing the use of information technology by nurses through a sociotechnical perspective

The introduction of IT in primary care means that nurses not only have to rethink and change their perceptions about computerisation and IT, but they also have to adapt to new working practices.

In order to have a better understanding of the impact of IT in primary care, especially for nurses, the nature of those changes needs to be assessed. This can be achieved by adopting a sociotechnical approach. Indeed, there is an increased awareness of the interactive relationships between users such as nurses and the technology, and there is an increasing recognition of social, organisational, political and non-technical factors surrounding IT use and access (Herbert 1998, Kaplan 1997).

Although the social interactionist perspective proposed by Kaplan (1997) still remains largely at a research level, this approach provides a useful framework for examining the impact of IT for nurses in primary care. This framework allows us to reflect on and raise questions about issues of communication, care, control and context that occur in primary care. For example, one may ask whether communication within the primary care team (as well as between the primary care team and the primary care group) improves, and whether the delivery and quality of care is better. It is also important to identify who owns the electronic patient record and who controls the updates of the patient database.

Need for empirical investigation

In order to help nurses to change and improve their attitudes towards computers and IT, it is necessary to have details of the nurses' current situation in this area. It is important to investigate not only nurses' IT skills but also their understanding of information management using those skills. However, as stated above, there is little empirical evidence in the literature. It is acknowledged that more empirical investigation is needed to assess the situation (Marin et al 1998, Negron 1995, Strachan 1996). At the Open University in the UK, the work in progress in the project PRACTIS (**PR**imary care nurses **A**ccess to **C**ommunications **T**echnology and **I**nformatics **S**kills), led by the first author of this chapter, aims to collect empirical evidence on the current levels of access to and use of IT by practice nurses in Buckinghamshire, UK. The project also aims to assess nurses' educational needs and to investigate their perceptions of the proposed benefits of IT to their practice and lifelong professional development.

Adequate nursing training programmes

Changes, either of attitudes or of work practices, brought about by the introduction of IT into primary care need to be complemented

Information technology for nurses in primary care

by comprehensive IT training programmes (Fullerton & Graveley 1998, Lynn 1995). Although courses in information technology that are offered to health care professionals are usually satisfactory for teaching the use of specific software packages, they fail to provide a broader overview of the potential of IT (Saranto 1998). Nurses need support as they develop their understanding of the benefits of IT for patient care and of the complexity of using information technology. More attention is now given to metacognition and cognitive tools to facilitate higher-order thinking skills required for the effective use of IT in nursing education (Ribbons 1998). Furthermore, educating nurses in IT ought to act as a bridge between the learning needs of the nurses and the needs of the care setting (Lindner 1998). For example, understanding the fundamentals of IT can help nurses to apply evidence-based nursing by accessing computerised databases (Kessenich et al 1997).

The situation with regard to IT training for nurses is now slowly evolving (Barnett 1995, Nagelkerk et al 1998). In the UK, a number of initiatives have supported nurses in identifying their own training and development needs, such as the NHS Enabling People programme (NHSTD 1995). Furthermore, the new NHS information strategy, Information for Health (DoH 1998a), has set out specific objectives to address these issues for nurses. At an international level, recent recommendations on education in health and medical informatics, including information technology, have been put forward by the working group of the International Medical Informatics Association (IMIA) (IMIA Working Group 1 1999). In the USA, an informatics agenda for nursing education has been put in place to prepare nurses to develop and use IT (Gassert & Salmon 1998).

Successful IT training for nurses requires not only that the subject matter be prepared adequately to meet nurses' learning needs but also that IT be taught by carefully selected educators. There is a need for a more humanistic approach to teaching informatics in nursing continuing education (Negron 1995).

A further issue associated with IT training centres around information contents. There is a growing view that, in order to be of practical value for nurses, IT training ought to be complemented by adequate training in information management (English National Board for Nursing, Midwifery and Health Visiting 1998).

CONCLUSION

It is clear that the future development of health care will be increasingly underpinned by sophisticated use of information technology.

Nurses in primary care are faced with the challenge of making IT a valuable tool in their practice. Drawing from current literature, this chapter has as its focus some aspects that hinder successful access to and use of IT by nurses in primary care, namely attitudes towards computerisation and IT, changes in work practices and education and training needs in IT. Although solutions to these difficulties are under way, there are still discrepancies between the reality of today and the ultimate vision of the 'IT-skilled' nurse. It is by actively addressing these challenges, recognising the benefits of IT coupled with adequate information management, and by taking charge of their future that nurses in primary care will be equipped to meet the technological advances of the 21st century with confidence.

Acknowledgement

This chapter is reproduced from Alpay L, Needham G, Murray P 2000 The potential of information technology for nurses in primary care: a review of issues and trends. Primary Health Care Research and Development 1: 5–13, with kind permission of Arnold Publishers, London.

References

Ahmed A, Berlin A 1997 Information technology in general practice: current use and view on future development. Journal of Informatics in Primary Care November: 5–8

Alpay L, Heathfield H 1997 A review of telematics in health care: evolution, challenges and caveats. Health Informatics Journal 3: 81–92

Ball M, Douglas J, Hoehn B 1997 New challenges for nursing informatics. In: Gerdin U, Talberg M, Wainwright P (eds) Nursing informatics – the impact of nursing knowledge on health care informatics. IOS Press, Amsterdam, pp 39–43

Ballard E 1997 Important considerations about nursing intelligence and information systems. In: Gerdin U, Talberg M, Wainwright P (eds) Nursing informatics – the impact of nursing knowledge on health care informatics. IOS Press, Amsterdam

Barnett D 1995 Informing the nursing professions with IT. In: Greenes R, Peterson H, Protti D (eds) Proceedings of the Eighth World Congress on Medical Informatics (MEDINFO '95), Vancouver. Healthcare Computing and Communications Canada Inc., Edmonton, Alberta, pp 1316–1320

Brown J 1998 The computer in the general practice consultation: a literature review. Health Informatics Journal 4: 106–108

Carlile S, Sefton A 1998 Healthcare and the information age: implications for medical education. Medical Journal of Australia 168: 340–343

Crudele M, Binetti P, Serio A, Tartaglini D 1996 The teaching of informatics to first-year students of medicine and nursing, through an interdisciplinary

Information technology for nurses in primary care

innovative methodology. In: Brender J, Christensen J, Scherrer J-R, McNair P (eds) Proceedings of Medical Informatics Europe (MIE '96). IOS Press, Amsterdam, pp 823–827

Department of Health 1997 The new NHS: modern, dependable. Stationery Office, London

Department of Health 1998a Information for health – an information strategy for the modern NHS 1998–2005. NHS Executive, Wetherby

Department of Health 1998b A first class service: quality in the NHS. Stationery Office, London

English National Board for Nursing, Midwifery and Health Visiting (ENB) 1998 Information for caring. ENB, London

Fogarty L 1997 Primary care informatics development: one view through the miasma. Journal of Informatics in Primary Care January: 2–11

Fullerton J, Graveley E 1998 Enhancement of basic computer skills – evaluation of an intervention. Computers in Nursing 16: 91–94

Gassert C, Salmon M 1998 Setting a national informatics agenda for nursing education and practice to prepare nurses to develop and use information technology. In: Cesnik B, McCray A-T, Scherrer J-R (eds) Proceedings of the Ninth World Congress on Medical Informatics (MEDINFO '98), Seoul, South Korea. IOS Press, Amsterdam, pp 748–751

Glen S 1998 The tension between 'IT' and 'values thinking': implications for health and social care education. Proceedings of the Second National Conference of the CTI Centre for Nursing and Midwifery, 'Communications across professional boundaries – can technology help?'. CTINM Publications, Sheffield, pp 39–50

Hall L 1996 Health informatics in general practice. In: Hovenga E, Kidd M, Cesnik B (eds) Health informatics: an overview. Churchill Livingstone, Melbourne, pp 303–312

Hall G, Hord S 1987 Change in schools: facilitating the process. State University of New York Press, New York

Hasman A 1994 Education and training in health informatics. Computer Methods and Programs in Biomedicine 45: 41–43

Herbert M 1998 Impact of IT on health care professionals: changes in work and the productivity paradox. Health Services Management Research 11: 69–79

IMIA Working Group 1 1999 Recommendations of the International Medical Informatics Association (IMIA) on Education in Health and Medical Informatics. Report of IMIA Working Group 1. International Medical Informatics Association, Göttingen

Kaplan B 1997 Addressing organisational issues in the evaluation of medical systems. Journal of the American Medical Informatics Society 4: 94–101

Keen J, Malby R 1992 Nursing power and practice in the United Kingdom National Health Service. Journal of Advanced Nursing 17: 863–870

Kessenich C, Guyatt G, DiCenso A 1997 Teaching nursing students evidence-based nursing. Nurse Education 22: 25–29

Lacey D 1993 Nurses' attitudes towards computerisation: a review of the literature. Journal of Nursing Management 1: 239–243

Lewis D 1997 Implementing instructional technology – strategies for success. Computers in Nursing 15: 187–190

Lindner R 1998 A framework to identify learning needs for continuing nurse education using information technology. Journal of Advanced Nursing 27: 1017–1020

Lock K 1995 Primary health care: using computers to enhance care in a GP practice. Nursing Times 91: 36–38

Lynn Z 1995 Change and technology in nursing education. In: Greenes R, Peterson H, Protti D et al (eds) Proceedings of the World Congress on Medical Informatics (MEDINFO '95). Elsevier, Amsterdam, pp 1357–1361

Mantas J 1998 Advances in health telematics education – a Nightingale perspective. Studies in Health Technology and Informatics. Vol 51. IOS Press, Amsterdam

Marin H, Cunha I, Safran C 1998 Nurses' requirements for information technology in the next millennium. In: Cesnik B, McCray AT, Scherrer J-R (eds) Proceedings of the Ninth World Congress on Medical Informatics (MEDINFO '98), Seoul, South Korea. IOS Press, Amsterdam, pp 1314–1317

Miller A, Jeffcote R 1997 Practice nurses and computing: some evidence on utilization, training and attitudes to computer use. Health Informatics Journal 3: 10–16

Moritz P 1990 Information technology – a priority for nursing research. Computers in Nursing 8: 111–115

Murray P 1996 Research and the Internet: some practical and ethical issues. Nursing On-line 10, http://www.nursing-standard.co.uk/week28/ol-art.htm

Nagelkerk L, Ritola P, Vandort P 1998 Nursing informatics: the trend of the future. Journal of Continuing Education in Nursing 29: 17–21

Negron J 1995 The impact of computer anxiety and computer resistance on the use of computer technology by nurses. Journal of Nursing Staff Development 11: 172–175

Nelson R 1997 Nursing informatics education and opportunities disguised as problems. In: Barnett D (ed) Sharing information: key issues for the nursing professions. Vol 1. INFOrmed Touch Series. The British Computer Society, Swindon, pp 88–92

NHSTD 1995 Education and training programme in IM&T for clinicians: a framework for nurses. Vol 5. NHSTD, Bristol

Procter P 1998 Responses within the virtual conference. Action One: culture change. Proceedings of the Second National Conference of the CTI Centre for Nursing and Midwifery, 'Communications across professional boundaries – can technology help?', University of Sheffield. CTINM Publications, Sheffield

Ribbons R 1998 The use of computers as cognitive tools to facilitate higher-order thinking skills in nurse education. Computers in Nursing 16: 223–228

Roberts J, Peel V 1997 Getting IT into shape – external factors affecting the potential benefits from health informatics. In: Pappas C et al (eds) Proceedings of Medical Informatics Europe (MIE '97). IOS Press, Amsterdam, pp 825–828

Ronald J 1991 The computer as a partner in nursing practice: implications for curriculum change. Lecture Notes in Medical Informatics 46: 149–153

Information technology for nurses in primary care

Managing knowledge in health care

Saranto K 1998 Outcomes of education in information technology at nursing polytechnics. Health Informatics Journal 4: 84–91

Saranto K, Leino-Kilpi H, Isoaho H 1997 Learning environments in information technology – the view of student nurses. Computers in Nursing 15: 324–332

Scarpa R, Smeltzer S, Jasion B 1992 Attitudes of nurses towards computerization: a replication. Computers in Nursing 10: 72–79

Shepherd S 1999 Primary care groups are a catalyst for change. Windows on Healthcare 5: 20–22

Simpson G, Kenrick M 1997 Nurses' attitudes towards computerisation in clinical practice in a British general hospital. Computers in Nursing 15: 37–42

Simpson L, Nestor G, Bojke C, Purves I 1998 Gender issues in primary care computing. Proceedings of the Primary Health Care Specialist Group Annual Conference, Cambridge

Strachan H 1996 Nursing informatics: a Delphi study. In: Brender J, Christensen J, Scherrer J-R, McNair P (eds) Proceedings of Medical Informatics Europe (MIE '96). IOS Press, Amsterdam, pp 867–871

Swanson T, Dostal J, Eichhorst B et al 1999 Recent implementations of electronic medical records in four family practice residency programs. In: van Bemmel J, McCray A (eds) Yearbook of medical informatics. Schattauer, Rotterdam, pp 377–382

Torn A, McNichol E 1998 A qualitative study-utilizing group to explore the role and concept of the nurse practitioner. Journal of Advanced Nursing 27: 1202–1211

Travis L, Hoehn B, Root A, Youngblut J 1992 In: Lun K et al (eds) Proceedings of the World Congress on Medical Informatics (MEDINFO '92). Elsevier, Amsterdam, pp 998–1003

Vanderbeek J, Ulrich D, Jaworski R 1994 Bringing nursing informatics into the undergraduate classroom. Computers in Nursing 12: 227–231

Whitecross L 1999 Collaboration between GPs and nurse practitioners: the overseas experience and lessons for Australia. Australian Family Physician 28: 349–353

Wright G 1994 A review of current IM&T provision within pre- and post-registration nurse training. Health Services Management Unit Centre for Health Informatics, University of Manchester

Application **11:1**

Judith James

Information technology in primary care

INTRODUCTION

Over the past 20 years computers have become an increasingly important tool in primary care. The majority of primary care staff use them to print prescriptions and an increasing minority use fully computerised patient records. As a GP working in a fully computerised practice I see the benefits that information technology brings to patients. Computers can:

- generate computerised prescriptions
- make patients' medical records easier to assimilate
- facilitate audit to improve patient care
- facilitate recall systems for patients
- allow patients access to good quality written information
- allow health care professionals access to good quality medical information
- improve communication between primary and secondary care.

It is, however, alarmingly easy for health care professionals to appear to, and even to take, more interest in the computer than the patient and this is a disadvantage of their use.

The other problem is that computers fail. Systems need to be put in place to minimise the effect of this on patient care and indeed primary health care team stress levels.

BENEFITS FOR THE PRIMARY CARE TEAM

Computerised prescriptions

Computerised prescriptions are legible and therefore safer – the pharmacist is more likely to dispense the correct medication. Having computerised prescriptions also enables us to search to find patients on a particular medication. For example, when general practitioners were advised that cisapride, a medicine to improve stomach emptying, might cause arrhythmias and had therefore been withdrawn, it took only a few seconds for us to find the patients who were taking it. This would have been much more difficult if we had been using hand-written notes.

Computerised patient records are easier to assimilate

The records are legible which is a huge benefit. Numerical readings like blood pressure and cholesterol levels can be displayed in a graphical form.

Computerised records facilitate audit to improve patient care

There is a nationally recognised coding system for primary care, the Read code, named after Dr Read who devised it. Each different medical condition has a code (e.g. G3 for ischaemic heart disease and A1 for tuberculosis). Using these codes we have been able to audit the care of patients with ischaemic heart disease, to ensure that they are taking aspirin and that their cholesterol and blood pressure levels are well controlled.

Computers facilitate recall systems for patients

Diabetic care has been shown to be as good in primary care as in secondary care provided that computerised central recall systems are used. Computerised diary systems are also used for cervical smear recall.

Computers allow patients access to good quality written information

Using Prodigy, a primary care information system, we can print out information leaflets for patients. There are over 100 such leaflets, on subjects as diverse as advice on diet for pregnant women, management of blepharitis (sore eyelids), treatment of asthma and eczema. This means that we no longer have to try and keep printed leaflets in our desks. This was very hard to do as the leaflets all came from different sources and had to be ordered; the reality was that often patients were not given printed information.

Managing knowledge in health care

Computers allow health care professionals access to good quality medical information

Having access to the NHSnet means that we can access the NHS library for health (www.nelh.nhs.uk). This is a wonderful resource. We can read the latest in Clinical Evidence, search the Cochrane database, MEDLINE and Bandolier and look things up in the Merck medical textbook. Prodigy allows us to have the text of the Oxford Handbook of Clinical Medicine on our desktop without having to access the Internet.

Practice nurses and health visitors have access to systems that connect them, via the internet, to the latest advice on immunisations and travel vaccinations. This means that the information that they give (e.g. on malaria prophylaxis) is easier to access and more reliable than in the past.

The NHSnet could improve communication between primary and secondary care

We receive our blood test and cervical smear results directly through a computer link with the hospital. This means that they arrive the day after they have been tested – much faster than paper. We hope that soon we will be able to email consultants to ask their advice on patients – when they want to see them, when they would like us to arrange further tests. The hope is that this will make the waiting list for outpatient appointments shorter, which will be better for all of us.

THE FUTURE: A SINGLE ELECTRONIC PATIENT RECORD

The NHS IM&T (information management and technology) strategy aims to have a single electronic patient record for use by primary and secondary care that can be accessed by patients themselves. This is some way off, although the aim is to have it up and running by 2005, but it will make a real difference to quality of care when it arrives. A universal coding system will need to be adopted by all hospital departments and by primary care – several are currently in use. Difficulties with maintaining confidentiality with such a system need to be overcome before it can be fully implemented.

Computers allow us to manage the growing mass of information about medicine and link that to our own patients' needs. They can also improve communication throughout the health care system. If well used they can give our patients access to a world of medical information and to an effectively communicating health service.

Information technology in primary care

Application 11:2

Mary Hollins

Aide 2 Health: an innovative use of information technology in school health

INTRODUCTION

In October 1997, the Government wrote to schools and chairs of governors and informed them of the intention to have all schools – infant, junior, primary, middle, senior and special – connected to the Internet by 2002. As a school nurse and school governor, I began to think about how I could use this intention to inform school children about the issues around keeping fit and healthy. School nurses are ideally placed to give accurate, up-to-date and appropriate health information to children and to the school population as a whole. However, this is mostly undertaken as and when school nurses have managed to identify the time outside their core programme of work. I began to think about creating a website which could be used at any time, by anybody, which was age appropriate and which was fun to use.

Technology holds no fears for children and young people, not like many adults who often have a distrust of things technological. Right from reception class, children begin to learn mouse skills which help to develop their fine coordination as well as begin to familiarise them with computers generally.

FUNDING

As I began to clarify my thoughts for the site, I started to think about how to fund this development. I had the ideas and knew what I wanted the site to achieve but I did not have the technical knowledge to put it into practice.

I decided to apply to the Queen's Nursing Institute (QNI) Innovation and Creative Practice Award Scheme for funding. I put forward the proposal and costings. I was then short-listed and, following an interview, I was granted almost £4,500 to enable me to carry the project forward.

PROJECT OUTLINE

The task was to identify someone who could help me with this. I looked in Yellow Pages under 'Computer Consultants' and was amazed at the number of local companies listed. I picked, at random, a company called Wizard I.T. because I liked the name. It sounded young and imaginative. I was not to be disappointed.

At our first meeting, their enthusiasm for the project was almost palpable. They could see what I wanted to create and had the ability to translate my ideas into reality via their technological expertise. 'Aide 2 Health' is the end product.

I divided the content into three age groups – infant, junior and senior – and selected the topics that school nurses are most asked to talk about, namely:

- smoking
- diet
- exercise
- feeling good about yourself
- allergies
- growing up.

Infants

For the infant pages, I saw a cartoon character speaking to the children through speech bubbles. The print would be bold and large and the text simple so that as the reading skills of the 5–7 year olds developed, they could follow the print as the character spoke to them. I also wanted the message to be reinforced with actions wherever possible because these days, whether we agree with it or not, children watch a lot of television, go to the cinema and play computer games. They expect to be entertained. I felt very strongly that this was an opportunity to show that health messages could be given in an entertaining way. We also know that a child's attention span is quite short and so a talking and moving character would be more likely to engage a child for longer than purely still pictures. Each message for each topic is short and simple and allows further development as the children move through into older age groups.

Throughout the whole website, children only need to be able to use a mouse to access the information rather than the computer keyboard itself. The only exception to this is if they want to email the school nursing service with a specific individual query.

The icons on the infant and junior pages are fairly self-explanatory. This mean that the children do not even have to be able to read the topic words to access the information pages that they want.

Juniors

The junior pages start to take on a more formal look. The speech bubbles have gone and the text looks more like the pages of a book. The information becomes more detailed and begins to link into the key stages of the national curriculum. The text is supported by pictures and in every topic there is the facility for the children to email a school nurse with specific questions.

Seniors

The senior pages concentrate more heavily on giving accurate, factual information which is designed to support the personal, social and health curriculum as well as the science curriculum. Again, there is the facility to contact the school nursing service for specific, individual health advice. The email facility is more heavily used after school nurses have delivered a health education programme in a school and this is a good way of monitoring just how effective we have been.

Parents/teachers

There is also a section for parents and teachers to access which explains what the site is about and recommending that parents and teachers look at the site as it may encourage questions from their children/pupils.

THE WAY FORWARD

This piece of work can go some way towards encouraging schools to look at the whole ethos of the way they approach health and healthy lifestyles. It could be used as a building block to begin to fulfil the standards in the Healthy Schools Scheme. The concept of these standards is to promote healthy lifestyles by encouraging the whole of the school community – pupils, teachers, parents and governors – to question what it is about their school that specifically does this. By identifying what is relevant to their school, they can identify the gaps and begin to look at how these can be filled. To get

Managing knowledge in health care

children and young people involved in this way, they have to feel empowered enough to want to take part. I think that anything that encourages them to look at the way they live, the way they use their bodies and the way their bodies work will begin to stimulate them to ask questions and, more importantly, want the answers. The website can go some way to help them achieve this.

Because children and young people can access the web from school, home and now, of course, from their mobile phones, they have the opportunity to access instant information. Our responsibility is to ensure that the information we are supplying them with is as accurate, up-to-date and evidence based as possible.

The potential of web-based health information is as yet in its infancy. I think a lot more could be developed to reach those vulnerable children and young people who cannot or will not engage with health professionals for whatever reason. We need to look at chat rooms and how they could be used to put youngsters in touch with each other to provide mutual support for specific conditions or problems. I know this may be contentious and there are issues around confidentiality and accessing sensitive information, but as information technology develops and we become better at building in firewalls to our systems to protect individuals as well as organisations, then I think these issues will be overcome.

Website

'Aide 2 Health' can be accessed on
www.southessex-trust.nhs.uk/aide2health

Chapter **Twelve**

Research and development: implications for nurse managers and leaders

Cynthia Thornton

- ● Nursing research, historical perspectives, recent developments and the challenge for the future
- ● Opportunities and challenges for successful integration of research and development

- ● Paradigms, philosophical approaches and nursing research
- ● Action research, a tool to facilitate practice-based research and development

OVERVIEW

Research and development are essential to the developing knowledge base of any organisation involved in the provision of health care. This chapter will focus upon critical issues that challenge nurses who are concerned with the innovation of research activity and development within their field of nursing practice.

The first part of this chapter will briefly review the historical development of research within nursing, consider the implications of the introduction of *A Strategy for Research in Nursing, Midwifery and Health Visiting* (DoH 1993), examine the concept of evidence-based practice and argue that the broad dimension of nursing requires a variety of research approaches in order to create an effective research base. Part 2 will explore a variety of approaches that may be considered when designing a research project. Finally action research will be discussed, as a possible option, for nurse leaders to promote at a local level, in order to encourage creativity and development that is evidence based within their own field of practice.

PART 1: HISTORY, RESEARCH, DEVELOPMENTS, FURTHER CONSIDERATIONS

Historical perspectives

Historically research has not been prominent in the development of nursing practice and it is only in recent years that a link between research and management has evolved. Trayner & Rafferty (1997) drew attention to the significance of three initiatives within the public services: managerialism (DHSS 1983), the market reforms of the NHS (DoH 1989) and the NHS research strategy (DoH 1991). Together they have created a situation in which the work of health professionals, including nurses, is more transparent and open to scrutiny than ever before. The potential for improvement in the quality of the services provided and the cost effectiveness is obvious but less so the implications for professional autonomy and accountability. An evidence base for nursing is no longer an optional extra but is an essential ingredient which must be acknowledged in both the development and management of nursing practice.

The change to a Labour government in 1997 heralded a shift from the competitive market to a more collaborative approach to the provision of health care. However, the emphasis on quality and accountability remains. The White Paper, *The New NHS: Modern, Dependable* states that 'The new NHS will have quality at its heart' (DoH 1997). The introduction of clinical governance is central to this strategy and is described as 'a framework through which NHS organisations are accountable for continuously improving the quality of their services and safeguarding high standards of care by creating an environment in which excellence in clinical care will flourish' (DoH 1999, p. 3).

The innovative nature emphasised within this legislation is that accountability is related not only to financial efficiency and effectiveness but also to the provision of excellence in clinical care. Sacket & Haynes (1995) suggest that evidence-based care is concerned

R&D: implications for nurse managers and leaders

with the incorporation of evidence from research, clinical expertise and patient preferences into decisions that determine the health care of individuals. This view is supported by Warner et al (1998) who point out that although health care decisions are currently dominated by the health care provider, trends such as choice as a fundamental of political ideology, greater consumer knowledge, empowerment of an increasing number of older people (half of the population of the UK will be 45 and over by 2025) and the challenging of professional autonomy are increasingly likely to influence the future balance of power within the health service.

Nurses who wish to contribute to the health care debate will depend upon the availability of scientific knowledge to support their arguments. This knowledge will be a fundamental requirement for nurse leaders who are promoting nursing within the development of collaborative approaches to health care.

Research and nursing

The scarcity of research-based knowledge which relates directly to nursing practice has long been acknowledged. Lahiff (1998) points out that although Florence Nightingale is often quoted as a pioneer in research she did not include research mindedness in the nursing foundation that she established. Sadly the emphasis on obedience to superiors and above all to doctors was the most dominating and enduring feature.

The Briggs Report (DHSS 1972) recommended that nursing should become a research-based profession and that every nurse should understand and value research in relation to their practice. Nursing research prior to 1972 was very sporadic and limited to a few pioneers including Norton (1957) and Hockey (1966, 1968). Research was rarely addressed within the education and training programmes for nurses. However, during the last decade a number of changes have occurred: the move of nurse education into institutions of higher education where research is an integral part of the culture of the organisation, and the introduction of a new curriculum that incorporates research awareness and the development of critical evaluation skills. These changes have prompted an increasing number of experienced nurses to study for higher degrees by research. Simultaneously projects such as the nursing development units, initiated by the King's Fund, have provided nurse leaders with the resources required to introduce a research-based approach to innovation, change and development within nursing practice (Marsh & Macalpine 1995).

A world-wide perspective shows the publication of an increasing number of international nursing journals, which aim to disseminate research findings for consideration by members of the wider profession. National journals, which traditionally focused upon practice and news items, have incorporated sections for refereed research-based papers. These developments within the nursing literature suggest a growth in awareness of the value of research, not only for the nurse perceived as academic but also for the majority of nurses in the front line of practice.

Research and development

Although there is a long history of medical research it is only very recently that the NHS has acknowledged responsibility to initiate its own research programme. *Research for Health* (DoH 1991) presented the government's research and development strategy and focused upon the research and development needs of the NHS. The 14 Regional Health Authorities were each responsible for appointing a director, funding was to be ring fenced and the research activities were to relate to the current priorities of the NHS. A Central Research and Development Committee that included two nurse members was established. Lorentzon (1998), although welcoming the introduction of a strategic approach to research, was sceptical of the opportunities that were likely to evolve for nurses. She believed that the dominance of the medical profession and the previous emphasis on biomedical research would prohibit the opportunities afforded to nurses. Others had shared this concern. In 1992 a task force was appointed by the Chief Nursing Officer Yvonne Moores to formulate a strategy for research in nursing, midwifery and health visiting, which was published in 1993 (DoH 1993).

Recommendations which arose from the report focused upon:

- structure and organisation
- research, education and training
- funding for research
- integrating research and development.

Structure and organisation

Royle & Blythe (1998) point out that the utilisation of research is dependent upon the commitment of the organisation. They suggest that evidence-based practice has been realised most effectively when it has been adopted as a policy at all levels of the organisation. Kitson et al (1996) support this view and emphasise that, if

R&D: implications for nurse managers and leaders

adopted, it will lead to substantial change for the organisation. This will include the integration of research within policies and procedures, increases in the provision of resources, supportive administration and information technology systems, the introduction of senior staff to promote research and the development of innovative forms of continuing education. The need for collaboration between the clinically focused organisation and a research unit within a university is evident. This may be promoted by the development of joint appointments. The recent introduction of nurse consultants has been heralded as an innovation to promote the status of nursing within the wider field of health care. It is anticipated that the nurse will have a strong clinical base and also engage in education, audit and research. The broad spectrum of the role, however, is likely to prohibit any serious research activity. If effective research is to be accomplished, then resources must be a management priority for the organisation at both a national and a local level.

Research, education and training

The shift of nurse education into universities and the increasing number of qualifying courses at degree and postgraduate level will strengthen the research awareness and expertise of many nurses. The NHS Research and Development (R&D) fellowships offer financial support to potential nurse researchers, allowing them to take time out from clinical posts in order to complete a supervised research programme. The project may be singularly focused or may include a programme of study leading to a doctorate or skills in managing a multidimensional research programme. There has also been a plethora of short courses, promoted as a result of the research and development strategy, that are easily accessible and are designed to provide the nurse in practice with critical appraisal skills.

Funding for research

Funding for major research is available through the NHS R&D programme, from a variety of charitable and commercial organisations and a limited amount from professional bodies. Examples are the Medical Research Council, the Rowntree Foundation, the Wellcome Trust and the Nursing and Midwifery Council. The focus of the research is often politically driven and proposals of a collaborative nature are submitted for review by an expert panel. Nurses can submit proposals but would normally be members of multiprofessional teams including academic researchers as well as clinicians. Since the

Culyer Report (DoH 1994) each trust has been required to ring fence a percentage of their budget for research and this may be one avenue for funding for nurse leaders who aim to engage in localised projects within their own field of practice.

Competition for research funding is intense and some would argue that the allocation is heavily biased towards medicine and studies that represent the positivist research design. However, the increase in the number of nurses with research expertise and the political emphasis upon the service users' view may lead to increased funding being made available to nurse researchers.

Integrating research and development

Kitson et al (1996, p. 432) suggest that the considerations outlined in Box 12.1 are necessary in order to promote the integration of research and development within nursing practice.

Royle & Blythe (1998) describe the Iowa Model and point out that, in this instance, the infrastructure supporting research encompasses both high level managers and front line nurses. Research was included in all job descriptions and evidence-based practice was linked to quality assurance. Educational support was provided, staff who used research to solve clinical problems were recognised and rewarded and clinical nurses were allocated time and resources to engage in all aspects of research, including the identification of problems, assessment of evidence and the planning, implementation and evaluation of change. They suggest that when the organisation makes research a number one priority then nurses will be motivated to get involved.

> **Box 12.1** Integrating research and development into nursing practice
>
> - Implementing research into practice is an organisational as well as an individual issue.
> - The research evidence must be strong (that is it must be based on a systematic review of methodologically sound studies) before implementation is justified.
> - Strategies for implementation require careful planning and need to comprise a range of interventions including components of education, audit and the management of change.
> - Criteria for evaluating the impact of the intervention must be identified and agreed before implementing any change.
> - There are few descriptions of roles or organisational models that have successfully combined research and practice.

R&D: implications for nurse managers and leaders

The integration of research and development will also be dependent upon numerous links and a networking system that includes institutions of higher education, centres of excellence, international libraries via the internet, professional bodies and consumers of health and social care services.

Further considerations for leaders and managers

The brief discussion above illuminates the increasingly high priority awarded to research and development and therefore the associated opportunities for creative management and leadership skills in promoting the successful integration within practice. Although the overall implications of research and development are positive there are some associated issues that warrant further discussion.

Accountability

The R&D strategy supports the increasing importance of research in nursing as a necessary base for practice but also for professional accountability, particularly in relation to current health service reforms with their emphasis on clinical governance, cost-effectiveness and measurable outcomes. Tierney (1995) draws attention to the significance of accountability because of the sizeable percentage of the NHS budget that is utilised by nursing. The overall R&D strategy is to promote the use of research within strategic health care planning, day-to-day decision making and the ongoing evaluation of performance.

The increased emphasis on accountability and the associated challenge to professional autonomy have not been restricted to nurses alone. All those engaged in the provision of health care, including medical doctors, have been challenged. Warner et al (1998) suggest that a scandal concerning the death of a number of children in Bristol following heart surgery, fuelled by considerable public and political concern, has brought to a head the requirement for clinical transparency concerning clinical judgements and the rationale for decisions relating to health care practice. One outcome has been the reinforcement of the relevance of evidence-based medicine which has become the focus of increasing attention during the last decade.

Evidence-based medicine/practice

Evidence-based medicine (EBM) is described by Haynes et al (1996, p. 71) as 'the conscientious, explicit and judicious use of current

Managing knowledge in health care

best evidence in making decisions about the care of individual patients . . . evidence based medicine means the integration of individual clinical expertise with the best external evidence available from systematic research'. Coyler & Kamath (1999) suggest that although the literature relating to evidence-based practice is dominated by medicine this situation is changing as there is a growing awareness that health care is seldom singular but dependent upon a multiprofessional team. Evidence-based practice (EBP) is therefore more congruent with the government's current emphasis on collaboration in the provision of health care and incorporates nursing as a major contributor within the process.

Accessing and evaluating evidence

Accessing and evaluating evidence has resource implications. It demands expertise in critical appraisal skills and a considerable amount of time. An acknowledgement that time is always a problem for health care practitioners prompted the establishment of the Cochrane Collaboration. This was followed by the NHS Centre for Reviews and Dissemination at the University of York where systematic reviews of existing information are prepared as part of the R&D provision. A systematic review may be undertaken in its own right but may also be used to develop a meta-analysis or an evaluation of best evidence. This evidence may be an essential resource in the development of clinical guidelines, which in turn may be used to influence clinical decisions in relation to individual clients or to facilitate clinical audit.

Research methods

There was an assumption that when a systematic review or meta-analysis was conducted in relation to EBP that the results would be expressed quantitatively. This may be normative within medicine where a reductionist view of clinical problems may be appropriate and where the randomised control trial (RCT) is dominant as a research method. The RCT is promoted as a benchmark in EBM because objectivity is high and bias almost non-existent and from which the positivist school of research perceive a gold standard of research evidence is derived. However, a number of professionals are recognising that complexity is a characteristic of the work of many health care practitioners, including nurses, and are expressing concern at the limitations of quantitative research methods (Coyler & Kamath 1999, Lorentzon 1998, Swale 1998).

Lemmer et al (1999), when conducting a systematic literature review to 'explore and uncover an evidence base for decision making

R&D: implications for nurse managers and leaders

in health visiting', discovered characteristics which appeared to confound conventional measurement. These characteristics arose from the multidimensional nature of the work that is influenced by social and economic factors, including:

- anticipation and prevention of ill health
- protracted and/or intermittent periods of involvement
- working in relative isolation
- a mix of physical and psychological care
- a gate-keeping or containing role, i.e. assessing whether to work with the client or refer to an appropriate specialist.

These issues illustrate the complexity of nursing and the wide variety of factors that contribute to the culture and context in which nursing practice takes place. On the one hand, there is the intensive care nurse working with high technology in a health care system that is dominated by the medical model of care. On the other hand, the primary health care nurse working within the community setting is dependent upon skills of personal interaction and communication and working in a health care system that acknowledges the needs of the carers and the characteristics of the local environment. Both require evidence on which to base and develop their practice.

Swale (1998) points out that research has been used for at least 50 years as a method of evaluating health care. He tells us that the birth of the NHS in 1948 coincided with the fruition of the first randomised control trial. This trial demonstrated that streptomycin was effective in treating tuberculosis, which considerably increased the scope of the NHS to cure that particular disease and to prevent death. Swale emphasises that health care requires the information provided by clinical trials but suggests that they have a limited role when complex care involves several professional disciplines. He identifies social care as a particular example and promotes the value of qualitative research in these instances.

Shapiro (2001) supports this view and suggests that traditional medical research is failing to meet the overall needs of health care for two reasons. First, the dual complexities of health issues, such as determining the causes of the high rate of teenage pregnancy, and the complexity of the many changes within the health care system, such as improving GP corporacy, by linking them to out-of-hours cooperatives. Neither of these could be effectively evaluated by adopting reductionist cause-and-effect research. Second, the time scale in reaching a conclusion; a 5-year programme is of little use in a politically dominated environment in which the goalposts are continually sliding objects. He suggests that evaluation programmes are emerging that meet the challenge and highlights the increasing acknowledgement of action research as a credible approach that breaks larger projects into smaller parts, uses a people-orientated approach and results in change within the life-time of the project.

Factors in implementing research and development strategies

It appears that the complexity of health care issues and the multi-faceted dimension of nursing practice must be acknowledged when implementing research and development strategies. Three factors need to be considered: historical culture, medicine/nursing overlap and professional artistry.

Historical culture in which nursing has evolved

Wedderburn Tate (1998) points out that nurses are not a homogen-ous group. They are composed of practitioners, educators, man-agers and researchers and although collectively they are the largest employee group within the NHS, nursing remains a marginalised professional group. This may be attributed primarily to the fact that the majority of nurses are women but also to the perception of subservience to the doctor and the persisting association of nursing with low level tasks.

Medicine/nursing overlap

Mulhall (1998) suggests that the increasing tendency for medicine and nursing to overlap is promoting both increased interprofes-sional working and nurses undertaking tasks that have previously been done by junior doctors. However, it is important to note that in their practice, nursing and medicine are very different. Doctors are normally concerned with diagnosis and treatment. The focus is reductionist and based upon a specific medical problem. The rela-tionship with patients is maintained through timed appointments and the balance of power is almost always heavily weighted in the doctor's court. The nurse–patient relationship however is often characterised by more lengthy periods of interaction when the focus of care is holistic and deals with intimate and sometimes untidy issues such as feelings and emotions. Nursing care may be concerned with diagnosis and treatment as in the management of wounds, but equally it may be concerned with the adaptation and changes precipitated by the health problem which Lawler (1991) describes as the interface between the biological and the social, as people reconcile the lived body with the object body in the experience of illness. The nurse's relationship may not be restricted to the patient but may also include carers and close relatives or friends. Nursing is concerned with the whole person and empowerment and partnership are important factors when developing and implementing programmes of nursing care.

Professional artistry

When implementing R&D strategies there should be an acknowledgement of what Schon (1983) described as professional artistry. Fish & Coles (1998) suggest that there are two views of professional practice. First the technical rational view (TR) which believes that health care is developed by applying a predetermined set of clear-cut routines and behaviour to specific tasks in order to develop a package which is easily accounted and costed. This package should not be tampered with by the health care professional in the process of delivery. A contrasting view is that of professional artistry (PA) in which the professional practitioner working within the real world will need to make many complex decisions. These will be dependent upon a combination of professional judgement (which includes research-based evidence), intuition and common sense. These activities cannot be broken down into absolute routines, or be made visible in simple terms, and are therefore difficult to measure, cost and teach.

The development of theory in each approach differs; technical rational views theory as 'formal theory' which is produced by researchers who often work apart from the practitioners. Fish & Coles (1998) consider this approach to be in tune with present trends in that it produces evidence and encapsulates an element of certainty.

Alternatively professional artistry, they suggest, recognises the value of uncertainty, humility and critical scepticism. Professional practice is viewed as an art in which risk is inevitable in order to promote creativity. Learning to do is achieved by engaging in the doing and then reflecting upon the doing. When this process results in improvisation, enquiry into action and the acknowledgement of insight by the practitioners involved, then a knowledge base will be generated. This process is commensurate with the notion of praxis 'which Aristotle described as action in which the end product is not an object but is the realisation of morally worthwhile good' (Fish & Coles 1998, p. 38).

PART 2: RESEARCH METHODS AND ACTION RESEARCH

Research methods

Research programmes are conducted at a macro and a micro level. The former requires a team of experienced researchers and attracts substantial financial support. Nursing research at this level has been sparse but the recent emphasis on and inclusion of nursing within the R&D strategy, combined with a greater political awareness of the importance of nursing to the provision of health care, has led to an increase in the number of nurse-led projects sponsored by the government and the professional bodies.

At the micro level there is evidence of research which is related to specific service provision and evaluation as well as to specialist groups of nurses and individuals whose interest in research is primarily to further their own professional development. Nurses aspiring to develop as creative managers and leaders will need to use research and development in order to initiate innovation and change. Action research has already been noted for its facilities in this regard (Shapiro 2001).

Polit et al (2001, p. 5) state that 'nursing research is systematic inquiry designed to develop knowledge about issues of importance to the nurses, including nursing practice, nursing education and nursing administration'. They suggest that the purpose of the research is for the development of the profession, to promote accountability, to highlight the social relevance of nursing within the delivery of health care services and to facilitate decision making when planning and providing patient care.

Research studies that focus upon a practice situation, and which are dependent upon practitioners who are members of the nursing team, must be rigorous in their application of the research process. The methodology must be transparent and open for validation by members of the profession. This type of research can be undertaken as part of a masters or higher degree programme when supervision will be provided by an experienced researcher. Alternately a research consultant may be brought in during the initiating stage to provide support and research expertise. It may be introduced as part of a management strategy to evaluate the effectiveness of practice or to introduce innovation and change within the practice environment.

Although research demands that the application of the research cycle or process to a specific problem is systematic and transparent,

R&D: implications for nurse managers and leaders

313

the researcher is not restricted to the use of one specific method. The methodology or research design is developed by the researcher to accommodate the philosophical concepts that are sensitive to the type of investigation required, the beliefs and values of the researcher and of the respondents who are integral to the study. A further important consideration is the availability of resources including finance, time and expertise of the personnel involved.

Research is often considered as either quantitative or qualitative. These terms are, in fact, descriptive of the type of data that are collected rather than the philosophical beliefs that have influenced the research design. An alternative is to consider the term 'paradigms' which Polit & Hungler (1993, p. 442) describe as 'a way of looking at a natural phenomenon that encompasses a set of philosophical assumptions and that guides one's approach to inquiry'. Two paradigms – positivist and interpretative – will be briefly explored and the relevance of each to nursing research evaluated.

The positivist paradigm

This approach to science encapsulates the traditional methods which are based upon a belief in universal laws and an insistence on objectivity and neutrality. The research is deductive, theories and hypotheses are tested and the search is for cause and effect. This is most often accomplished by the use of experiments or surveys, the researcher's role is perceived to be objective, the data are numerical (quantitative), measurable and are presented in a statistical format. The researcher's role is perceived to be purely objective and control is important in relation to the theoretical framework, the sample and the research design. Quantitative research is normally evaluated in relation to its objectivity and is measured in relation to validity and reliability. Validity is described as the extent to which an inquiry actually measures what it set out to measure. Reliability is concerned with the consistency and repeatability of the data collecting tool (Stevens et al 1993).

The randomised control trial, which is central to the concept of evidence-based medicine, is an example of the positivist, scientific approach.

Holloway & Wheeler (1996) suggest that many researchers consider that numerical measurement, statistical analysis and cause and effect are the basic components of all research. Concerns that the researchers were treating perceptions of the social world as objective and absolute and were neglecting everyday subjective interpretations and the context in which the inquiry occurred resulted in a paradigm shift in the 1960s.

Managing knowledge in health care

The interpretative paradigm

The interpretative (or humanistic) paradigm is associated with the work of Kuhn (1970), although it has its origins in philosophy and the human sciences, particularly history and anthropology. Holloway & Wheeler (1996) point out that Kuhn was drawing upon the work of Weber (1886–1920) and his concept of 'Verstehen' (understanding something in its context). Acceptance of this approach for research has grown considerably and the philosophical assumptions on which it is based are similar to those that have influenced developments within nursing practice since the 1970s.

This type of research is often described as qualitative and is particularly useful when little is known about the phenomenon under review. Morse (1992) suggests that it is characterised by the three main features outlined in Box 12.2.

The research is almost always descriptive, the data are textual, the role of the researcher is subjective and a degree of reflexivity may be required as the respondent leads the research. In some forms of qualitative research a partnership is established between the researcher and the researched and it is anticipated that both parties will benefit from the process in which they are engaged. Data collection is usually by observation, interview or documentation (e.g. diaries, letters) and data analysis is developed by the use of codes, categories and themes. This type of research is evaluated in terms of credibility, transferability, dependability and confirmability. The transparency of the 'decision trail' throughout the research is of paramount importance to allow the reader to make judgements regarding its credibility, rigour and quality (Guba & Lincoln 1989, Holloway & Fulbrook 2001).

Smith's (1992) ethnographic, doctoral study, *The Emotional Labour of Nursing: How Nurses Care*, conducted over a period of 3 years in a city hospital, is one example of a qualitative study which

---

Box 12.2 Main features of qualitative research

- The emic perspective, which means that meaning, experience or perception are elicited from the participant's point of view. This is in contrast to the etic (world) view that is characteristic of the positivist paradigm.
- The holistic perspective in that the approach to the phenomenon of interest considers and includes underlying values and the context in which it occurs.
- There is an inductive and interactive process of inquiry between the researcher and the data.

R&D: implications for nurse managers and leaders

has illuminated important issues in relation to nursing practice and the needs of nursing students. Smith & Gray (2000), reporting on a recent update of the original study, purport that emotional labour is an integral aspect of nursing care and yet it still remains largely implicit at the level of the national nursing agenda. Interviews with doctors (GPs) and nurses suggest that doctors avoid emotional labour and perceive it as the work of nurses, to be avoided by doctors to allow them to get on with the work of diagnosing and cure. Both studies illuminate the importance of education and make a plea for the development of specific holistic competencies within the nursing curriculum. They also place emphasis on the importance of the clinical nurse leader, both as a role model and in facilitating support for nurses as they develop competency in the area of emotional labour. An evidence base is urgently required on which to develop educational and professional support systems for this important area of nursing care. In order to achieve this a research programme which draws upon research methods that are sensitive to the problem being investigated will be required. It will demand creative and innovative research that is unlikely to incorporate RCTs or large scale surveys.

The interpretative paradigm embraces a variety of theoretical approaches that may be adopted when considering research design:

- anthropology
- grounded theory
- ethnography
- phenomenology
- case studies
- action research.

A researcher should be familiar with the theory that underpins each approach before engaging in research design. It is impossible to explore all of these approaches within the confines of this chapter but many texts have been published that will provide a description and an evaluation of each. Action research will be addressed in more detail in order to demonstrate the potential that this method offers the nurse leader to facilitate the creativity and development that evolves from nursing practice.

Action research

The complexity of nursing care and the many factors that influence nursing practice produce a constant agenda of challenges, to which the nurse leader is expected to respond. Research often involves a lengthy time schedule before results are available to inform practice. Hunt (1996) suggests that this may be a reason for the reluctance of nurses to integrate research evidence within practice. The process of activity that constitutes action research has been described by Seale (1999) as a struggle between practice, the formulation of a research question and the reporting of the research findings, which will in turn inform further practical struggle. Creative management and leadership will involve struggle, not only for the leader but also the respondents involved in the change process. Action research is practice based, reflects the reality of the real world and produces timely results that are validated by the respondents. Its potential as a tool to facilitate the generation of practice-based evidence on which to promote nursing development is worthy of further exploration.

Action research is defined by Carr & Kemmis (1986, p. 162) as 'a form of self reflective enquiry undertaken by participants in social situations in order to improve the rationality and justice of their own practices, the understanding of these practices and the situation in which these practices are carried out'. It has become increasingly attractive to nurse researchers during the last 20 years. Hart (1996, p. 455) suggests the following reasons for this popularity:

● It offers a means of improving quality of care by narrowing the gap between researching and doing, theory and practice. It therefore produces an immediate spin off for practice.
● It defines individuals as active participants in the change process and not as passive subjects. It therefore promotes a sense of recognition and ownership on the part of the participants.
● It incorporates a cyclical process that mirrors stages of the nursing process and the quality cycle. There are therefore similarities with nursing practice, thus reducing any reticence that might exist about research.
● It is directed towards the implementation of change and improvement. It therefore provides a vehicle for development, which may incorporate the introduction of innovation and change as well as an evaluation process designed for a specific practice environment.
● It is non-exploitative, collaborative and offers the medium, through reflective practice, for emancipating the nurse as an autonomous practitioner.

Action research is therefore a form of research that provides a useful and immediate tool for managers and leaders of nursing practice to

R&D: implications for nurse managers and leaders

use in the implementation of innovation and change. It has the potential to involve all who will be affected by the change within the process, to promote the development and growth of those individuals and to improve the quality of the service that is under review. It is responsive to the development aspect of the R&D programme and also provides a tool whereby nursing knowledge which is generated in the reality of practice can be rigorously recorded, analysed, evaluated and disseminated for the benefit of the whole.

Examples of action research projects include changing medication programmes in a home for older people (Bond 1990), empowering users in a care programme approach (Loveland 1998), improving standards of care in a district general hospital (Hart & Bond 1995), investigating and implementing change within the primary health care nursing team (Galvin et al 1999) and evaluating the effectiveness of a community nurse education programme in preparing nurses for practice (Ewens et al 2001).

Kurt Lewin, a Prussian social psychologist working in the USA, is generally acknowledged as the founder of action research. He is possibly better known in relation to his 'field theory' from which 'force field analysis' is derived and often used in management as an aid to the implementation of innovation and change. Hart (1996) points out that Lewin's work related to the social problems of the day, including racism and industrial unrest. He believed that social problems were no less real than physical problems and could therefore be investigated within the positivist school of inquiry using the experiment as the research method.

Action research today, however, is most often viewed under the umbrella of the interpretative paradigm and emphasis is placed upon its educational potential and ability to promote empowerment and emancipation. In the early days, a consensus model – characterised by rational social management – dominated society. This was replaced by a conflict model that had the potential to produce structural change. Action research was adapted appropriately but was criticised by the positivists who considered it to be scientifically weak. In an attempt to promote the academic rigor associated with action research, Hart & Bond (1995, pp. 40–43) provide a typology that demonstrates how action research has developed along a continuum to meet the needs of a changing society. The continuum demonstrates that action research may be adapted to fulfil a variety of aims: experimental, organisational, professionalising or empowering. The distinguishing criteria include the educative base, the individuals in groups, the problem focus, the change intervention, improvement and involvement, the cyclical processes and the research relationship and degree of collaboration.

Managing knowledge in health care

Stringer (1996) suggests that action research is now understood to be a disciplined research method which attempts to improve the quality of people's organisational, community and family lives. He also points out that it is allied to the recent emergence of reflection and practitioner research. Greenwood (1994) associates the nursing research communities' acknowledgement of action research as a recognition that nursing is a social practice that aims to bring about positive change in the health status of individuals and communities. Stringer (1996, pp. 9–10) purports that the following four characteristics should be encapsulated within action research:

- it is democratic, enabling the participation of all people
- it is equitable, acknowledging people's equality of worth
- it is liberating, providing freedom from oppressive, debilitating conditions
- it is life enhancing, enabling the expression of people's full human potential.

Evidence and enthusiasm to support the use of action research as a tool to promote innovation and change in nursing in both its traditional and more recently emphasised public health role are apparent. The following section will therefore consider the process that facilitates action research and proceed to critically evaluate issues that may arise.

Action research: the process

The similarities between the nursing process, the reflective cycle and action research has already been noted and can be seen within the cyclical nature of them all. Ewens et al (2001) explain that action researchers today continue to acknowledge the Lewinian notion of planning, acting, observing and reflecting but include two further elements within the process: participation and policy development. They suggest that there are three minimum requirements for action research and that the project should:

- explore social practice as a form of strategic action susceptible to improvement
- proceed through cycles of planning, acting, observing and reflecting, each of these activities being systematically and self-critically interrelated and implemented
- involve those responsible for the practice in each activity, widening participation gradually to include relevant others.

R&D: implications for nurse managers and leaders

Bowen (1998) adopts the following activities for structuring an action research project:

- the statement of the problem
- the imagination of the solution
- the implementation of a solution
- the evaluation of a solution
- the modification of practice in the light of evaluation.

Action research is dependent upon the identification of a problem which should be acknowledged and owned by the whole of the immediate workforce (the nursing team). The project may include a number of stakeholders, for example patients, informal carers, managers and doctors. If empowerment is one of the aims of the research then collaboration of all those involved is essential. A leader may be appointed, either from within the contributing team or as a consultant who is invited to fulfil an independent role and who may withdraw once the research process is established. An advantage of the latter option is that the action research will be a priority for the researcher and the project will not risk being lost in the demands of an increasingly busy workplace.

All participants will need to have a clear understanding of the aims and objectives of the research and will be required to sign informed consent forms. The research question will be defined as information relating to the research problem to be reviewed. A hypothesis may be generated and tested. A variety of data collecting techniques may be used including observation, questionnaires, individual or group interviews, diaries and reflective journals and the use of patient records. These may produce a mix of both quantitative and qualitative data but the latter are likely to dominate. The research should be evaluated and the criteria outlined in Box 12.3 may be applied. Gomm et al (2000, pp. 311–313) also provide a useful guide to questions that should be applied when evaluating action research.

Critical issues

The action research cycle itself is not difficult to comprehend but the process may trigger issues of greater complexity. Ethical issues are important and must be of prime consideration when the research is enacted within the environment of health care delivery. Lathlean (1996) draws attention to a number of circumstances that may raise ethical tensions.

> ## Box 12.3 Criteria for evaluating research
>
> **Credibility** Those identified as participating in the research must be described accurately and all of the participants must agree that the results are presented correctly.
>
> **Transferability** This depends on the theoretical framework and details of the study being made explicit to allow readers to make their own judgements regarding the transferability of the findings to their own sphere of practice.
>
> **Dependability** This depends upon the decision-making trail being evident and open for auditing
>
> **Confirmability** This depends on the three previous criteria each contributing to the degree of confirmability. Holloway & Wheeler (1996) confirm that transparency of the audit trail provides rigour and is the key element in evaluating qualitative research (Guba & Lincoln 1989).

Power and equity

The first is the relationship between action and research and the question of power and equity. Problems may arise if there is a partnership between independent researchers, for example a university research team and nurses working in the practice setting. Galvin et al (1999) recorded difficulties of this nature in their study that investigated and implemented change within the primary health care nursing team. They attribute the problems to poor communication that led to difficulties in maintaining true collaboration over an extended period of time and poorly defined group boundaries and responsibilities within the research. Also, the time restrictions introduced by the funding bodies proved to be unrealistic and the overall outcome left the nursing team feeling unsupported by the researcher team from the university.

Informed consent

As in all participatory research, evidence of informed consent from all participants must be obtained. In action research, there may be a fine line between activities that are part of a nurse's routine work and those that become part of the research project. Patients or clients may unknowingly or unexpectedly become involved with the action. The actual dimensions of the research may become opaque and care will therefore be needed in order to prevent ethical discrepancies occurring.

Confidentiality and anonymity

Concerns may also arise in relation to confidentiality and anonymity, particularly if the research takes place in a service area that is easily identifiable, even without a name being divulged. Lathlean (1996) draws from her own experience when writing an action research report for publication. The final draft was offered to all those who had participated for comment, resulting in only one critical response. Lathlean believes that in the effort expended to be fair, to retain confidentiality and anonymity, the presentation of the findings had become too bland and that possibly some of the reality of the experience may have been lost.

Ownership

A further consideration maybe the issue of ownership. If the research is participatory the rights of ownership belong equally to the researcher and the participants. A misunderstanding regarding the final outcome of the research may become an issue. If the study aims to emancipate then the ownership may transfer as the research proceeds. It is possible, if claims for publication rights have not been clarified in the planning stages, that the collaborative principles that underpin action research may be jeopardised.

Transparency and action in the practice setting

Hart (1996) raises two further points that may have pragmatic consequences. Important attributes of action research are the transparency of the process and the potential to bring immediate action to the practice setting. The former may highlight shortcomings in the practice arena that in the current culture of critical accountability may cause embarrassment or even the incitement of penalties within the organisation. The latter point reflects the purpose of action research but conflict might arise if resources are not available for the implementation process. The research may, on the one hand, enhance the autonomy of the nurses involved but, on the other, this may be counteracted by the frustrations and dissatisfaction that may occur if they have no control in the allocation of the resources that are needed to implement the research findings. Existing tensions between efficiency by cost cutting and the provision of resources to improve the quality of patient care may be considerably increased.

Action research clearly is not a guaranteed panacea for success but in spite of the above constraints it has many characteristics that promote its value for nurses who are intent upon developing and managing nursing practice.

One important aspect is the philosophical values on which action research is normally based. They include democracy, enabling the participation of all people; equality, acknowledging the worth of all people; liberty, offering a pathway towards freedom from oppressive, debilitating conditions; and life enhancing, enabling the expression of people's full human potential (Stringer 1996). These values juxtapose with the value base on which nursing is built and which should form a foundation from which developments in nursing practice may evolve.

Attention has been drawn to the dominant role that medicine has historically been awarded in health care and the struggle that nurses experience in developing a knowledge base that is independent of the medical model of care. Medical research predominantly rests within the positivist paradigm and is intent upon discovering cause and effect. Nursing is rarely reductionist in nature but rather deals with many complex issues that are part and parcel of the real world experience of patients and their carers. Action research is situated within the interpretative paradigm, the research adopts a bottom-up approach, is practice based, focuses upon problem solving and values reflection as an important aspect of the data collecting process. It is therefore one way that is open to nurse leaders to create a knowledge base that is generated from nursing practice and which acknowledges the complexities of nursing practice and the professional artistry in which nurses engage. It may also encourage an increase in the utilisation of research in nursing that, as Hunt (1996) suggests, has been hampered in the past by problems relating to ownership and acceptance.

There will be struggles and some risks facing the nurse leader who adopts action research to introduce innovation and change within nursing practice. It does, however, provide a research tool that meets the systematic rigour required by the research community, is based in the practice setting and enhances the possibility of developments that are both creative and progressive.

CONCLUSION

This chapter has introduced research and development as an integral component of the current health care debate and suggested that it has strong political alignment and must be a central element of any innovation and change strategy. A brief review of the relationship between research and nursing raised a number of controversial issues that remain critical to the development of an evidence base on which to build nursing practice. The relationship between nursing and medicine is a key factor and Kitson (2001) emphasises the urgent need for nursing to conceptualise its relationship with medicine and redefine and develop a unique epistemological base. If this is to be achieved then action research may prove to be one approach that becomes a key facet in the strengthening and development of a profession.

References

Bond M 1990 Changing medication practices in a home for older people. In: Hart E, Bond M 1995 Action research for health and social care: a guide for practice. Open University Press, Buckingham

Bowen R 1998 Graphic approaches to describing action research methodology. Educational Action Research 6(3): 507–526

Carr W, Kemmis S 1986 Becoming critical: education knowledge and action research. Falmer Press, London

Coyler H, Kamath P 1999 Evidence-based practice. A philosophical and political analysis: some matters for consideration by professional practitioners. Journal of Advanced Nursing 29(1): 188–193

Department of Health 1989 Working for Patients, Cmnd 555. HMSO, London

Department of Health 1991 Research for health: a research and development strategy for the NHS. Department of Health R&D Division, London

Department of Health 1993 Report of the task force on the strategy for research in nursing, midwifery and health visiting. Department of Health R&D Division, London

Department of Health 1994 Supporting research and development in the NHS (The Culyer Report). HMSO, London

Department of Health 1997 The new NHS: modern, dependable. Stationery Office, London

Department of Health and Social Security 1972 Report of the Committee on Nursing (The Briggs Report). HMSO, London

Department of Health and Social Security 1983 National Health Service management enquiry (The Griffiths Report). HMSO, London

Ewens A, Howkins E, McClure L 2001 Fit for purpose: does specialist community nurse education prepare nurses for practice? Nurse Education Today 21: 127–135

Fish D, Coles C 1998 Developing professional judgement in health care. Butterworth-Heinemann, Oxford

Galvin K, Andrews C, Jackson D et al 1999 Investigating and implementing change within the primary health care nursing team. Journal of Advanced Nursing 30(1): 238–247

Gomm R, Needham G, Bullman A (eds) 2000 Evaluating research in health and social care. The Open University, London

Greenwood J 1994 Action research: a few details, a caution and something new. Journal of Advanced Nursing 20: 13–18

Guba E, Lincoln Y 1989 Fourth generation evaluation. Sage, Beverly Hills, California

Hart E 1996 Action research as a professionalizing strategy; issues and dilemmas. Journal of Advanced Nursing 23: 454–461

Hart E, Bond M 1995 Action research for health and social care; a guide to practice. Open University Press, Buckingham

Haynes R, Sackett D, Gray J et al 1996 Transferring evidence from research into practice. APC Journal Club 125(A): 14–16

Hockey L 1966 Cited in Lelean S, Clarke M 1990 Research resource development in the United Kingdom. International Journal of Nursing Studies 27(2): 123–138

Hockey L 1968 Cited in Lelean S, Clarke M 1990 Research resource development in the United Kingdom. International Journal of Nursing Studies 27(2): 123–138

Holloway I, Fulbrook P 2001 Revisiting qualitative inquiry: interviewing in nursing and midwifery research. Nursing Times Research 6(1): 539–550

Holloway I, Wheeler S 1996 Qualitative research for nurses. Blackwell, Oxford

Hunt E 1996 Barriers to research utilization. Guest editorial. Journal of Advanced Nursing 23: 423–425

Kitson A 2001 Does nursing education have a future? Nurse Education Today 24: 86–96

Kitson A, Bana Ahmed L, Harvey G, Seers K, Thompson D 1996 From research to practice: one organisational model for promoting research based practice. Journal of Advanced Nursing 23: 430–440

Kuhn TS 1970 The structure of scientific revolution, 2nd edn. University of Chicago Press, Chicago

Lahiff M 1998 Nursing research: 'the why and why not'. In: Smith P (ed) Nursing research setting new agendas. Arnold, London

Lathlean J 1996 Ethical dimensions of action research. In: de Raeve L (ed) Nursing research; an ethical and legal appraisal. Baillière Tindall, London

Lawler J 1991 Behind the screens nursing. Churchill Livingstone, Edinburgh

Lemmer B, Greller R, Stevens J 1999 Systematic review of nonrandom and qualitative research literature: exploring and uncovering an evidence base for health visiting and decision making. Qualitative Health Research 9(3): 315–328

Lorentzon M 1998 Where do ideas come from? Setting research agendas. In: Smith P (ed) Nursing research setting new agendas. Arnold, London

Loveland B 1998 The care programme approach: whose is it? Empowering users in the care programme process. Educational Action Research 6(2): 321–336

Marsh S, Macalpine M 1995 Our own capabilities; clinical nurse managers taking a strategic approach to service improvement. King's Fund, London

Morse J (ed) 1992 Qualitative health research. Sage, Beverly Hills, California

Mulhall A 1998 Nursing research and the evidence. Evidence-Based Nursing 1(1): 4–6

Six Steps to **Effective Management**

Managing knowledge in health care

Norton D 1957 Cited in Lelean S, Clarke M 1990 Research resource development in the United Kingdom. International Journal of Nursing Studies 27(2): 123–138

Polit F, Hungler P 1993 Essentials of nursing research. Methods, appraisal and utilization, 3rd edn. Lippincott, Philadelphia

Polit D, Beck C, Hungler B 2001 Essentials of nursing research: methods, appraisal and utilization, 5th edn. Lippincott, Philadelphia

Royle J, Blythe J 1998 Promoting research utilisation in nursing: the role of the individual, organisation and the environment. Evidence-Based Nursing 1(3): 71–72

Sackett D, Haynes B 1995 On the need for evidence-based medicine. Evidence-Based Medicine Nov/Dec: 5–6

Schon D 1983 The reflective practitioner. Basic Books, New York

Seale C 1999 The quality of qualitative research. Sage, London

Shapiro J 2001 Soft changes, hard work. Health Service Journal March 1: 22

Smith P 1992 The emotional labour of nursing: how nurses care. Macmillan, London

Smith P, Gray B 2000 The emotional labour of nursing: how student and qualified nurses learn to care. A report on nurse education, nursing practice and emotional labour in the contemporary NHS. South Bank University, London

Stevens P, Schade A, Chalk B, Slevin O 1993 Understanding research. Campion Press, Edinburgh

Stringer E 1996 Action research; a handbook for practitioners. Sage, Thousand Oaks, California

Swale J 1998 The National Health Service and the science of evaluation: two anniversaries. Health Trends 30(1): 20–22

Tierney A 1995 Accountability in nursing research. In: Watson R (ed) Accountability in nursing practice. Chapman & Hall, London, pp 209–231

Trayner M, Rafferty A 1997 The NHS R&D context for nursing research: a working paper. Centre for Policy in Nursing Research, London School of Hygiene and Tropical Research, London

Warner M, Longley M, Gould E, Picek A 1998 Welsh Institute for Health and Social Care, University of Glamorgan

Wedderburn Tate C 1998 'B' road or motorway?: charting a future for nursing research. In Smith P (ed) Nursing research: setting new agendas. Arnold, London, pp 8–29

Application **12:1**

Pam Denicolo

Action research to improve services

BACKGROUND TO THE PROJECT

The project was focused on the planned resettlement, into 24-hour nursed care homes in the community, of people with severe or enduring mental health problems prior to the closure of a local hospital, predicted to take place early in 2003. The people concerned in the resettlement had all been in long-term care in the hospital.

The resettlement plan and principles demonstrate the considerable care taken to ensure that the hospital did not close without appropriate new services being established. The documents also include information on the chosen site for the first cohort of patients. The reasons identified for the development of the facility at the chosen site include recognition of proposed residents' expressed wishes about location and of aspects of the environment/community that would facilitate the continuation of care.

The Trust board had discussed a variety of evaluation mechanisms to provide feedback on the success or otherwise of different aspects of resettlement. It was of particular concern that those engaged with resettlement at the primary level, i.e. the patients and their immediate carers, were also engaged as fully as possible with significant parts of the evaluation. Amongst other considerations, it was important that factors that impinge on the quality of life of patients should be identified by the patients and their immediate carers while factors that impinge on the ability of staff to provide quality of care should also be identified by those people directly involved. Equally it was considered important that the primary level participants should be engaged in identifying ways in which the required environment and activities (those that would contribute further to quality of life and quality of care) could be achieved. This was considered crucial in engaging them in any change processes that would be required.

The Trust board approached the university team who had commitment to and experience of action research projects that

Action research to improve services

327

fulfilled Stringer's (1996) four characteristics, as described in Chapter 12. Each member of the team values the opportunity to help individuals or groups to reflect on current ideas and practices so that they might consider alternatives and may engage in emancipatory praxis (Denicolo & Pope 2001). The team, together with a steering group who had frequent and immediate contact with the participants in the home, devised a pilot project to meet the aims outlined below. These aims were based on the premise that, though the resettlement programme itself is intended to provide enhanced living conditions for patients and working conditions for staff, the anticipation of change and the process of adjustment to the new environment may be stressful to all concerned. Thus the project sought to support and encourage both staff and patients to take an active role in developing new methods of engaging with each other and the community. The group involved in this project was the first cohort to be resettled and had been in residence in the community for only a few months before the project started.

AIMS OF THE PROJECT

1. To develop a framework process model for future evaluation and development of resettlement
2. To identify factors within the changing environments which enhance and inhibit quality of life for the patients in the first cohort
3. To identify factors within the resettlement programme and the new working context which enhance and inhibit the ability of staff to provide quality of care for those patients
4. To inform continuously the development of practice during and beyond resettlement by exploring and evaluating processes of dynamic interchange of the views and perspectives of patients, staff and managers

TERMS USED IN THE PROJECT

- *House* refers to the locus of the project, a residential facility.
- *Patients* are those eight patients living in the house who volunteered to take part in the study. The term selected is the one that the patients most frequently use to refer to themselves and each other, although the resettlement team would prefer them to see themselves as residents, rather than patients.
- *Staff* are the seven qualified nurses and eight support staff working in the house on various shift patterns. All staff volunteered to take part in the study.

- Patients and staff combine to form the core *participants* in the project.
- *Peripheral informants* is the term used to indicate the eight members of the hospital multidisciplinary team who, while providing care and services of great importance, are not involved in the house on a regular, day-to-day, extended capacity. Two relatives of patients also contributed perspectives that are included in the data from this group.

All participants and peripheral informants gave informed consent in a form agreed with the local Trust Ethics Committee.

IMPLEMENTATION OF THE RESEARCH

This involved five aspects:

- Initial discussion with a range of key staff to obtain background information and assess feasibility
- A detailed literature review to guide topic areas for the fieldwork
- Development of a code of practice
- Data collection using a multimethod approach
- Review of findings and development of a process model for implementation with this and future cohorts.

Fieldwork undertaken

Undertaking a study in a complex environment in which the participants either lived or worked was bound to be fraught with unpredictable difficulties, though it provided an unparalleled opportunity to illuminate the situation in which they found themselves. Equally, opportunities arose for a more detailed study of some issues than was expected.

An extended preliminary period performed the valuable function of allowing all the participants to become increasingly familiar with the researchers and to accept, and be comfortable with, their presence in the house. The researchers, in turn, got to know all the participants by name and were able to develop a basic knowledge and understanding of the routines over a normal day and normal week.

This period also enabled the participants to question and comment on the intended process and procedures for the research. For instance, it became clear that some amendments had to be made to the original research plan (e.g. the variable availability of both staff and patients and the small size of the space available for meetings made it apparent that engaging in full focus group activities would be impractical).

The researchers also recognised that the core participants were more relaxed and open when 'chatting' with the researchers

Action research to improve services

while they jointly undertook domestic tasks such as washing up than they were when attending a formally arranged interview, either individually or in a small group. The researchers thus used these informal opportunities for discussion to raise points of clarification or to probe particular points. They also resolved to explore other opportunities to talk in informal circumstances with the participants, although assiduously reminding them of their research role and checking back with them that they had understood and interpreted adequately the ideas presented.

Over 3 months, the researchers made a total of over 60 visits to the house and the surrounding area, including visits to occupational facilities provided at the hospital. The researchers took the patients on short trips to shops and cafes and attended house meetings and menu meetings. The researchers helped the staff with some domestic chores, attended their staff meetings and had coffee and tea breaks with them as well as engaging in the various interview activities. In this respect the collaborative intent of the research was recognised and generally fulfilled.

Interviews were arranged with peripheral informants to suit their busy schedules, while the researchers were provided with guided tours of wards when on site in the hospital. On these visits they were allowed to take photographs as probes to use with patients. Both the staff and peripheral informants provided access to useful background documents which aided understanding of the final data. Information provided by the peripheral informants helped in making sense of historical references made by participants and thus allowed conversations with the latter to flow more naturally.

This general approach and combination of methods could justifiably be termed 'immersion in the situation' and certainly it provided a very rich data set. The collection of data was iterative in nature with each intervention or visit being reviewed rigorously for links with previous data, helping to clarify or extend previous understandings. This process also stimulated further questions about previously unconsidered issues.

A great deal of consideration was given to the process of feedback of the results. It had been intended to do this regularly throughout the project and then to have a formal feedback session at the end of the project. However, getting the relevant people together in the same place at the same time posed a practical hurdle, for which others engaged in similar research should be prepared.

Discussions were held with the staff about the fruitful ways of organising the formal feedback session. In the end a compromise was reached with the researchers providing cakes and drinks during a period when a house meeting would take place, closely following the patients' lunch, so that the information could be discussed with two mixed groups.

Methodological issues derived from fieldwork experience

It is clear from the wealth of data collected that an in-depth study using a variety of techniques is appropriate for research in contexts in which the participants are unused to expressing their opinions about their lives/work, or who have disabilities which restrict their communication abilities. They form a vulnerable group and the efforts made, and time devoted, to establish trust and rapport were critical to the success of the project. Some of the techniques used to collect data were more fruitful than others and details of each technique employed are outlined below.

Participant observation

Participant observation was the most valuable data collection method with this group of patient participants, because it:

- facilitated the development of relationships/familiarity of the group with the researchers
- facilitated the collection of other data, e.g. photographic, counting, conduct of formal or informal interviews
- was the most useful method in overcoming communication difficulties.

It aided in building rapport with staff participants because:

- they were able to get to know the researchers in informal circumstances
- they recognised the efforts of the researchers to be unobtrusive
- they could see that the actual life within the house was valued in an holistic way.

Informal open-ended interviews

This was a useful method for this patient group but, because of limited concentration span and other constraints, it needed to be used flexibly, with attention paid to the non-verbal signals of interviewees that indicated tiredness, distraction, etc. Sometimes it was possible to explore only one question or theme per visit. However, this technique combined well with participant observation.

Open-ended 'chats', fitted in between work or conducted while simple chores were jointly engaged in, allowed the researchers to respect the busy lives of the staff and identified issues of salience before formal interviews. Similarly, staff were able to raise as illustration, during these activities, recent events that related to points made in the formal interviews.

Action research to improve services

331

Managing knowledge in health care

Table 12.1.1 Data collection techniques – benefits and drawbacks

Technique	Benefits	Drawbacks
Picture/flashcard prompts	Generated some interest amongst patients; had a novelty value related to introducing something new into the house	Interest in the different tools was not sustained for long periods
	Stimulated some discussions with some patients; one patient was especially interested to look at prints	Communication difficulties remained a barrier for this method
Diary records	Useful tool for this project, where researchers were only able to attend the house for limited periods at a time	Offers a snapshot in time only, which may or may not be representative
	Highlight areas for further consideration, e.g. heavy reliance on hospital-based activities for some patients, limited participation in chores, reduced activity options for some patients at weekends	Relies on staff observation of patients' activities
		Does not give an accurate record of the amount of time spent on activities
Community profiles	Elicited additional qualitative data in several cases, including description of experiences, preferences and reasons why certain venues were/were not used	Patients appeared to experience difficulty in reflecting back over a specific time period; comparisons of past with present use of community venues may therefore be inaccurate

Table 12.1.1 *(contd)*

Simple format
Flexible, could be adapted to patient capacity/
need; could be done in stages
Useful as: method to engage patients; prompt
to further discussion regarding use of venues
and facilities outside the ward/house; vehicle
to collect additional qualitative data
Appropriate for use with the majority of
participating patients

staff found it difficult to isolate specifics for
individual patients, tending to view them as a
whole group. However, they were able to add
some venues not included by the patients

Large group interviews with staff

It was difficult to implement large group interviews given how this service, and those like it, operate. Care and safety issues related to patients have to take precedence over research meetings.

Formal interviews with staff

These were held in private in a quiet area because it had been apparent during the informal interviews that the staff were continuously observing the patients and would, therefore, have their attention divided during the interview.

Picture prompts, diary records, community profiles

The benefits and drawbacks of these data collection techniques are outlined in Table 12.1.1.

Photography

Patients were asked to participate in creating a photographic record of aspects of community life and home life. Two patients volunteered and were provided with disposable cameras and instruction on how to use them. One later returned the camera, saying he had changed his mind. The second continued to appear keen but ultimately did not carry out the task.

Multimethod approach

One problem that arose from using this approach and this combination of methods was that the resulting data were substantially greater in volume, and richer, than had been anticipated for a pilot study. A great deal more time was therefore required for data analysis and discussion of results than had been initially expected. This should be borne in mind when designing and costing future research. In this case, the researchers gave up personal time to the project but such generosity should not become the expected norm.

Other results

It is not the purpose of this study to provide details of the results, rather it is to illustrate the process of research in action. However, it is worth mentioning that the participants were enabled to identify, and draw heart from, the successes they had achieved. They were

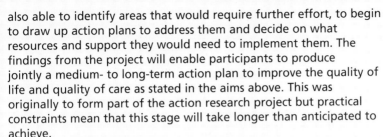

also able to identify areas that would require further effort, to begin to draw up action plans to address them and decide on what resources and support they would need to implement them. The findings from the project will enable participants to produce jointly a medium- to long-term action plan to improve the quality of life and quality of care as stated in the aims above. This was originally to form part of the action research project but practical constraints mean that this stage will take longer than anticipated to achieve.

It is notable that some diverse understandings of policy and procedure were clarified and communication channels improved. It was recognised that tradition can sometimes be an insidious anaesthetic to change, both the staff and patients needing to challenge their reliance on institutionalised patterns of behaviour. In contrast, each participant found that being empowered to make decisions about life and work style can motivate transformation, while peripheral informants were provided with new perspectives on life and work in the house which enabled them to provide an improved service.

Readers who would like further information on the project and its results should contact the author by email: p.m.denicolo@reading.ac.uk.

POINTS FOR REFLECTION

Before undertaking such action research, it is important to consider whether enough time can be set aside for all participants to engage in the process. This is an important resource issue because the quality of output is dependent on quality of input. Similarly the preliminary period when trust is developed and ideas exchanged should not be underestimated. The use of facilitators, as the researchers were in this project, can help to overcome problems and facilitate honest and focused reflection but it does usually mean an additional financial outlay. Finally, everyone engaged in action research should recognise that flexibility is a key concept. This includes being adaptable to changes in the process of the research as unexpected issues arise and being open to the challenge of new ideas and alternative understandings.

Acknowledgement

The author of this text represents the Research Team which included Ann Harwood, Susanna Yeomans, the Steering Committee and, most importantly, the patients and staff of the 24-hour nursed care home.

Action research to improve services

Six Steps to **Effective Management**

References

Denicolo PM, Pope ML 2001 Transformative professional practice. Whurr, London

Stringer E 1996 Action research: a handbook for practitioners. Sage, Thousand Oaks, California

Action research to improve services

Section **Five**

OLD PROBLEMS, NEW SOLUTIONS

OVERVIEW

In the final section of the book suggestions are offered to provide new solutions for change. Throughout the book the issues of managing change, changing attitudes and shifting the culture in health care have been addressed in a variety of ways. Two very important and significant aspects are raised in these final chapters: one of quality and the other the creative potential in health care.

Ben Thomas and Chris Flood discuss quality, but take a creative approach. Quality has to become an integral part of a coherent system that continuously involves the whole organisation in planning, delivering and evaluating quality health care. All kinds of systems have been put in place to monitor and measure outcomes of quality. Ben and Chris argue that there is a need to move away from an approach that merely prevents failing services to one that encourages development, innovation and excellence. Again the issue of local ownership is seen as essential, as is the need for staff and users to be involved to shape their own local services. However, as staff strive for uniformity to conform to government standards there is a danger that this will only become the norm. Ben and Chris encourage an approach that reaches for the optimum, one that requires individual initiative, vision, enthusiasm and determination. Application 13.1 by Thoreya Swage gives an illustration of quality, using integrated pathways in providing patient-centred care.

The last theory chapter by John Turnbull tackles the concept of creativity and examines how the workforce can be helped to realise their potential. Future trends in the organisation of health care are discussed as a way of setting the scene and some key steps are identified to transform relationships and promote creativity. The drive to improve the capacity to expand creative thinking can to some extent be achieved through a systemic view of organisations which frees people to think outside their buildings and organisations and to question assumptions. But John argues that there is a further approach which has the potential to improve the quality of thinking in an organisation. This he describes as 'time to think' (Kline 1999). John develops this approach in Application 14.1 in which he relates his experience of an NHS Trust board that set out to promote the value of partnership working and person centredness in its organisation. A key component was to improve the quality of thinking amongst staff in the Trust, with the intention of providing better quality services for users and more equitable relationships between staff in the Trust. It is a personal account based on John's reflections of the process.

Reference

Kline N 1999 Time to think. Listening to ignite the human mind. Ward Lock, London

Old problems, new solutions

Chapter Thirteen

Creative solutions to the issue of quality improvement in the NHS

Ben Thomas and Chris Flood

- Traditional approaches to evaluating quality in health care
- Definitions: quality assurance, continuous quality improvement and total quality management
- Clinical governance and the National Service Frameworks

- Local initiatives
- Raising quality
- User and carer involvement
- Performance monitoring and outcome measurement
- Professional quality

OVERVIEW

This chapter aims to introduce readers to the traditional approaches of evaluating and improving the quality of health care in the NHS. These include quality assurance programmes, quality accreditation, total quality management and continuous quality improvement. The chapter examines the various definitions of quality and acknowledges that often people's understanding of the terms differ. The introduction of many quality initiatives is critically analysed and some of the reasons why they have to meet expectations identified. There is no doubt that the determination to improve and measure quality in the NHS continues. The present Labour government proclaims that every part of the NHS and every member of staff must take responsibility for improving quality.

The government defines quality in its broadest sense: doing the right things, at the right time, for the right people and getting things right first time. They are not purely interested in clinical results but also in the quality of the patient's experience. The government proposes that quality be measured in terms of prompt access, good relationships and efficient administration. The current drive for quality is addressed in detail, including the new system of clinical governance, the National Institute for Clinical Excellence (NICE), the Commission for Health Improvement (CHI) and the new National Service Frameworks (NSF). The chapter concludes by identifying three areas that need to be addressed if the delivery of high quality care is to become a reality and suggests that there needs to be a move away from approaches that merely prevent services from failing, to one that encourages development, innovation and excellence.

WHAT IS QUALITY IN HEALTH CARE?

Quality is a fundamental concept in health care and much has been written both about its importance and its use strategically to improve services within the NHS. The present government has set out detailed plans for a new focus on quality in their White Paper *A First Class Service: Quality in the NHS* (DoH 1998) and which has been reinforced in *The NHS Plan* (DoH 2000a). They aim to develop a National Health Service that strives continuously to improve the overall standard of clinical care, to reduce unacceptable variations in practice and to ensure that patient care is based on the most up-to-date evidence and what is known to be effective. In a nutshell, the NHS will continuously improve its efficiency, productivity and performance.

However, definitions and interpretations of quality vary according to societal and professional values and the meanings people attach to the terms. Ovretveit (1998) suggests that quality is political, and apparently various professions have used objective definitions of quality to advance their own interests. Detailed explication of quality in health care can be found in Marr & Giebing (1994) and Stricker & Rodriguez (1988). For the purposes of this chapter, no particular single definition of quality has been chosen, although those definitions and frameworks that are service-user focused are favoured. Maxwell (1984) suggests that quality health care includes the following dimensions:

- access to services
- relevance (to need for the whole community)

- effectiveness (for individual patients)
- equity (fairness)
- social acceptability
- efficiency and economy.

The discourse around quality is explained by Charles Shaw in his brief history of quality management in the UK (Shaw 1993). Quality gained its popularity because of promises to resolve a number of problems that trouble the modern NHS. In addition to ensuring professional responsibility for clinical competence, it recognised patients as customers and the appointment of senior managers with the specific remit for quality in service delivery. Undoubtedly the debate about quality and its potency to bring about change will continue. In the meantime it is incumbent on all of us to stand by our principles and ensure service users and carers are at the forefront of such an important debate.

TERMS COMMONLY USED

Despite the multiple definitions of quality that now exist, there is a common vocabulary which has grown over the past 10 years and which provides some joint understanding.

Quality assurance (QA)

QA is a popular term which covers all the activities and systems for assessing and improving quality. Ovretveit (1998) suggests that quality assurance not only involves measuring and evaluating quality but also covers other activities to prevent poor quality and ensure high standards. Within the NHS there are numerous ways of assessing and monitoring professional practice, including risk management and service accreditation. However, clinical audit seems the most popular method of evaluating care. Standards and criteria are set to give a baseline measurement against which actual quality can be measured. Marr & Giebing (1994) suggest that as quality systems have developed within the NHS, the complex dynamic nature of quality and its assessment, together with the inability to guarantee excellence, have led to a move towards quality improvement systems and away from quality assurance. In fact some would go as far as to say that assurance is impossible and improvement is a more accurate and realistic description of what goes on in health care.

Continuous quality improvement (CQI)

CQI is an organisation-wide approach, which attempts to improve quality by addressing the attitude, approach and processes within an organisation. The basic principle of CQI is that the workforce can only be as good as the organisation allows them to be. The CQI paradigm maintains that most quality problems are not caused by employees' lack of effort but by the way the work is organised. Upgrading the work system is therefore more productive than creating procedures to catch a few employees who are not trying to do their best. The saying often heard is that CQI is about growing better apples rather than weeding out the bad ones (Bull 1992).

However, there have been difficulties in implementing this approach. Hutchins (1990) argues that in state-owned organisations such as hospitals and trusts, the characteristics associated with a mechanistic way of working are often displayed. These include:

- lack of clear leadership from the top
- spirit of departmental working rather than company mindedness
- low morale and significant levels of demarcation
- managers who are defensive, aggressive and operate a 'blame culture'
- 'blame culture' extends downwards right through the organisation.

It is no wonder that organisations which have experienced this type of culture for decades find it difficult to change to a continuous quality improvement environment.

Total quality management (TQM)

Koch (1992) defines TQM in the NHS as an approach that strives to achieve several benefits including good and better services, delighted customers, satisfied staff, staff working well across agencies and reduced operating costs. TQM therefore involves the interweaving of culture, teamwork and techniques.

TQM was yet another approach developed in the manufacturing services and transferred to the NHS. The process is management led and has three essential elements: employees, the work system and customer results. It is based on the following principles:

- continuous quality improvement
- customer satisfaction

● continuous and relentless cost reduction
● all staff working together for a common purpose.

For TQM to succeed in the NHS, line managers, clinicians and support staff must be committed and take responsibility for its implementation – a tall order considering the inherent conflict between
managers and professionals, status-consciousness of different clinical groups, specialism-mindedness and the different cultures
which operate in most hospitals and trusts. TQM required breaking
new ground and completely changing old ways of working and
relating. It also meant an enormous outlay on education and training which was rarely forthcoming. Finally, although the intention
was to put the service user first and to treat their needs as paramount, for the most part these remained an aspiration rather than
a practical reality.

PROBLEMS PREVIOUSLY ASSOCIATED WITH THE QUALITY MOVEMENT

There is no doubt that quality assurance has had a widespread
influence on service delivery throughout the NHS. Its promotion is
evident by the increasing number of books, articles and policy documents aimed at making quality integral to every organisation and
the core of every health professional's business. Despite quality
assurance being enthusiastically embraced by many health professionals, others continue to view it cynically, believing it has been
forced upon an unwilling, over-burdened health community. Like
many other reforms it has had very little effect on what is happening on the ground. For example, it is widely recognised that older
people are the main users of health services. However, care and
treatment for this particular group often fall short of the ideal. Not
only do services sometimes fail to meet their needs but scandals of
ill-treatment of patients continue to exist (Camden & Islington
Community Health Services NHS Trust 1998)

The following quotes are taken from an independent inquiry
(Health Advisory Service 2000, p. 6) into the care of older people on
acute wards in general hospitals:

> It was not unusual to find her lying in wet bedding, or sitting in a
> chair without even a blanket over her. The excuse given was that
> the laundry did not arrive until the afternoon and all clean supplies
> had been used.

> Her toe nails had not been cut for weeks. They were horrendous
> and hurt. Nurses were asked to cut them, but didn't do so.

Creative solutions in quality improvement

Without being too negative about the concept of quality assurance it is certainly the case that long after its introduction, services across the country still do not meet the high standard of quality care expected. Reports of service inadequacies and failures are only too common (Health Service Ombudsman for England 2001). The focus of many complaints investigated by the Health Service Ombudsman remains on essential aspects of nursing care including insufficient attention to patient nutrition, hydration and bladder and bowel care. The continual highlighting of failures in standards of care inevitably begs the question: Why have measures taken so far to assure and improve the quality of care not always worked? The following section explores some of the reasons why quality assurance initiatives may have failed.

IMPOSED NOT OWNED

Like the introduction of any type of change or innovation, quality assurance initiatives are most likely to succeed if planned, organised and 'owned' by the staff. However, historically there has been a tendency for some staff to see quality initiatives imposed from above, as just one more short-lived management strategy which will have little or no bearing on their day-to-day work. Similarly some staff may have been inclined to take the view that some quality assurance activities had little or nothing to do with improving the standard of the service but were form-filling exercises and nit-picking excursions to control costs (Byalin 1992).

There is also the belief held by many staff that the NHS is constantly being changed and reorganised and that quality assurance is just another new idea which, given time, would fade away. The lukewarm reception given to the Department of Health's publication *Essence of Care* (DoH 2001a) by some staff is typical of this kind of attitude. Rather than make use of the evidence-based benchmarks provided in *Essence of Care* to improve clinical practice, many staff take a defensive stance, proclaiming that the benchmarks only describe care as already provided by them.

FAILURE TO INCLUDE SERVICE USERS

If staff did not feel involved in the decision-making processes around quality assurance initiatives and held such cynical viewpoints there was certainly little evidence of involving service users in the exercise. The last decade has seen a growing awareness on the part of managers and professionals to listen and respond to the views of service users, primarily through formal complaints procedures and patient satisfaction surveys. Such processes have begun to give service users and carers a voice in the standard of care that is provided. However, these are not enough and service users still regard many NHS services as lacking in quality. They suggest that quality could be radically improved by genuinely involving service users in planning new services, policy formulation, training professionals, educating the public and providing advocacy (Beeforth et al 1990).

Rose et al (1998) provide an example of the type of genuine involvement required. Their report describes a set of interviews with people with severe and enduring mental health problems. The interviews were carried out by eight other local service users who had been trained and supported throughout the work. As a result of the feedback, services have begun to change in line with the users' views expressed. The work clearly shows that service users can have a voice in decisions about the health care they receive.

LITTLE PREPARATION, POOR SELECTION AND TRAINING

Quality improvement necessitates an organisational culture committed to providing high quality services. It also requires the identification of those areas which need to change or improve. Failing to select the right opportunities for improvement often leads to discouragement and disillusionment. The best opportunities are those that motivate managers, staff and service users towards change. Change is more likely to take place if a staff and service user consensus is reached on the problems that should be tackled. Previously quality endeavours may have failed due to poor selection, prioritisation and/or timing. Selecting topics linked to organisational priorities which are of the right size in terms of time and resources available is crucially important. Projects that are viewed as either too trivial or unmanageable within the available resources will lead to failure. If a project is too trivial or does not fit in with the organisational priorities, commitment and enthusiasm from staff will not be forthcoming.

Complex changes can also be accompanied by practical difficulties, such as consensus, evaluation and measurement, especially when examining complex issues such as standards and quality of care. For example, despite the widespread adoption of quality assurance programmes in the 1980s there is very little empirical

Creative solutions in quality improvement

data formally evaluating these programmes. In a literature review Wells & Brook (1988) found only one study that evaluated the effectiveness of quality assurance activities in mental health care using a control group and a prospective design.

Previously there has been a tendency for the process of quality assurance to be overvalued with the result that it becomes an end in itself. Much activity around quality initiatives has meant simplistic counting rather than data being analysed and synthesised to reveal underlying lessons (DoH 2000a). Many quality endeavours have fallen foul of this in the past, especially where there has been little professional consensus as to what constitutes good practice and treatment, a clear idea of the organisation's vision for change and a sharing of fundamental values. Where there is lack of clarity and consensus of a firm value base quality improvement initiatives invariably become stuck. Many health organisations allegedly value the promotion of independence, choice and inclusion of service users. Nowhere is this of greater importance than for people with learning disabilities. However, numerous reports continue to show that even with this government's drive to social inclusion many NHS services fail to provide flexible, individually tailored care, leaving many people with learning disabilities with little choice or control over their lives (DoH 1999a).

A NEW COMMITMENT TO QUALITY

Quality assurance initiatives over the past decade have been piecemeal, unpredictable and variable. In a way it is reassuring that current government policy is focused and full of the rhetoric of quality care. *A First Class Service: Quality in the New NHS* (DoH 1998) sets out a vision for a modernised health service with quality at its heart. The government argues that without guaranteed quality, there is unacceptable variation in health care provision, which will result in inequality. The policy makers argue that every patient who is treated in the NHS wants to be assured of receiving high quality care, when and where this is needed. Every part of the NHS, and everyone who works within it, should take responsibility for working to improve quality.

This all sounds very familiar, so why should the public believe that quality care will materialise under the present government when previous attempts have often failed? Already the old arguments are appearing. Policies and performance indicators are being imposed top down; they are far removed from the pressures and reality of day-to-day work where staff bear the brunt of continual reorganisation and overwhelming change. However, the government argues that its drive to ensure excellence in health care will transpire because it recognises that continuous improvement is a long haul, not a quick fix, and for the first time there will be focused targeted action on service improvement directed at a national level (DoH 1998).

The government's agenda to drive up quality and reduce unacceptable variations in health services depends on three main strands (Fig. 13.1):

● Standards across the NHS will be set by the newly formed National Institute for Clinical Excellence and National Service Frameworks
● The standards will be delivered through clinical governance, underpinned by self-regulation and lifelong learning
● The standards will be monitored by the Commission for Health Improvement and new National Framework for Assessing Performance and the National Patient and User Survey.

By now most staff in the NHS will be familiar with these concepts. However, their importance and centrality to the improvement of quality improvement calls for a brief description.

The National Institute for Clinical Excellence

The National Institute for Clinical Excellence (NICE) was set up as a special health authority in 1999 and is intended to provide the

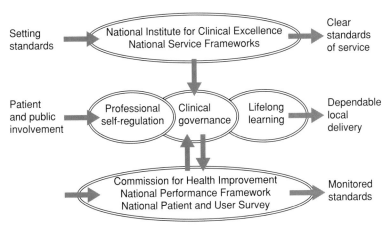

Figure 13.1 Setting, delivering and monitoring standards (reproduced with permission from DoH 1998)

347

NHS with authoritative, robust and reliable guidance on current 'best practice'. The three types of guidance provided by NICE are:

- the results of appraisals of new and existing health technologies
- clinical guidelines for the management of specific conditions
- simple methods of clinical audit (these will support both the Institute's guidance on the use of individual technologies and on adoption of clinical guidelines).

Since the Institute's work has the status of guidance it is crucial that what it does is recognised by service users, clinicians and managers as directly relevant and useful to direct care. Within its limited resource it is also important that its guidelines are those agreed as the most needed and which have the greatest benefit.

National Service Frameworks

National Service Frameworks (NSFs) provide the NHS with explicit standards of care and principles for the pattern, model and level of services required for specific client groups (e.g. mental health, coronary heart disease and older people). The aim of NSFs is to reduce unacceptable variations in the care and standard of treatment, using evidence-based practice and cost-effectiveness.

Each NSF sets out where care is best provided and the standard of care service users should be offered in each setting. Each Framework is developed with the help of an expert reference group bringing together the views of professionals, service users, carers, managers and other relevant groups. NSFs will also have supporting programmes including workforce planning, education and training and information development.

Built into the NSFs are performance measures against which their introduction and progress is measured. The measures are monitored through the new National Framework for Assessing Performance, the independent rolling programme of spot checks by the Commission for Health Improvement and its systematic reviews and the National Patient and User Survey.

Clinical governance

Clinical governance is a key part of concerted 10-year programme of work throughout the NHS to improve the quality of patient care. Clinical governance is defined as a framework through which NHS organisations are accountable for improving the quality of their services and safeguarding high standards of care by creating an

Old problems, new solutions

environment in which excellence in clinical care will flourish (DoH 1998).

The development of the principle of clinical governance is inextricably linked to keeping quality at the centre of health care provision. At a local level this means bringing together all current activities for assessing, monitoring and improving quality into a single coherent programme. Where necessary it also involves changing organisational culture in a systematic way, moving away from a culture of 'blame' to one of open learning where staff continually expand their capacity to deliver a quality service.

Much of the detail of clinical governance arrangements has been left to local implementation. However, there are a number of core steps which every NHS organisation should undertake:

- Identification of a senior clinician to lead the process
- Setting up a clinical governance committee with professional and service user representation
- Baseline assessment of the strengths and weaknesses of the organisation
- Using the information gathered in developing a plan to introduce clinical governance and clinical audit to bring about improvement
- Developing ways of collecting information and monitoring changes
- Linking clinical governance plans to research and development, lifelong learning and personal and organisational development
- Providing regular progress reports to the organisation's board and producing annual reports.

Commission for Health Improvement

The Commission for Health Improvement (CHI) is an independent body. It is part of the government's programme to modernise the NHS with the remit of raising the quality of care and reducing unacceptable variations in standards of care. To achieve its aims the CHI will visit every NHS organisation and undertake clinical governance reviews on a rolling programme every 4 years, including providing feedback into the National Service Frameworks.

The CHI is meant to provide independent reassurance to service users that effective systems are in place to deliver high quality care throughout the NHS. It also has a supportive role for NHS organisations who need to urgently resolve particularly difficult problems.

Over the next 4 years the CHI intends to visit and assess clinical governance arrangements in 500 NHS organisations in England

Creative solutions in quality improvement

and Wales. Already the impact of their visits and hard-hitting reports are being felt throughout the NHS and are brought to the attention of the public through media interest.

MAKING IT HAPPEN

Time and time again it has been emphasised that successful implementation of clinical governance and quality improvement throughout the NHS depends on the commitment of the workforce and the development of a culture that fosters learning. However, not only do organisations need to develop the capacity to measure and analyse quality but they also need to encourage experimentation, risk-taking, change, empowerment and teamwork (Elliott 1994). How such a culture would sit alongside the principles of clinical governance remains to be seen. Clinical governance may well reduce variation in practice, improve quality and promote evidence-based practice. However, in the government's drive to standardise the health care system, organisations need to take care that individual initiative, creativity and inquiry are not stifled. Similarly, that the bureaucracy involved and the techniques of surveillance and monitoring are not counterproductive in terms of clinical staff's commitment and internal motivation, with increased costs and time not spent on direct patient care (Lugon & Secker-Walker 1999).

Although the drive to improve the quality of health care services is widely welcomed, the government's new initiatives are not without their critics. Godfrey (1997) argues that it is questionable whether a clinical effectiveness approach takes account of the perspective of patients other than to seek their level of satisfaction with the extent to which services achieve goals set by professionals. What is often perceived by staff as quality health care and how best to evaluate it may be quite different from the views of service users. Brooker & Dinshaw (1998) found that generally patients were more positive about the physical environment and standards of professional care than staff, but less positive about issues of privacy, social interaction and empowerment.

Despite the rhetoric about providing services that are responsive to patients' needs, the reality is often insufficient and inflexible service provision. Sometimes this is due to lack of resources but often it is due to the traditional viewpoint that the 'professional knows best'. For example, the debate around the extent of mental health care that should be provided at primary care level continues, mainly between general practitioners and psychiatrists. However, patients care little about who does what. Their principal concern is that somebody will respond appropriately and as quickly as possible to their needs at the time, preferably someone with the appropriate skills, knowledge and attitude.

RAISING THE QUALITY OF HEALTH CARE

If high quality health care is to become a reality, then a number of deficits must be addressed and the various quality assurance threads brought together into a fully functioning system. The government's vision for successful implementation of an integrated programme of quality improvement (DoH 2001c, p. 6) can be summarised as follows:

- Patient-centred care is at the heart of every organisation
- Variation in process, in outcome and in access to health care (where not in patients' interest) are greatly reduced
- Health organisations continuously assure and improve quality of their services
- The quality programme enhances the achievement of the goals of major clinical programmes
- Teams of health professionals practise safely, to a consistently high standard and develop and improve, in both primary and secondary care
- Risks and hazards to patients are reduced to as low a level as currently possible
- Emerging problems are identified at an early stage and appropriate action taken
- Good practice and research evidence are systematically adopted (where prioritised for implementation)
- Information systems are in place which, with other underpinning strategies (such as human resources), contribute effectively to the quality programme and improved quality care.

The reforms proposed by the present government go some way to addressing the variation in performance and improving the quality of service for patients. However, the following section provides examples of three areas that need to be successfully implemented if the high quality health care promised by the government is to become a reality. As stated previously, service user and carer involvement is fundamental to high quality health care. The focus on outcome measures and performance measuring also presents a challenge to clinicians and managers and all of these are intricately linked to the recruitment of sufficient high-calibre staff.

Creative solutions in quality improvement

Strong user and carer involvement

The role of service users and carers in promoting quality is central to improving health services. The government recognised the need for active participation and partnership of patients throughout the NHS in its document *A First Class Service: Quality in the New NHS* (DoH 1998). However, despite many organisations and care staff actively involving service users, their involvement and participation is not happening universally across the NHS. Paternalistic attitudes and behaviour still prevail and many organisations have a long way to go to make services truly patient centred. *Valuing People* (DoH 2001b) shows how users and carers are not informed or supported so that they can be empowered to be involved in decision making and make choices about the care and treatment they receive.

As part of a quality and audit programme the views of services users need to be sought through questionnaires, interviews and participation in routine monitoring. The government's introduction of the National Patient and User Survey goes some way to meeting this need. However, the problems with simply surveying people's opinions have been well documented. A recent inquiry commissioned by the secretary of state for health into the care of older people on acute wards in general hospitals identified the following problems with self-completed questionnaires:

> It is notoriously difficult to obtain valid, 'uncontaminated' reports from patients regarding their satisfaction with care. Measures of satisfaction depend very much on what questions are asked, who asks them and how. Satisfaction with care also reflects individual expectations and, if patients (and relatives) have very low expectations, then it is easy to confuse high levels of satisfaction with good quality care. (Health Advisory Service 2000, p. 9)

The involvement of service users is a complex process and often calls for creativity and new ways of working. Following the publication of the National Service Framework for Mental Health (DoH 1999b), with its emphasis on the involvement of service users and their carers in the planning and delivery of care, the NHS Executive South West funded a short course at the University of Plymouth. The course is part of a wider development programme to explore models of carer and user involvement. The impact of the course is being evaluated independently of the teaching team but as a condition of accepting a place, participants are expected to be involved in the evaluation and to be interviewed at the beginning, during and after the course.

The course organisers recognised that previous attempts to involve service users and carers have often been perceived from within the user movement as tokenistic. The interprofessional module aims to help health and social care staff, service users and carers learn from each other and develop more genuine participation for all. In addition to examining the development and politics of user involvement and survivors groups, the module includes work on advocacy and empowerment, social exclusion, dependency, autonomy and responsibility, 'normalising' services, employment issues and rights.

The course is interprofessional, intended not only for anyone involved in mental health care with the relevant academic prerequisites, but also for service users and carers who are especially welcome. For professionals the course may be undertaken at either degree or diploma level, depending on the academic background of the participant. Participants in the course will be expected to demonstrate a commitment to extending user and carer involvement in mental health care, to the continuing improvement in mental health care and the quality of local services.

Participants completing the course will be able to:

- participate in the development of user-centred services
- incorporate user perspectives to improve the quality of mental health services
- demonstrate the development of relationship and therapeutic skills
- work collaboratively with users, carers and a range of professional groups.

The course consists of a 10-day programme and covers the areas outlined in Box 13.1. Teaching and learning methods include lectures, discussions, student-led seminars, workshops, facilitated reflection on practice and learning sets. Personal revelation and preparedness to share uncomfortable feelings are a key aspect of some elements of the course.

The premise for the programme is 'the notion that participants will undertake real health improvement projects using continuous quality improvement techniques'. Throughout the course, participants are encouraged to seek solutions to local needs and problems.

One local area in which it proved particularly difficult to involve service users and carers was that of children and adolescents with mental health problems. To address this problem the health community worked in partnership to put on a series of evening consultation meetings with parents and carers in the first

Creative solutions in quality improvement

> **Box 13.1** User and carer involvement in mental health – course content
>
> - User involvement
> - Advocacy and empowerment
> - Prejudice, stigma, social exclusion and inclusion
> - The politics of user involvement
> - Power and control
> - Survivor groups, user groups and self-help groups
> - Service users' rights
> - Dependency, institutionalisation
> - and support versus dependence
> - Autonomy and responsibility
> - Employment
> - Relationships, boundaries
> - Confidentiality, information and access
> - User groups
> - Service users as workers and professional 'coming out'

instance. The meetings covered major disorders for this particular group, the available treatment and descriptions of the services provided. Following the presentations parents and carers had ample opportunity to ask questions, voice their concerns and offer alternative ideas and approaches. The meetings were held at local venues across the county, kept as informal as possible and free refreshments were served. The presentations included self harm, eating disorders, autism, Asperger's syndrome, behavioural/conduct disorders and attention deficit hyperactivity disorders. Concerns raised included poor communication, long waiting lists and lack of resources.

Performance monitoring and outcome measurement

Shaw (1997) suggests that health care outcomes are slippery concepts that challenge definition and measurement. Despite a decade of standard setting and the improvement of monitoring systems, little headway has been made with the regular linking of clinical practice and outcomes. Barrell et al (1997) identify a general lack of outcome evaluations and point out that many clinical specialists have not yet incorporated formal outcome evaluations in their day-to-day practice.

The government recognises that the routine data currently collected are not accurate or perfect. Nevertheless it has developed clinical indicators based on existing information with a view to their improvement as new systems develop. The past few years have seen a proliferation of performance indicators including *Quality and Performance in the NHS: Clinical Indicators* (DoH 1999c) and *Quality and Performance in the NHS: High Level Performance Indicators* (DoH 1999d).

Each of the 41 high level performance indicators is meant to demonstrate changes in performance within the NHS. The most publicised indicator is that of hospital waiting times but others include deaths following surgery and emergency psychiatric re-admission rates. Indicators are meant to show performance at the wider level including finance and efficiency within the NHS. However, at a more practical level, a set of clinical indicators has been developed to allow the study of quality and outcome of 'real' health care and cover:

- deaths in hospital following surgery
- deaths in hospital following a fractured hip
- deaths in hospital following a heart attack
- readmission to hospital following discharge
- returning home following treatment for a stroke
- returning home following treatment for a fractured hip.

The indicators are meant to serve a number of purposes including the comparison of performance between trusts and health authorities, raising standards of care, charting improvements and informing the public about how local health services are performing. There is no doubt that clinical indicators give a more balanced picture of performance. However, as the government emphasises, the indicators should not be seen as a direct measure of quality but rather should be used to raise questions about patient care and prompt further investigation. For example national implementation of easy-to-measure indicators is a welcome initiative in attempting to improve performance in the NHS. However, indicators such as emergency psychiatric readmission rates are by no means simple and, as Lyons et al (1997) point out, their use may well have untoward consequences, particularly if the indicators are used to influence service reconfiguration and the reallocation of resources.

Whether or not measurement of the clinical indicators will provide the information needed to raise standards and meet the government's determination to deliver high quality care remains to be seen. There is a danger that like other indicators attention will be focused on the process rather than the outcome and unless feedback to staff is given high priority the process may be seen as a means of control rather than a means of communication. Many staff still view any type of monitoring in the NHS not only as data gathering to measure progress but also as an element of control by the Department of Health (Doll 1973). Current indicators are also limited in that they measure outcomes of past actions, which may result in organisations inevitably rectifying current problems and improving short-term performance. Unfortunately, this may be at the expense of future performance and long-term value. By basing the future on current problems means we are stuck with what currently exists, rather than thinking imaginatively about how things could be provided differently.

In an attempt to transcend the narrow management concerns of activity and finance Somerset Health Authority in collaboration with Somerset Partnership NHS and Social Care Trust has adopted the 'balanced score card' approach as developed by Kaplan & Norton (1996) which captures not only a broad range of performance objectives but also engages clinical staff, service users and carers. The balanced score card is represented graphically in Figure 13.2.

Each element contains objectives and measures used in the performance management process. The model can be used at different levels within the organisation to capture both an organisation-wide strategy and locally at unit or team level.

Professional quality

If quality care in the NHS is to become a reality, recruitment and retention of high calibre staff must be addressed. Staff shortages across the NHS has been a growing problem for a number of years (Thomas 1998). These shortages have major implications not only in terms of the quality of services provided but in some instances have resulted in ward closure and reduction of service provision. The government recognises the seriousness of the problem and acknowledges that the biggest constraint currently facing the NHS is the shortage of human resources, particularly front-line staff including doctors, nurses and therapists (DoH 2000a).

Over the next 5 years the government has planned a massive increase in the number of clinical staff. These include:

- 7500 more consultants
- 2000 more GPs
- 20 000 nurses
- over 6500 more therapists and other health professionals.

Not only does the government plan to expand the workforce but it also plans to modernise education and training, improve work-

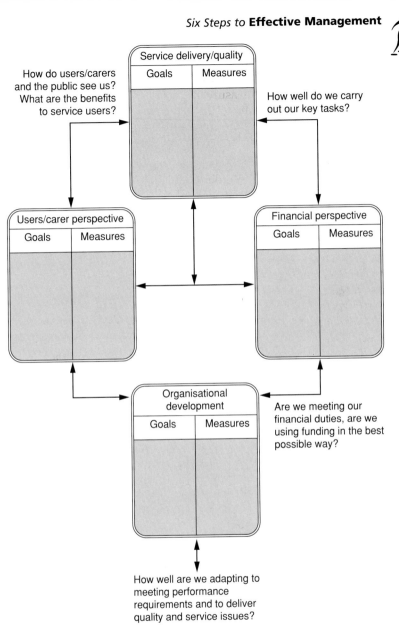

Figure 13.2 Balanced score card diagram

force planning and boost staff morale through more flexible careers and improved working lives. The government recognises that by improving the working lives of staff it will have a direct knock-on

Creative solutions in quality improvement

effect on the quality of patient care. Improved recruitment and retention means a more motivated and committed staff.

As with many of the new monitoring systems introduced, the government intends to measure the way NHS employers treat staff against performance targets and the new 'improving working lives' standard. The standard means that all NHS staff are entitled to belong to an organisation which can prove that it is:

- investing in their training and development
- tackling discrimination and harassment
- improving diversity
- applying a zero tolerance to violence against staff
- reducing workplace accidents
- reducing sick absences
- providing better occupational health and counselling services
- conducting annual attitude surveys and acting on key messages.

In return for this investment the government expects to see changes in the way staff work and the way the NHS is run and emphasises the need for reform in order to deliver a patient-centred service. For the first time it seems that much of the work around quality improvement is more systematic and balanced, i.e. the implementation of national standards and quality care is matched with workforce planning, education and training, service satisfaction, research and development and staff morale. However, the complexity of such an undertaking must not be underestimated and tensions in the system are inevitable. For example in mental health the national Workforce Action Team (2001) has identified the considerable gap between the demand for nurses and current supply. The Workforce Action Team (WAT) also recognises the time lag with recruitment and the implications that this will have on implementation of the NSF.

A positive outcome from the WAT report has been the national mapping exercise of all current education and training provision required to deliver the standards outlined in the NSF and the requirements of the NHS Plan. Some of the main findings include obvious gaps in the teaching of key skills and knowledge, a greater need to make better use of service users and their carers at all levels of education and training and a requirement to provide more opportunities for shared learning. Despite these deficits for the first time there is a national database of information regarding current training in mental health nursing which can inform workforce development confederations.

Old problems, new solutions

CONCLUSION

Since being introduced, quality assurance activities have developed at an uneven pace across the NHS. Despite nearly 20 years of quality initiatives, poor practice, inconsistency and inefficiency are evident in many NHS organisations, although there are numerous examples of excellent practice and quality care. A cursory look at the *NHS Beacons Learning Handbook* (DoH 2000b) provides real examples of organisations that are making improvement to the way health care is delivered, driving up standards and introducing innovative and effective ways of caring for patients.

The government is determined that there is uniformity and consistent high quality health care for all. There is a great deal to commend this approach to quality improvement, particularly the whole systems approach and the long-term haul rather than any quick fix solutions. However, time is ticking away and the new approach should be making its impact felt with clear signs that the health service is changing for the better.

It has been argued throughout the chapter that despite the government's commitment to influence the quality agenda, a centrally driven and controlled system may well fail to deliver the major changes expected. There has to be local ownership, interpretation and implementation to engage staff and to generate the enthusiasm and commitment required to bring about the improvements sought. The government acknowledges the importance of both staff and service user involvement in shaping services and bringing about change. The introduction of the National Patient and User Survey goes some way towards this goal. However, since so much importance is attached to active involvement of service users and carers there would have been great benefit from such measures being part of the National Framework for Assessing Performance.

As previously discussed many of these ideas are not new – the top-down approach was seen as one of the reasons quality assurance never lived up to its expectations in the 1980s. This time the unified approach may stand a better chance of succeeding because there is an expectation that professionals will realign themselves with service users. The majority of professionals are willing to work in partnership or at least engage and work alongside service users and carers to improve standards of care. Users and carers must be given opportunities to make sure local needs are effectively voiced. Professionals must ensure that, in the drive for uniformity, quality not only conforms to the standards set by the government but also

Creative solutions in quality improvement

that they continually strive for the optimum rather than settle for the norm. This will require individual initiative, vision, enthusiasm and determination, not just the ability to meet expectations.

References

Barrell LM, Merwin EI, Poster EC 1997 Patient outcomes used by advanced practice psychiatric nurses to evaluate effectiveness of practice. Archives of Psychiatric Nursing 11(4): 184–197

Beeforth M, Conlan E, Field V, Hoser B, Sayce L (eds) 1990 Whose service is it anyway? Users' views on co-ordinating community care. Research and Development for Psychiatry, London

Bull MJ 1992 Quality assurance: professional accountability via continuous quality improvement. In: Meisenheimer CG (ed) Improving quality: a guide to effective programs. Aspen, Gaithersburg, Maryland

Brooker DJR, Dinshaw CJ 1998 Staff and patient feedback in mental health services for older people. Quality in Health Care 7: 70–76

Byalin K 1992 The quality assurance dilemma in psychiatry: a sociological perspective. Community Mental Health Journal 28(5): 453–459

Camden and Islington Community Mental Health Services NHS Trust 1998 Beech House Inquiry: report of the internal inquiry relating to the treatment of patients residing at Beech House, St Pancras Hospital during the period March 1993–April 1996. Camden and Islington Community Mental Health Services NHS Trust, London

Department of Health 1998 A first class service: quality in the new NHS. Department of Health, London

Department of Health 1999a Facing the facts: services for people with learning disabilities – policy impact study of social care and health services. Department of Health, London

Department of Health 1999b National Service Framework for Mental Health: modern standards and service models. Department of Health, London

Department of Health 1999c Performance assessment framework: quality and performance in the NHS: clinical indicators. Department of Health, London

Department of Health 1999d Quality and performance in the NHS: high level performance indicators. Department of Health, London

Department of Health 2000a The NHS plan: a plan for investment, a plan for reform. Department of Health, London

Department of Health 2000b NHS Beacons learning handbook: spreading good practice across the NHS. Department of Health, London

Department of Health 2001a Essence of care: patient focused benchmarking for health care practitioners. Department of Health, London

Department of Health 2001b Valuing people: a new strategy for learning disability for the 21st century. Department of Health, London

Department of Health 2001c A commitment to quality: a quest for excellence. A statement on behalf of the government, the medical profession and the NHS. Department of Health, London

Doll R 1973 Nuffield Lecture, Monitoring the National Health Service. Proceedings of the Royal Society of Medicine 66(8): 729–740

Elliott RL 1994 Applying quality improvement principles and techniques in public mental health systems. Hospital and Community Psychiatry 45(5): 439–444

Godfrey M 1997 The user perspective on managing for health outcomes: the case of mental health. Health and Social Care in the Community 5(5): 325–332

Health Advisory Service 2000 Not because they are old. An independent inquiry into the care of older people in acute wards in general hospitals. Health Advisory Service, London

Health Service Ombudsman for England 2001 Annual report 2000. Stationery Office, London

Hutchins D 1990 In pursuit of quality, participative techniques for quality improvement. Pitman, London

Kaplan RS, Norton DP 1996 The balanced scorecard: translating strategy into action. Harvard Business School Press, Boston

Koch H 1992 Implementing and sustaining total quality management in health care. Longman, Harlow

Lugon M, Secker-Walker J 1999 Clinical governance: making it happen. Royal Society of Medicine, London

Lyons JS, O'Mahoney MT, Muiller SI et al 1997 Predicting readmission to the psychiatric hospital in a managed care environment: implications for quality indicators. American Journal of Psychiatry 154(3): 337–340

Marr H, Giebing H 1994 Quality assurance in nursing: concepts, methods and case studies. Campion Press, Edinburgh

Maxwell R 1984 Quality assessment in health. British Medical Journal 13: 31–34

Ovretveit J 1998 Evaluating health interventions. Open University Press, Buckingham

Rose D, Ford R, Lindley P, Gwaith L, KCW Mental Health Monitoring Users' Group 1998 In our experience: user-focused monitoring of mental health services in Kensington & Chelsea and Westminster Health Authority. The Sainsbury Centre for Mental Health, London

Shaw C 1993 Quality assurance in the UK. Quality Assurance in Health Care 5(2): 107–118

Shaw I 1997 Assessing quality in health care services: lessons from mental health nursing. Journal of Advanced Nursing 26: 758–764

Stricker G, Rodriguez AR 1988 Handbook of quality assurance in mental health. Plenum Press, New York

Thomas B 1998 Stressed staff: implications for staff selection. In: Hardy S, Carson J, Thomas B (eds) Occupational stress: personal and professional approaches. Stanley Thornes, Cheltenham

Wells K, Brook RH 1988 Historical trends in quality assurance for mental health services. In: Stricker G, Rodriguez AR (eds) Handbook of quality assurance in mental health. Plenum Press, New York

Workforce Action Team 2001 Unpublished document. Department of Health, London

Creative solutions in quality improvement

Application **13:1**
Thoreya Swage

Quality issues relating to integrated care pathways

Old problems, new solutions

As clinical care becomes more complex it is increasingly important to have a method or system by which the quality of the delivery of care can be assessed. The process needs to be flexible enough to be modified to allow the incorporation of new research evidence as this comes to light, to test the implementation of clinical guidance and to be amenable to audit. One tool that is capable of tackling this is integrated care pathways. In 1999 around 250 organisations in the NHS and independent sector were piloting the use of pathways or were fully implementing them in all kinds of medical, surgical and mental health specialties. Pathways are also being developed in the general practice setting.

WHAT ARE CARE PATHWAYS?

The concept came originally from the United States of America where critical paths were developed for charting the care patients received in the hospital setting and for assessing the clinical and cost effectiveness of various specific treatments or procedures. This was then introduced in the United Kingdom in 1989 as part of a resource management initiative undertaken by North West Thames Regional Health Authority and adapted for the NHS setting. Various names have been used to describe the tool, for example multidisciplinary pathways of care, protocols, integrated care pathways, critical care paths, anticipated recovery pathways and pathways of care. Nowadays, the term 'care pathways' is used.

DEFINITION OF A CARE PATHWAY

An integrated care pathway determines locally agreed, multidisciplinary practice, based on guidelines and evidence where available, for a specific patient/client group. It forms all or part of the clinical record, documents the care given and facilitates the evaluation of outcomes for continuous quality improvement. (National Pathways Association 1998)

Essentially care pathways are developed using the best available evidence and current clinical practice, including the use of guidelines, by the multiprofessional team that provides the care of the specific patient group identified. The pathway charts the various interventions made by different health professionals over a specific period of time. The process used in the development and refinement of care pathways is illustrated in Figure 13.1.1 (Swage 2000) and the use of care pathways in Box 13.1.1.

STEPS TO DEVELOP INTEGRATED CARE PATHWAYS

Selection of a topic area of practice

Selection of the topic area includes:

- common or costly conditions
- where there is a high level of interest amongst clinical staff
- variations in practice or national imperatives such as the National Service Frameworks (NSF) or NHS Plan (NHS Executive 2000).

These areas may have been identified in the clinical governance action plan of individual organisations.

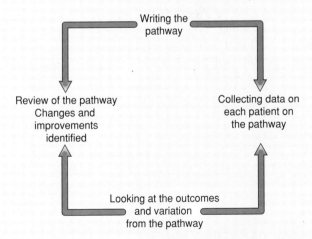

Figure 13.1.1 Development and refinement of care pathways (from Clinical Governance in Health Care Practice, Swage T 2000 reproduced with permission from Elsevier Science Ltd)

> **Box 13.1.1** Use of care pathways
>
> - Facilitate the introduction of guidelines and audit into clinical practice
> - Develop multidisciplinary methods of working, communication and planning of care
> - Achieve or exceed set quality standards
> - Reduce unwanted variation in clinical practice
> - Improve communication between clinicians and patients
> - Improve patient/carer satisfaction
> - Identify research and development questions
> - An aid for managing risk
> - Identification of training needs
> - A performance monitoring tool – outcomes
> - Implement evidence-based practice

Gain commitment to the project

As with the introduction of any new ideas, obtaining support is vital for the pathway to work effectively.

Review of current practice

This will begin the debate among the different professional groups that provide an input into the care of patients; a good method is through clinical audit.

Defining the multidisciplinary team

This is the multidisciplinary team who are involved in providing the care for the identified topic area. It is this team that will be responsible for developing and implementing the pathway.

Identifying the case type or client group

Once the topic area is selected, then agreement on the exact patient condition for which a pathway is to be developed should be reached (e.g. management of an acute myocardial infarction in A&E or diagnosis and treatment of asthma in primary care). To enhance the likelihood of success it is better to begin with a small, well-defined case type or client group.

Agreement of the time frame

This defines the beginning and the end of the pathway, for example a door-to-needle time for thrombolytic therapy would be minutes in timescale whereas a pathway for a total hip replacement would be admission to discharge, a period of days. Community pathways can be up to a year to reflect the chronic nature of some conditions (e.g. diabetes or management of depression).

Agreement of the goals or outcomes of care

These can be determined by the team or from nationally set standards (e.g. NSF). Outcomes can be categorised as clinical, managerial or administrative, for example ensuring that every patient has adequate postoperative pain relief; looking at the use of resources such as unnecessary treatments or duplication of effort by different clinical staff; is the right equipment available at the right time to treat patients requiring an emergency caesarian operation? Keeping the number of outcomes or goals low facilitates easier assessment of the effect of the pathway on the condition selected.

Putting together the pathway

Once the team has gone through the above steps it is time for the pathway to be written. The process is to identify, in a systematic way, the tasks or input each member of the team provides for a patient presenting with the condition selected and to determine the timescales in which each should be done. The essential method is to document what is actually done by the team members together with the standards the team has identified. At this point, national guidelines, such as those produced by the National Institute for Clinical Excellence, or critical appraisal of the research evidence can be helpful. The endpoint is a grid, on one sheet of paper, outlining the interventions that the team has identified in the agreed time frame.

Increasingly pathways are being developed with the input of patients and/or carers. As people have become more comfortable with the use of pathways, the documentation has become part of the patient's notes used by all the health professionals involved.

Training

To ensure that the use of the pathway is successful when it 'goes live' all the staff involved need to be trained on the appropriate use of the tool.

Piloting the pathway

It is helpful to 'test out' the pathway on a small sample of patients or for a short period of time (e.g. 3 or 6 months). This is to iron out possible inconsistencies and ensure that staff are confident in using the pathway.

Quality issues relating to integrated care pathways

Six Steps to **Effective Management**

Pathway implementation

The pathway can now be implemented. In the early stages there needs to be a close check to assess the level of recording of information on the pathway by the staff.

NOTING THE VARIATIONS FROM THE PATHWAY

Patients are different in their reactions to the treatments they receive. For the majority of patients the pathway will chart the expected course of treatment. However, there will be occasions when the course of a patient's treatment will not follow the pathway. This is normal and these variations can be classified as avoidable, unavoidable or a combination of both:

- Avoidable, e.g. a delay in instituting postoperative physiotherapy following orthopaedic surgery which may then delay discharge, resulting in a longer stay in hospital.
- Unavoidable, e.g. further clinical complications such as the development of an infection postoperatively.

It is important to note that variations to the pathway are to be expected and documenting these forms the basis of clinical audit. Reasons for variation from the pathway (Campbell et al 1998) are outlined in Box 13.1.2. Each pathway will have a variation sheet attached to it.

Assessing the variations that occur will provide a guide to the main issues that need to be examined. This corresponds to the review section of the audit cycle where the standards or outcomes that have been set are appropriate. Any changes that need to take place should then be incorporated into the next version of the pathway when it is next reviewed.

Box 13.1.2 Reasons for variation from the pathway

- Patient's clinical condition
- Patient's social circumstances
- Associated conditions
- Changing technology or techniques
- Clinician's decision not to follow the pathway
- Internal system: services or consultations from other departments within the organisation
- External system: services or consultations from social services or other health care sectors

FURTHER SUPPORT FOR CARE PATHWAY DEVELOPMENT

The National Pathways Association is a national organisation whose members have developed care pathways in a number of settings. Further details can be found on the web site
http://www.the-npa.org.uk

References

Campbell H, Hotchkiss R, Bradshaw N, Porteous M 1998 Integrated care pathways. British Medical Journal 316: 133–137

National Health Service Executive 2000 The NHS plan: a plan for investment, a plan for reform. NHS Executive, London

National Pathways Association 1998 Care pathways definition. Spring Newsletter. National Pathways Association, http://www.the-npa.org.uk

Swage T 2000 Clinical governance in health care practice. Butterworth-Heinemann, Oxford, ch. 5

Quality issues relating to integrated care pathways

Chapter **Fourteen**

Managing to change the way we manage to change

John Turnbull

- What prevents a skilled and intelligent workforce from using their best thinking and realising their creative potential?
- What are the main organisational theories and do they encourage or discourage creativity and innovation?

- What can be learned from the way that these theories have been applied in health care organisations?
- What else needs to happen to release the creative potential of people working in health care organisations?

OVERVIEW

Throughout this book, the contributors have emphasised the critical role of creativity and innovation in improving health care. This final chapter will move on the discussion by exploring the four key issues detailed above that relate to how creativity can be encouraged further in health care organisations.

The chapter begins by identifying some of the barriers associated with making change in the NHS. It moves on to stress the critical role played by creativity in making change and, given its importance, explores the meaning of creativity as both an intellectual act and a symbol of freedom for those working in the NHS. If creativity is central to making change, a key question is: How well has the NHS used the creative talents of those working in it? In order to respond to this, the middle section of this chapter explores the main theoretical perspectives on organisations and their capacity to encourage creativity and to identify how these theories have been applied to the NHS. Of particular concern in this section is the need to identify trends in the organisation of health care in the future. The concluding section makes a judgement about the likelihood of the NHS improving its capacity to encourage creative thinking and sets out the further steps it needs to take to achieve this.

THE CHALLENGE OF CHANGE

The popular image of the NHS is one of a bureaucratic organisation paralysed by paperwork and policy imperatives and incapable of lasting change. Politicians are often heard blaming professional self-interest for the apparent inertia in health services. Professionals will blame politicians for 'initiative overload' and a lack of resources to effect change and both groups blame ineffective management when things go wrong. Against this background, it is not surprising that staff are often mistrustful of change, and Finger & Burgin-Brand (1999) rightly observe that the case for change in public services nearly always has to be made more vehemently than in other organisations.

Several reasons have been put forward to explain why change seems so difficult to bring about in the NHS. Stewart (1986), for example, points out that public services such as the NHS were designed to be permanent features of the political and social landscape in order to give the population a sense of security and well-being. The structure and management of public services was therefore designed for survival as a symbol of the state's commitment to its population rather than change. Garrett (1994) suggests that public sector organisations simply do not face the same pressures for change compared to private sector companies. Expanding on this, James (1994) points out that the potential reward for commercial sector organisations changing and improving their services is extra income, thus providing a powerful motivator for change. In contrast, she points out that additional income for services to fund change is largely a decision in the hands of politicians that often follows high profile failure rather than success. According to Butcher (2000), a major problem for the NHS is its sheer size and complexity, which provide significant logistical problems for anyone contemplating change. Over the years of the NHS' existence, several authors, including the government (Griffiths 1983), have also criticised the low calibre of managers and leaders in the NHS, in particular their ability to manage the change process.

Managing to change the way we manage to change

369

Following on from this analysis, many solutions have been put forward to improve the effectiveness and efficiency of the NHS. Firstly, Brown (1994) and James (1994) note how successive governments have sought to limit the power of professionals in the NHS in their effort to effect change. Ham (1992) also points to the many changes since the inception of the NHS in 1948 that have been introduced in order to simplify the structure of health services in the hope of making it easier to manage change. A consistent theme has been one of introducing commercial sector practices into the NHS, the most prominent example of which was the creation of managed competition introduced by the Thatcher government (DoH 1990). Preceding this, the concept of general management had been introduced to the NHS in the 1980s, following Sir Roy Griffiths' inquiry into NHS management (Griffiths 1983). More recently, the government announced the creation of a Modernisation Agency (DoH 2000a) for the NHS, in which a stated aim is to learn from good management practice in the commercial sector. In contrast, other authors (Hudson 1995, James 1994) believe that the NHS' problems have been compounded by these attempts to see it as yet another organisation. James (1994) believes that the NHS needs to rediscover its original purpose and founding principles and refocus management activity on achieving social change rather than seeking to 'fix' the population's medical ailments and conditions.

From this brief account, it can be seen that there is no shortage of remedies for the ills of the NHS. However, the purpose in this chapter is not to comment on the merits of one of these specific ideas for change over another. Rather, the rest of this chapter will explore ways to improve the conditions that influence the change process itself. The main proposition that will be put forward is that ideas for change, and the way change is brought about in organisations, depend for their success upon creative thinking. Few management and leadership theorists have given serious attention to improving the quality of thinking in organisations which is surprising since, as Kline (1999) asserts, almost everything that happens depends upon someone's thinking. She goes on to emphasise her point by saying:

> Every minute, while you sleep, groups known as organisations are meeting to decide how you will live. They are deciding whether you will work or not; whether you will suffer or luxuriate; what you will be allowed to know and when; where you should put your faith; what you will put in your body; and how much all of this will cost. These groups are deciding who matters and how much. In fact, most of what affects each of our minute-to-minute individual

Old problems, new solutions

lives is decided by groups meeting without us. We have to trust them. And when *we* are in one of those organisations making some of those decisions, we have to be trusted. But just how good can the thinking of these groups be? Their decisions will be as good as their thinking. (p. 100)

THE MEANING AND IMPORTANCE OF CREATIVITY

Despite the availability of dictionaries and encyclopaedias, the dynamic nature of society brings with it the need to continually reflect upon and clarify the meaning of words. True to the title of this book, all the contributors have given examples of how the creative talents of people have been harnessed to bring about improvements for individuals who use health care services. In this chapter, the word 'creativity' will be used in a literal as well as a symbolic way and time will be spent clarifying some of the key assumptions about the meaning of the word.

Creativity and the environment

If a representative sample of the population were asked to define creativity and to rate how creative they felt they were, the chances are that many would give examples of works of art or music and, consequently, would probably rank themselves as not very creative people. Although few of us could aspire to the heights attained by a Salvador Dali or a John Lennon, social psychologists such as Brotherton (1999) would assert that human beings are almost constantly engaged in creative activity, mostly through their ability to problem solve and to form and sustain relationships. The fact that creativity is an innate characteristic is a key assumption in this chapter. Another assumption is that creativity, like other human qualities, needs the right environment in order to flourish. To illustrate this, consider what would happen if the representative sample was asked whether it was bothered that they were creative or not. The chances are that most people would not be too concerned, suggesting that society may not place a high value on everyone being creative. This is not to say that society actively discourages creativity but rather that it shapes attitudes towards it in more subtle ways. For example, someone admitting that they cannot write would be greeted with shock and disdain sufficient to make the person feel ashamed and embarrassed. On the other hand, someone

Six Steps to **Effective Management**

admitting that they cannot draw would be greeted with sympathetic amusement. From this, it can only be concluded that creative thinking depends more on the capacity of the environment to encourage it than on the power of a person's intellect.

Creativity and individual freedom

Expanding on the importance of the environment and the society in which people live, several authors have made the link between creativity and concepts such as individual freedom and democracy. Fromm (1966), for example, believed that creativity, evidenced by individuals thinking for themselves, was more than an intellectual activity but a symbol of individual freedom and responsibility. Paulo Freire's (1972) educational approach enabled poor and illiterate individuals and communities in Brazil to create and develop their own solutions to their powerlessness rather than rely upon the ideas and strategies of others. He referred to this as a process of 'conscientization'. Foucault (1984) developed a similar concept called 'enlightenment', which he described as being the outcome of a social process in which a people were free to think for themselves and under no pressure to accept the ideas of more powerful groups and individuals. Translating these ideas into the field of health care, Traynor (1999) explored nurses' feelings of powerlessness and concluded that nurses have colluded in their own oppression by accepting others' views of nursing and health care. Traynor believes that a key role for nursing leaders is to create environments in which nurses can learn to think independently and reclaim nursing as a creative, humanistic enterprise. Elsewhere Binnie & Titchen (1999) described their efforts to change a leadership style in an acute hospital setting and its impact on nursing staff. Part of the difficulties they initially encountered related to nurses having to get used to the fact that others would no longer do their thinking for them. Thus, creativity will be used in this chapter to represent independent thinking, individual freedom and empowerment.

The view that creativity is more than original thought but symbolic of individual freedom could easily be misinterpreted as promoting some sort of anarchic vision of society in which the emphasis lies in outrageousness, eccentricity and self-interest. In terms of health service organisations, it also seems to be the antithesis of good organisation. In other words, how can tasks be planned and coordinated at the same time as encouraging independent thinking? The answer to this is simple, as outlined in the points below.

Old problems, new solutions

Working towards agreement

Creativity doesn't mean that everyone must think differently but that people are as free to agree as they are to disagree with each other. In a culture of respect for each other, people are more likely to want to work towards agreement. Commitment to any agreement is also stronger and longer lasting than in cultures in which people are instructed to agree with each other.

Thinking for oneself

The freedom to think *for* oneself should not be confused with thinking *about* oneself. People are more likely to think about themselves in an atmosphere in which they feel stressed, oppressed and threatened. In contrast, people are more likely to think for themselves and to be free with their ideas in a culture of equality and respect.

Organisational behaviour

A third answer to the criticism that individual freedom breeds chaos comes from our understanding of how organisations behave. Burns & Stalker (1996), for example, studied management approaches in Scottish engineering firms and noted a paradox in organisations that were striving for increasing efficiency and effectiveness. In the firms' efforts to discover, or produce, individuals whose creativity and inventiveness would give them the competitive advantage they desired, it was found that the centralisation of decision making in these organisations created a reliance on managers to solve problems. According to Burns & Stalker, this style of management had brought about a dysfunctional community within organisations in which creativity had come to be seen as a 'one-off' product of genius instead of a quality possessed by everyone. Thus, rather than interfering with the effectiveness and efficiency of an organisation, creativity is essential to it.

MANAGEMENT THEORY AND CREATIVITY IN THE NHS

If creativity is central to the process of change, a key question for the remainder of this chapter is whether current management practice in the NHS is a hindrance or a help in encouraging creative thinking within services. Given the complexity and size of the NHS, it is impossible to draw any firm conclusions on this issue.

Managing to change the way we manage to change

However, it is possible to develop a meaningful answer by exploring trends in management practice in the NHS and the theoretical perspectives that have underpinned them. In doing so, it is also possible to detect future trends in order to judge the ease or difficulty this presents in encouraging creative thinking in services. This exploration will begin with scientific management.

Scientific management

The scientific theory of management, sometimes referred to as the classic theory, was developed by F. W Taylor (1856–1917). Scientific management takes a highly mechanistic view of organisations: in fact, the literature on the subject will often describe organisations as machines. The scientific view believes that workers derive greater satisfaction when their jobs are clearly specified. This leads to high levels of demarcation and specialisation within organisations and, along with it, detailed job descriptions. This also brings with it the need to grade jobs according to difficulty and the level of discretion needed to carry them out. In turn, this creates the need for line management to monitor the work of those below in the hierarchy and to specificy the limits of others' authority. Given the high level of demarcation, larger organisations will create separate departments to manage their work more efficiently.

Another characteristic of scientific management is its view that workers are motivated mainly by the material benefits they receive. Together with the assumption concerning the need for clarity, this leads to the use of incentive schemes such as performance-related pay and management by objectives.

Many authors (Butcher 2000, Ham 1992, James 1994, Yeatman 1990) believe that the scientific approach to management has been the dominant influence in the NHS. This is evidenced by several characteristics of health services such as the high level of demarcation between professionals and departments, a chain of command stretching from the Department of Health to ward level, and large numbers of managers and administrators (Hunter 1994). The introduction of general management into the NHS in the 1980s (Griffiths 1983) went a long way to reinforce the scientific approach, bringing with it a concentration of decision making, specifying lines of accountability, as well as management techniques such as management by objectives, performance-related pay and the introduction of performance indicators. Although general management was superseded by the managed market in health services (DoH 1990), bringing with it potentially more free-dom for the new NHS trusts, Hoggett (1991) observes that, essen-tially, it was 'business as usual', with control by hierarchy simply replaced by control by contract. Furthermore, the political impera-tive to control expenditure remained and, along with it, the admin-istrators and managers whose task was now to specify and cost professional services. Although competition in the NHS has now been replaced by a more pluralistic approach under the current government, scientific management instincts and approaches remain. For example, the concept of governance, designed to safe-guard and improve standards in the NHS (DoH 1998), has brought with it the need to clarify accountability and comply with standard statements handed down from government. The increasing pres-sure to move towards an evidence-based culture within health services is also seen by some (Culshaw 1995) as a form of manager-ial control over professional activity.

The scientific approach to management has been subjected to much criticism, although the focus here will be on its capacity to promote creative and independent thinking.

Manufacturing versus service systems

James (1994) observes that scientific approaches are better suited to manufacturing systems rather than service systems. In service sys-tems, the customer, or user, needs to be part of the system in order to influence the quality and specification of the service. This brings with it the need for workers to be flexible and creative in order to meet the needs and requirements of the customer. In contrast, pro-duction systems are designed to manufacture a high volume of goods according to a predetermined specification. There is there-fore little room for discretion and, consequently, little need for workers to think creatively. James (1994) regards this as the prin-cipal reason why staff in the NHS cannot meet individual need and why the NHS finds it difficult to change.

Demarcation

Demarcation and the separation of responsibility for tasks bring other problems. Fish (1995) notes how individuals and depart-ments will develop a vested interest in holding onto their power base and thus resist change. The incentive for managers, in particular, is to spend more time 'policing' the boundaries of their department rather than thinking more creatively and laterally.

Managing to change the way we manage to change

Rules

Scientific management brings with it a large number of both formal and informal 'rules'. Formal rules consist of the job descriptions, policy and procedure manuals and departmental terms of reference that go with the specialisation and demarcation. Again, much management time needs to be spent on enforcing these rules, leaving little time to think independently. Rees (1991) also notes that the existence of formal rules can create a culture in which workers will fail to use their initiative, even when circumstances call for it. He refers to this as the exercise of 'anonymous authority' (p. 14).

Blame culture

Lastly, scientific management brings with it the separation of service delivery, or production, from monitoring and control. James (1994) claims that this creates circumstances in which blame can be attributed. Given the discussion earlier on the nature of creativity, this can lead to a culture of fear and mistrust in which people are more likely to think about themselves rather than for themselves. A further consequence of this is that those in a position of accountability have a greater incentive to control rather than liberate those below them, for fear of being blamed. This will encourage them to keep decision making and discretion to themselves. Bowman's (1995) study of the pressures on nurses revealed the impact of managerial dominance of this kind:

> There is little choice in nursing practice as everything is decided elsewhere by the nursing procedures committee and nursing management: there is little flexibility to alter what is decided. (p. 40)

Human relations management

At the same time as Taylor's ideas were being implemented, Elton Mayo (1880–1949) was conducting research into organisations that led to what has become known as the human relations theory of organisations. Whereas classic, or scientific organisational theory focuses on the formal and structural aspects of organisations, the human relations approach believes that work is dignifying rather than simply a means to an end. Consequently, Mayo believed that workers were motivated by the informal aspects of working life such as working in teams, participation and communication with other workers. Researchers into the human relations model discovered that workers felt more motivated when managers took an interest in them. For example, in the classic 'Hawthorne' experiment (Roethlisberger & Dickson 1939), apparently insignificant changes such as altering lighting levels in factories brought about improvements in productivity. Researchers also discovered that improvements in productivity occurred when extra attention was given to workers. Given this, the role of managers working within this model is to motivate workers rather than specify their tasks. The emphasis is also on personal development, achieved through techniques such as appraisal and supervision. More freedom is also given to communicate across any departmental boundaries and to develop team working.

Despite the attractiveness of the human relations school of thought, James (1994) points out that there has never been an organisation that has applied it whole-heartedly. However, many organisations, including the NHS, have sought to incorporate some of the ideas and techniques from the human relations school. For example, clinical supervision, continuing professional development, reducing workplace violence and, more recently, more flexible arrangements for employment in order to improve working lives (DoH 2000b) have all received increasing attention in recent years.

At first sight, the human relations model might be regarded as an antidote for the excesses of scientific management and to provide more freedom for people to be creative. However, the human relations model should not be confused with a humanistic approach to management. In other words, although attention is focused on meeting a broader range of human needs in the workforce, the model does not say who should define those needs. In practice, Mullins (1989) points out that it is nearly always management that decides what those needs are and how best they can be met (p. 41). Although workers might enjoy greater job satisfaction, this results in a paternalistic approach that does little to change power relationships. Consequently, it may do little to encourage creative and innovative thinking.

Systemic management

In recent years, a third approach to understanding organisations has been developed, known as systems theory. The systemic approach contrasts with the rational, predictable and controlling approach of scientific management by looking at organisations in a more organic, or ecological, way. Systemic approaches pay less attention to vertical lines of communication and accountability in

Managing to change the way we manage to change

organisations and, instead, focus more on relationships between different groups, or subsystems, within organisations. The systemic approach also encourages organisations to be more outward looking and see themselves as parts of a larger system made up of different stakeholders.

The learning organisation

In contrast to the other main theories of organisations, systems theory does not put forward a particular view of human need and motivation except that it views the world as a complex and sometimes chaotic and unpredictable place in which people are constantly readjusting their perspectives (Simon 1977). Therefore, individual and organisational success depends upon accessing and interpreting information (Argyris & Schon 1978, Senge 1990) in order to learn and adapt. The predominant expression of systems theory is the concept of the 'learning organisation' which now has a central position in contemporary thinking about organisations (Glynn et al 1994). A full discussion of the learning organisation can be found in Dodgson (1993) and Prange (1999). The learning organisation is primarily seen as a systemic response to a rapidly changing environment in which the organisation learns from its experience by processing information from within as well as outside its boundaries. Key authors such as Argyris & Schon (1978), Senge (1990) and Garrett (1994) have developed methods of enhancing the capacity of the organisation to learn from experience that closely resemble models of individual learning developed by Kolb (1984) in which reflection on action is a key principle.

The networked organisation

The influence of systems theory is relatively new to the NHS but Ferlie & Pettigrew (1996) note the development of interest in the concept of 'networked' organisations throughout the previous decade. Although the creation of the internal market within health care following the *NHS and Community Care Act* (DoH 1990) reinforced a scientific management approach, it also paved the way for the NHS to be seen as a system. For example, the present government's abolition of the internal market has not been accompanied by a return to a hierarchical relationship between Trusts and Health Authorities. Instead, the government has encouraged managers to see themselves working within a health system. Another initiative, the 'Health of the Nation' strategy (DoH 1991), could also be seen as one of the first attempts by government to recognise health care as a system by setting targets for health across different organisations within the NHS. The current Labour government's emphasis on partnership in both health and social care services, or 'joined up government', is a further indication of more systemic thinking in the NHS. In some regions, different organisations have developed more formal strategic alliances with each other whilst retaining their autonomy, in order to advance practice in areas such as cancer and learning disability (NHS Executive South East 2000, Oxfordshire Learning Disability NHS Trust 2000). The introduction of the concept of corporate governance into the NHS (DoH 1998) has also emphasised the need for organisations to learn from their practice and experiences in order to safeguard and promote standards. Despite these interesting developments, some authors (Dewar 1999) have warned that the wholesale adoption of a systemic approach requires massive cultural and organisational change. This suggests that the NHS has a long way to go but trends indicate that this approach may become a more prominent feature of ministerial and civil service thinking (Ferlie & Pettigrew 1996).

The partnership organisation

Because systems theory is a relatively new concept to the NHS, little consideration has been given to its implications for managers and leaders or its capacity to encourage creative and innovative thinking within organisations. However, Ferlie & Pettigrew (1996) note that systemic approaches inevitably call for a greater focus on forming relationships and networks between organisations and key stakeholders in the health care system. Therefore, organisations that work in partnership are more likely to value skills such as negotiating and persuading. This would place greater emphasis on creative and innovative approaches and more equitable relationships between organisations that are based on trust and mutual respect. However, if these values can be used to build different relationships between organisations, what are the implications for relationships within organisations?

Organisational cultures

As previously stated, the main symbol of the systemic approach to management is the concept of the learning organisation, yet there is still considerable theoretical confusion over the meaning of this phrase (Prange 1999). Most of the confusion centres around the question of whether the learning organisation is an intervention, a strategic objective or a process of organisational transformation

Managing to change the way we manage to change

(Nadler et al 1995, Prange 1999). Consequently, this makes it difficult to evaluate its impact on relationships within organisations. Certainly, experts can point to evidence that there is a great deal more individual and collective learning taking place in organisations (Dixon 1994). This suggests greater creative thinking and openness amongst the workforce. On the other hand, Finger & Burgin-Brand's (1999) experience of introducing the learning organisation to the public sector suggests that there is little fundamental change in power relationships between management, workforce and the customer. Their analysis of the learning organisation as an intervention, or strategic objective, suggests that the majority of learning that occurs in organisations is 'management learning' in which managers become 'keepers' of the system. Their experience of developing collective learning in organisations is only slightly more optimistic of its capacity to transform organisational cultures (p. 146).

Another doubt about systems theory comes from Quinn (1980). Although systemic theory undoubtedly encourages differentiation, the fact that each group or organisation is linked and dependent upon the other means that development can only occur at the pace of the slowest. Quinn prefers to see the decisions taken within systemic approaches as pragmatic and incremental, made according to circumstances rather than with reference to grand theory.

Summary

The purpose of this section was twofold: to explore the extent to which the main organisational theories have been applied in the NHS and to judge their capacity to promote creative thinking. In answer to the first question, it appears that the scientific model of management has dominated the NHS since its inception. However, because of its emphasis on control, doubts must now exist about its relevance amidst a growing culture of partnership and a focus on service user priorities. The NHS now appears to be on a course towards developing structures and processes that will encourage greater collaboration between organisations and groups that are more characteristic of a systemic approach to management. However, this does not necessarily mean that the principles and practice of systemic management are being pursued as an explicit aim of the Department of Health.

As far as the human relations approach to organisations is concerned, all that can be said is that its principles and techniques have been selectively applied to NHS organisations.

Old problems, new solutions

From the three approaches, it can be concluded that the scientific approach is the least likely to encourage creative thinking within organisations. Both the human relations and the systemic approach have aspects that have the potential to release creativity in the workforce. However, from what can be seen from their application so far, they have failed to address a fundamental issue in releasing creativity, which is the power imbalance between managers and the workforce. Legislative and policy changes have been introduced in the form of a duty of partnership on NHS organisations (DoH 1997) and greater flexibility for those managing health and social care services (DoH 2001). However, structural and legislative change is a necessary but insufficient condition to change behaviours and relationships between the numerous stakeholders within the health system. This is not surprising, since the introduction of general management into the NHS in the mid-1980s required at least a further 5 years before changing management behaviour (Glynn & Perkins 1995). In order to realise its potential to transform relationships and promote creativity, there needs to be considerably more reflection to identify precisely what else needs to happen. The concluding section will seek to identify some of the key steps that need to be taken.

THE VALUES-LED ORGANISATION

Despite the foundations for a systemic approach to management having been laid by the government in recent policy and legislative change, it is cultural change that transforms organisations. Cultural change is a much used (and possibly over-used) word, but the power of culture is undeniable. Peters & Waterman (1982), in their exploration of the meaning of excellence in American companies, concluded:

> The stronger the culture and the more it was directed towards the marketplace, the less need there was for policy manuals, organisational charts, or detailed procedures and rules. In these companies people way down the line know what they are supposed to do in most situations because the handful of guiding values is crystal clear. (pp. 75–76)

Culture has been described by various authors but is generally understood to be a 'set of shared beliefs, values, attitudes, traditions, language, rules, behaviours and ways of doing' (Wells 1999, p. 68) that exist in an organisation. It should not be confused with the concept of corporate identity. Corporate identity is more

Managing to change the way we manage to change

> **Box 14.1** Effecting cultural change
>
> - Cultural change is about changing behaviour as well as attitudes
> - Cultural change applies to managers as well as the rest of the workforce
> - Cultural change must be accompanied by a clear description of what is expected to change
> - Planning and bringing about cultural change must involve everyone in the organisation

concerned with developing and projecting a unified image and encouraging conformity with this image amongst the workforce. In contrast, a culture of an organisation could encourage independent thinking and the organisation could have developed ways of handling conflict and difference.

Although there might be general agreement on the components of organisational culture, there are several opinions on how best to effect cultural change, some of which are outlined in Box 14.1.

Assuming that this advice is followed, Peters & Waterman (1982) offer their observation of the power of culture by reminding readers that cultures can become dysfunctional as well as functional. Therefore, the central question, as far as the NHS is concerned, is: What represents a functional culture?

THE IMPORTANCE OF MISSION

In his excellent exploration of managing in voluntary and charitable organisations, Mike Hudson (1995) highlights a sense of mission as being one of the most important components in driving and changing organisational culture. Hudson believes that mission is more important in organisations that are motivated by social rather than commercial objectives because, in the latter case, the 'bottom line' is profit or loss. Whereas every organisation needs to be well run, socially motivated organisations will judge their success more on the extent to which lives are changed or campaigns are won. According to Hudson, the idea of mission has two elements: the organisation's mission will comprise the values held by people working in it and the mission is the organisation's raison d'être that explains why the organisation exists and who benefits from it. Thus, Hudson believes that mission is about both 'hearts and minds' (1995, p. 94), in that values represent the emotions and that the rationale represents the intellect of the organisation.

(side margin) Old problems, new solutions

Hudson is quick to explain that mission should not be confused with a mission statement. Although mission statements can encapsulate some of the elements of the mission, Hudson believes that they represent a danger in that they can often be 'a list of good intentions dreamed up by senior management' (p. 95).

Hudson's analysis was preceded by Hadley & Young's (1990) account of the transformation of a social service department in the 1980s from a bureaucracy to a responsive service, in which the importance of mission was emphasised. Hadley & Young go further than Hudson by describing the content of a public service mission in greater detail. Although they did not use the term 'mission' to describe their approach, the following quotation describes both the values and the raison d'être of a new public service:

> Responsive management has two main elements: a) belief in the value of public services and the recognition of the threat to their continued survival which has resulted, in part, from the failure of the administrative model. b) belief in the potential of a new orientation in public services which is enabling rather than disabling, user-orientated rather than producer-orientated, pluralistic rather than unitary, entrepreneurial and pragmatic rather than administrative and rule-bound. (p. 60)

Similarly, in the field of health care, James (1994) has argued for a rediscovery of the founding principles of the NHS. For Ann James, the NHS exists to enable and to empower those who use its services, based on shared values of equity and social inclusion. She justifies her belief in the following way:

> People who are ill or who have disabilities, people who are very old or very young, people who are unemployed or who live in poverty, people who are uneducated, or homeless, and people who care for them, people who have offended against the law: these are the people who make up the majority of the users of our care services ... managing this clientele is not about how to control but how to enable, not how to maximise profit but how to enfranchise. Empowerment of users is not a bolted on extra to managing welfare, but central to it. (pp. 1–2)

These are powerful examples of a mission that would, no doubt, provide inspiration and clarification for many working in public services about their purpose in a way that structures and policies could not. Their importance to a systemic approach to management is that an agreed sense of mission has the potential to unite the purposes of the different organisations and groups that comprise the health care system. Their importance to the process of driving creativity is that an agreed set of principles can be applied

Managing to change the way we manage to change

by individual staff or teams to the unique circumstances that they find themselves working in. In this way, mission becomes more effective than the controlling devices with which NHS staff are more familiar, such as policies, procedures and a sole reliance on managers to solve problems. This is not to say that there is no longer a need for these devices but that they become less important.

ACCOUNTING FOR PERFORMANCE

A reliance on mission and the loosening of the hold of traditional management devices such as policies, standards and detailed job descriptions may seem anathema in a service such as the NHS where people's lives, health and personal futures are at stake. The question is: Where is the accountability in a systemic approach? Proponents would claim that accountability is stronger in a systemic approach or 'networked organisations'. Firstly, accountability in scientifically managed organisations is vertical, since those who are accountable also demand the authority and resources to get the job done. Consequently, accountability rests with a small number of managers and the majority of the workforce is left believing that they are accountable for nothing. As far as the NHS is concerned, during the Thatcher government years of general management and market solutions, lines of accountability were simplified in the interests of efficiency (James 1994), thus leaving out accountability to service users, the wider community and interest groups, despite the rhetoric to the contrary. Given the emphasis on sound management of public finances, accountability in the NHS was synonymous with financial rather than clinical accountability. Therefore, what was left was accountability from NHS trusts to the government through local purchasers. A 'side effect' of this type of accountability is that strong allegiances can be built up to individuals and organisations to the detriment of users or key values and beliefs.

In contrast, the systemic view of organisations is based on a system of exchange between individuals and groups rather than instruction, information sharing rather than reporting. In systemically managed organisations, accountability is exercised through devices such as agreed quality assurance systems and published documents such as health improvement programmes and joint investment plans. If these initiatives are compatible with a shared vision and mission across organisations, and if they have been inclusive in their development, then all practitioners are account-

Old problems, new solutions

able for their delivery, not just a few managers. The impact of this is that allegiance to buildings, organisations or managers is broken and commitment to values and ideas can be developed. Its value is that this situation is more compatible with the prime reason why staff work for the NHS in the first place, which is to improve life for individuals rather than a desire to work in a particular building or NHS trust. A disadvantage is the length of time it takes to achieve agreement over key strategies or initiatives. However, this can be offset by improvements in the supply of accurate and timely information as well as making the best use of people's thinking when they meet. The value in terms of creativity is that a systemic view of organisations encourages practitioners to think beyond traditional allegiances and frees them up to think outside of their buildings, organisations and professions and to question assumptions.

IMPROVING THE QUALITY OF THINKING

Although the systemic approach has the potential to encourage staff to think for themselves, this can be enhanced further by making it a strategic aim to improve the quality of thinking in an organisation or across the health care system. A detailed description of how this can happen is illustrated in Application 14.1.

It may seem unusual that, within a health care system comprised of individuals with degrees, second degrees, doctorates and a host of other academic qualifications, it should be necessary to improve the quality of thinking among the workforce. However, the traditional hierarchical and controlling cultures in which most people work result in highly dysfunctional systems in which it is considered unusual, and sometimes dangerous, to think for oneself. Nancy Kline (1999) is someone who has spent much of her time helping to develop an approach to improving the quality of thinking in organisations called Time to Think.[1] She believes that thinking is a natural state but has become rare because of the effects of working in dysfunctional organisations. The essence of her approach is to restore this natural state by removing obstacles rather than importing a vast array of techniques or gimmicks. Kline's ideas are not specifically designed for a systemic approach to organisations, although her approach has a great deal of synergy with its beliefs and aims. As already pointed out, almost everything we do depends for its success on the quality of people's thinking. Within a networked health care system, if individuals are

---

[1] Time to Think is a registered trademark.

to become more accountable, then they need to take their responsibilities more seriously. This can begin by giving their best of themselves to others and demanding the same of their partners. Key to this is to improve the quality of their thinking and to encourage better thinking in others by improving the quality of their listening.

The other advantage of concentrating on the quality of thinking in organisations is that it helps people to cope better with the pace of change. It might sound paradoxical that taking time out to think can save time but this is achieved because better decisions are made. As Kline says, 'to take time to think is to gain time to live' (1999, p. 21). This advantage will also help counter the criticism that gaining agreement amongst a wide range of partners is time consuming.

The systemic approach is based on the notion that groups and organisations are connected in an interdependent system. In order for the system to develop solutions to problems, agreement needs to be reached amongst the partners. This calls for high-level negotiation and communications skills as well as respect for the views of the different partners. Improving the capacity to think and to listen could prove to be an efficient and effective strategy to assist this process. Kline (1999) emphasises this as follows: 'By taking steps to turn our world into a Thinking Environment . . . no human mind is wasted, and no human heart is trampled' (p. 21).

Finally, creating opportunities for people to think and to think well is underpinned by a belief in the value of others. Creating the conditions in which staff feel free to think for themselves and encourage others to do so will, inevitably, improve their motivation and commitment.

CONCLUSION

The pressures and demands of working within the NHS are greater than ever before and it is quite likely that this pace will increase. Gradually, organisations are having to change the way they interact with each other and with other key groups and individuals in the health care system in order to meet these demands. Although labels can be detrimental, it is apparent that the NHS is adopting a more systemic approach to its work and organisation and becoming a 'networked organisation'. Networked organisations can bring many opportunities and are probably more superior than their predecessors in their capacity to promote creative thinking. However, this capacity needs to be realised by changing the values, mission, responsibilities and accountabilities within organisations

> **Box 14.2** Working towards a networked organisation
>
> - If you knew that you were free to tell your manager about the one thing that would improve thinking in the organisation, what would it be?
> - If you were given the task of developing a new mission for your organisation, what would it need to contain?
> - What are the three most important changes you would make to enable your place of work to become a more networked organisation?

and, above all, to encourage everyone to give their best thinking. Perhaps this is easier said than done. However, the discussion points in Box 14.2 may help pave the way.

References

Argyris C, Schon DA 1978 Organisational learning: a theory of action perspective. Addison-Wesley, Reading, Massachusetts

Binnie A, Titchen A 1999 Freedom to practise: the development of patient centred nursing. Butterworth-Heinemann, Oxford

Bowman M 1995 The professional nurse. Chapman & Hall, London

Brotherton M 1999 Social psychology and management. Sage, London

Brown J 1994 The hybrid worker. Department of Social Policy and Social Work, University of York

Burns T, Stalker GM 1996 The management of innovation. Oxford University Press, Oxford

Butcher T 2000 The public administration model of welfare delivery. In: Davies C, Finlay L, Bullman A (eds) Changing practice in health and social care. Sage, London

Culshaw H 1995 Evidence based practice for sale? British Journal of Occupational Therapy 58: 233

Department of Health 1990 The NHS and Community Care Act. Department of Health, London

Department of Health 1991 The health of the nation. Department of Health, London

Department of Health 1997 The new NHS: modern, dependable. Department of Health, London

Department of Health 1998 A first class service: quality in the new NHS. Department of Health, London

Department of Health 2000a The NHS plan. Department of Health, London

Department of Health 2000b Improving working lives. Department of Health, London

Department of Health 2001 The Health Act. Department of Health, London

Managing to change the way we manage to change

Dewar S 1999 Clinical governance under construction: problems of design and difficulties in practice. King's Fund, London

Dixon N 1994 The organisational learning cycle. How we can learn collectively. McGraw-Hill, London

Dodgson M 1993 A review of some literatures. Organisation Studies 14(3): 375–394

Ferlie E, Pettigrew A 1996 Managing through networks: some issues and implications for the NHS. British Journal of Management 7: 81–89

Finger M, Burgin-Brand S 1999 The concept of the learning organisation applied to the transformation of the public sector: conceptual contributions for theory development. In: Easterby-Smith M, Burgoyne J, Aranjo L (eds) Organisational learning and the learning organisation: developments in theory and practice. Sage, London

Fish D 1995 Quality mentoring for student teachers: a principled approach to practice. Fulton, London

Foucault M 1984 The history of sexuality: an introduction. Penguin, Harmondsworth

Freire P 1972 Pedagogy of the oppressed. Penguin, Harmondsworth

Fromm E 1966 The heart of man. Penguin, Harmondsworth

Garrett B 1994 The learning organisation. Harper Collins, London

Glynn J, Perkins DA 1995 Managing health care: challenges for the 90s. Saunders, London

Glynn NA, Lant TK, Milliken FJ 1994 Mapping learning processes in organisations. In: Stubbard C, Meindl JR, Porac JF (eds) Advances in managerial cognition and organisational information processing. Sage, London

Griffiths R 1983 NHS management. Department of Health and Social Security, London

Hadley R, Young K 1990 Creating a responsive public service. Harvester Wheatsheaf, London

Ham C 1992 Health policy in Britain, 3rd edn. Macmillan, Basingstoke

Hoggett P 1991 A new management for the public sector? Policy and Politics 19: 243–256

Hudson M 1995 Managing without profit: the art of managing third-sector organisations. Penguin, Harmondsworth

Hunter D 1994 From tribalism to opportunism: the management challenge to medical dominance. In: Gabe J, Kelleher D, Williams G (eds) Challenging medicine. Routledge, London

James A 1994 Managing to care: public service and the market. Longman, London

Kline N 1999 Time to think. Listening to ignite the human mind. Ward Lock, London

Kolb DA 1984 Experiential learning. Prentice Hall, Englewood Cliffs, New Jersey

Mullins LJ 1989 Management and organisational behaviour, 2nd edn. Pitman, London

Nadler D, Shaw R, Walton E 1995 Discontinuous change. Leading organisational transformation. Jossey-Bass, San Francisco

NHS Executive South East 2000 Managed clinical networks. NHS Executive South East, London

Oxfordshire Learning Disability NHS Trust 2000 Strategic alliance in research and development in learning disability: statement of intent. Oxfordshire Learning Disability NHS Trust, Oxford

Peters T, Waterman R 1982 In search of excellence. Harper & Row, New York

Prange C 1999 Organisational learning – desperately seeking theory? In: Easterby-Smith M, Burgoyne J, Aranjo L (eds) Organisational learning and the learning organisation: developments in theory and practice. Sage, London

Quinn JB 1980 Strategies for change. Logical incrementalism. Irwin, Homewood, Illinois

Rees S 1991 Achieving power: practice and policy in social welfare. Allen & Unwin, St Leonards, NSW

Roethlisberger FJ, Dickson WJ 1939 Management and the worker. Harvard University Press, New York

Schon D 1983 The reflective practitioner. Basic Books, New York

Senge P 1990 The fifth discipline: the art and practice of the learning organisation. Doubleday, New York

Simon HA 1977 The new science of management decision. Prentice Hall, London

Stewart J 1986 The new management of local government. Allen & Unwin, London

Traynor M 1999 Managerialism and nursing: beyond oppression and profession. Routledge, London

Wells JSG 1999 The growth of managerialism and its impact on nursing and the NHS. In: Norman I, Cowley S (eds) The changing nature of nursing in a managerial age. Blackwell, Oxford

Yeatman A 1990 Bureaucrats, technocrats, femocrats. Allen & Unwin, Sydney

Managing to change the way we manage to change

Application **14:1**
John Turnbull

Thinking for a better future

Chapter 14 emphasised the need for NHS organisations to work increasingly as part of a health and social care system, pointing out that this would require a loosening of traditional power structures in order to bring about more equitable relationships between individuals within and across organisations. For managers and leaders of organisations, this brings with it the challenge of developing structures and systems that will encourage staff to work in partnership and to demonstrate accountability to jointly agreed strategies, principles and their outcomes instead of to managers alone. In turn, this opens up opportunities for more creative thinking amongst staff. However, some key issues need to be addressed: In what ways should managers and leaders change their everyday practice to encourage creative thinking? How can managers and leaders sustain creative thinking in their organisations? This application will explore these issues by describing the experiences of a NHS Trust board that set out to promote the value of partnership working and person-centredness in its organisation.

BACKGROUND

Oxfordshire Learning Disability NHS Trust became a trust in 1993. It is one of the very few NHS trusts in the United Kingdom providing services solely for people with learning disabilities. The Trust currently employs 848 staff and its services are entirely community based. Since 1993 it has doubled in size and now provides the following specialist health services:

● Three community learning disability teams, comprising learning disability nurses, occupational therapists, clinical psychologists, dieticians, speech and language therapists, physiotherapists and psychiatrists

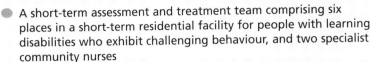

- A short-term assessment and treatment team comprising six places in a short-term residential facility for people with learning disabilities who exhibit challenging behaviour, and two specialist community nurses
- A medium secure facility, providing six medium-term therapeutic residential places for people with learning disabilities with severe challenging behaviour and mental health needs
- A secure facility for people with learning disabilities who have offended
- A children's respite service
- A child and adolescent community team

The Trust also provides social support in the form of:

- 155 places in residential care homes
- supported homes for 63 people
- a community development service, aimed at developing leisure opportunities and meaningful day-time occupation for people with learning disabilities
- an employment service, providing job coaches to support people with learning disabilities who want to work
- VOX, which is part of the millennium volunteers project and provides opportunities for people to undertake voluntary work with people with learning disabilities
- eight places for people with learning disabilities taking planned short-term breaks.

PHILOSOPHY

In the mid-1970s, the philosophy of supporting people with learning disabilities changed radically. Prior to this, it was believed that it was best to segregate people with learning disabilities from society because they would not 'fit in'. Services took the form of long-stay hospitals, usually built miles away from the facilities and amenities enjoyed by the general population. For those people who remained at home, cared for by their parents, services consisted mainly of social service day centres in which the goal was to occupy people with learning disabilities rather than provide them with meaningful activity.

The writings of people such as Wolfensberger (1972) in the United States and Scandinavian authors such as Nirje (1980) challenged people's understanding of learning disability and proposed that people with learning disabilities could enjoy a more 'normal' lifestyle if they were exposed to the opportunities and activities that the rest of the population enjoyed. These authors criticised the predominant medical view that located the 'problem' of learning disability in the individual rather than in the attitudes, stereotyping and behaviour of members of society. These ideas were later developed by people such

Thinking for a better future

Six Steps to Effective Management

as Oliver (1990) and Barnes (1991) into a social model of disability that put forward the view that the limitations experienced by disabled people did not result directly from their impairment but from the constraints imposed by society. Supported by legislation such as the Disability Discrimination Act 1996, the Human Rights Act 1999 and the recent White Paper on learning disability, *Valuing People* (DoH 2001), the current philosophy in services is that people with learning disabilities are equal citizens and should be enabled to exercise the same rights and responsibilities as anyone else in society.

A SERVICE WITH A MISSION

In 1999, the Trust developed and published a new mission statement (Box 14.1.1), the language of which was altered slightly in the light

---

Box 14.1.1 The trust's mission statement

Aims

The Oxfordshire Learning Disability NHS Trust has two main aims:
- To provide high quality health care and social support to people who have a learning disability and to those with related needs who live in Oxfordshire and the surrounding area.
- To promote the rights and opportunities of people who have a learning disability, working in partnership with service users, their families/carers and other agencies.

Commitments

These aims are supported by four commitments:
- *Listening to individuals* – We are committed, through skilled listening, to become informed and to understand the needs, wishes and aspirations of each service user about how he or she wants to live life now and in the future.
- *Providing person-centred services* – We are committed both to responding to information about each person's needs, wishes and aspirations and to delivering relevant, flexible and affordable services which are informed by best practice.
- *Working with others* – We are committed to working in partnership with families/carers, commissioners and other agencies, as well as with social networks and communities, to build a society in which all people who have a learning disability can participate as equal and valued citizens.
- *Investing in our staff* – We are committed to creating a working environment which celebrates diversity, promotes the active involvement of staff in the design and delivery of person-centred services and responds to their needs for training, development and support.

Old problems, new solutions

of the White Paper on learning disability in August 2001. According to Hudson (1995), a mission should set out what an organisation stands for. He makes an important distinction between a mission statement and a mission by claiming that a mission statement can simply be a collection of well-meaning words and phrases, whereas a mission is the philosophy that drives forward an organisation. Therefore, in setting out its four commitments, the Trust made some bold promises that, it was believed, would re-energise its commitment to people with learning disabilities, enhance the quality of its services, retain valuable staff and make its services fit for the future. A key question was: How could the Trust ensure that its commitments remained at the centre of everything that it did and, more urgently, where should it begin the journey?

Perhaps because it is a relatively young specialty or, as some would say, a profession, management seems vulnerable to fashion and initiatives that promise instant results. Although some of these initiatives are well meaning and well thought out, they frequently result in managers and staff adopting rules of interaction that do not apply to their lives outside the organisation. In other words, organisations can become quite unnatural environments. Another difficulty is that many solutions are management solutions that take as their starting point the problems that managers experience rather than those experienced by the workforce or users of the service. Finally, many organisational change strategies have been developed for the commercial rather than public sector organisations.

The Thinking Environment

Managers in the Trust began their search for improvement by taking a more fundamental approach to change and reflected firstly on the nature of organisations. As Mullins (1989) points out, many authors have put forward a definition of an organisation but, in pure terms, it is a collection of individuals working towards a common purpose: the individual and the organisation cannot truly be separated. Following this, further assumptions were made:

- Managers believed that the prime motivation of people who come to work with people with learning disabilities is to treat them as equals and support them to lead a life of their choice.
- It was believed that traditional ways of structuring and running organisations have resulted in power imbalances between managers and staff as well as staff and those who use services.
- Although management and leadership are essential components of organisations, their function is to create the optimum conditions for staff to do their job.

These beliefs and assumptions added up to an approach to change that would involve creating conditions in which more equal and

Thinking for a better future

393

natural relationships could exist. With this in mind, trust managers turned to the work of Nancy Kline, an international leadership consultant, whose experience in coaching in different organisations is described in her book *Time to Think* (1999). Nancy Kline's ideas and coaching are based on the belief that everything that we do depends on thinking. Therefore, if organisations want to improve the quality of their services, then they need to improve the quality of their thinking. To help organisations to do this, Kline has identified ten behaviours that form a system called a Thinking Environment.[1] The ten components will be described shortly, but Kline's ambitious and enticing vision is worth quoting first because it embodies the philosophy underpinning her ideas:

> I would like the whole world to become a Thinking Environment. I would like people to wake up each morning knowing that they are going to think for themselves without punishment; that they can be logical, eloquent, bold and imaginative; that their ideas count; that other people are going to pay attention to them, to appreciate them, be at ease with them, allow them to finish their thoughts and their sentences, help them to recognise and remove assumptions that are limiting them, acknowledge them as thinking equals. (p. 196)

The attraction of this vision is that thinking is seen as not only a cognitive function but also a symbol of individual freedom that belongs to people's lives in organisations as well as outside them. It also fits well with the mission of the Trust.

Box 14.1.2 The ten components of the Thinking Environment (Kline 1999)

- *Attention*. Listen with respect, interest and fascination
- *Incisive questions*. Remove assumptions that limit ideas
- *Equality*. Treat each other as thinking peers
  —give equal turns and attention
  —keep agreements and boundaries
- *Appreciation*. Practise a five-to-one ratio of appreciation to criticism
- *Ease*. Offer freedom from rush or urgency
- *Encouragement*. Move beyond competition
- *Feelings*. Allow sufficient emotional release to restore thinking
- *Information*. Provide a full and accurate picture of reality
- *Place*. Create a physical environment that says back to people, 'You matter'
- *Diversity*. Add quality because of the differences between us

---

[1] Thinking Environment is a registered trademark.

To enable people to think better for themselves, Kline has developed ten behaviours that form the Thinking Environment (Box 14.1.2). Space precludes a full description of each component here and interested readers are referred to Nancy Kline's book.

Nancy Kline's ideas were first introduced to the Trust board by one of the non-executive directors who was familiar with her work. Directors made an immediate connection between her philosophy and the mission of the Trust and agreed to learn more. Nancy was subsequently invited to present her ideas at a Trust board 'away day' that was attended by all the executive and non-executive directors. Following this, the Trust board decided to employ Nancy Kline to coach the board in the use of the Thinking Environment. The Thinking Environment has had a significant positive impact on the work of the Trust, but space is only available in this application for reflection on a small aspect of this. The remainder of this application therefore consists of a personal reflection by the author on its impact on meetings within the Trust board.

ATTENTION PLEASE

Although all of the ten components of the Thinking Environment are interrelated, the key that unlocks people's thinking is the quality of attention that others give to an individual. Much of this is concerned with learning how to listen and to provide the conditions for someone to think. Therefore, after explaining her philosophy and its components, Nancy Kline provided an early opportunity for Trust board members to practise listening and giving maximum attention to each other.

People think best when asked a question. Nancy asked people to get into pairs and take 5 minutes each to answer the question: 'Given what you now know about the Thinking Environment, how do you think it could help the work of the Trust board?'. Nancy Kline's approach to listening is different from the 'active listening' approach typically taught to health and social care staff. First of all, she asks listeners to adopt a neutral but 'interested' facial expression. This is because facial expressions can often influence the thinker, however positive and encouraging they seem. She also asks the listener to look at the person without deviating, even though the thinker is expected to break eye contact. This is because the thinker must feel that he or she has the listener's total attention. Interruption is never allowed and listeners must resist the temptation to finish off the thinker's sentence. This is because the listener should never assume that his or her words are better than the thinker's. For the same reason, paraphrasing is also banned. Silences should be considered spaces in which the thinker is searching for another thought and the temptation to speak should be resisted, except to prompt the thinker for further thoughts by asking: 'And what else do you think about this?'. When the 5 minutes were up, the listeners then took their turn to answer the question.

My first reaction to being asked to practise our listening skills was somewhat negative. After all, the board was made up of people from impressive professional, managerial and commercial backgrounds. It therefore seemed impertinent to ask us to do something that I assumed we were all good at. However, Nancy's approach felt quite different to the active listening approach that I was familiar with. I felt my facial expression changing. I felt my brow furrow as I tried to make sense of what the other person was saying. At other times I felt my eyebrows rising, indicating agreement with the other person. According to Nancy's reasoning, this could have influenced what the other person was saying. 'Would this really matter?', I asked. Nancy reminded us that the role of the listener is to create a space for the other person to think for themselves. Naturally, the listener will take in what the other person is saying and will want to make sense of it. The listener should not expect the thinker to utter perfectly formulated responses; this rarely happens. This can make it difficult for the listener to keep a neutral expression but it is essential that they do so. Nancy's views are supported by research literature into interpersonal behaviour that suggests that non-verbal behaviour, however subtle, can provide cues for others to think and behave in different ways (Abraham & Stanley 1992, p. 194).

Shortly after practising my listening skills, I began to contrast Nancy's approach with my experience as a nurse listening to people with learning disabilities and their carers. There was a difference, I thought, between this situation and my previous experience because my clients had expected me to offer advice, to give an opinion and, in some cases, to tell them what to do. Was this a correct assumption to make? After all, many people seemed pleased with my advice and I could recall, on many occasions, feeling pleased with the help that I had given someone. However, Nancy's philosophy had now made me reflect on the appropriateness of my assumptions concerning my helping role. In her book, Nancy discusses the nature of help and the importance of listening:

> Real help, professionally or personally, consists of listening to people, of paying respectful attention to people so that they can access their own ideas first. Usually, the brain that contains the problem also contains the solution – often the best one. This is not to say that advice is never a good thing or that your ideas are never needed. Sometimes, your suggestions are exactly what the person wants and needs . . . But don't rush into it. Give people the chance to find their own ideas first. (Kline 1999, p. 39)

(side tab) **Old problems, new solutions**

Contrasting my knowledge and experiences with Nancy's explanation of helping reinforced many comments and criticisms made by people about the nature of professional help, namely that professionals are socialised to behave as experts and to provide all the answers to problems. This criticism could also be applied to traditional management approaches in which decision making is concentrated in the few managers in organisations. It seemed to me that Nancy's approach might provide a means of developing more equitable relationships between professionals, their clients, managers and their staff.

MEETING OF MINDS

Listening is key to Nancy Kline's approach because it changes the nature of interactions in organisations. Nancy recommends that good listening should be applied to informal interactions in organisations but she spends a great deal of time in her book discussing meetings. Meetings are the main medium through which the business of an organisation is transacted. If asked to describe their experience of meetings, most people would report a mixture of feelings of boredom, frustration and exasperation. Many meetings are dominated by a few individuals who appear to have a lot to say for themselves and an ineffective chair means that meetings often become sidetracked. Sometimes the agenda does not adequately describe what is going to be discussed and there seems little time to discuss the most important items.

Nancy's approach to running meetings is radical and refreshing and our 'away day' gave us the first opportunity to put her ideas to the test. Meetings are based on the same principles of good listening but the task of running effective meetings starts before the meeting takes place. Nancy believes that the human mind works best in the face of an incisive question. Therefore, agenda items must be expressed in the form of questions. For example, the agenda item 'To receive the quarterly performance report' becomes 'What do you think are the most significant aspects of this quarter's performance report?'. The other task that belongs to the chair is to organise the agenda to give the most time to the most significant items as well as to let people know how much time they should devote to each item. Therefore, agenda items should appear with an approximation of the time at which the item will be discussed. Two hypothetical trust board agendas are shown in Boxes 14.1.3 and 14.1.4 in order to contrast the differences in agenda construction.

The most important principle of the Thinking Environment is that each person is listened to. Therefore, in meetings, everyone should have a turn to speak, even if they decline the offer. Meetings begin with an opening round. The chair should phrase a question that will

Thinking for a better future

Box 14.1.3 Hypothetical agenda using a typical approach to agenda construction

OXFORDSHIRE LEARNING DISABILITY NHS TRUST
Trust Board Meeting 11th September 2001, 2pm

AGENDA

1. Apologies for absence
2. Minutes of the last meeting
3. Matters arising from the minutes
4. Chief Executive's report
5. Finance report
6. Quarterly performance report
7. Finance committee report
8. Vision statement
9. Trust Board away day
10. Time and date of next meeting

enable the meeting to start on a positive note, such as 'Tell me about something at work that is going well' or 'What are you most looking forward to discussing at this meeting?'.

Each person is asked the question, in turn, and is listened to without interruption. My own reflection on this and in subsequent meetings is that the opening round certainly has the effect of clearing negative thoughts. So many people arrive at meetings thinking about what is not going well at work. Although an opening round does not deny anyone an opportunity to express negative thoughts (if people really want to express their feelings, they will!), I have found that it sets a constructive tone for the rest of the meeting. There was some anxiety amongst myself and my colleagues about the time that it would take to complete this opening round. On reflection, we were simply displaying our previous learning and had not yet recognised that the opening round was an integral part of the meeting and not a frivolous extra.

In the same way that the opening round requires a question, the meeting ends with a closing round. This could be 'Tell me about something that you are looking forward to doing after the meeting' or 'What have you found the most interesting aspect of our meeting today?'. To me, this had two effects: it helped us to focus on our achievements and it helped us to feel that the business had been completed. Sometimes people leave meetings feeling that something hasn't been said. A badly run meeting can also mean that business is hurried and conversations are still being held as people are rising out of their chairs or packing away their papers.

This approach to running meetings is designed to help people to think and to approach their discussions constructively. Occasionally participants may not seem to be making progress and the meeting

Box 14.1.4 Hypothetical agenda using Thinking Environment guidelines

OXFORDSHIRE LEARNING DISABILITY NHS TRUST
Trust Board Meeting 11th September 2001, 2pm

AGENDA

1. Opening round   2pm
   What is going well in your work at the moment?
2. Minutes of the last meeting   2.10pm
   Are you satisfied that the minutes are an accurate recording of our previous meeting?
3. Chief Executive's Report   2.15pm
   What do you think is the most significant aspect of the Chief Executive's report?
4. Performance Report   2.35pm
   How would you change the quarterly performance report to ensure that the Trust Board is better informed about the performance of the Trust?
5. Finance Committee Report   3.05pm
   Does the Finance Committee report give you confidence that the financial targets for the Trust will be met?
6. BREAK   3.30pm
7. Vision statement   3.45pm
   In the light of the new White Paper on learning disability, in what way do you think that we need to modify the Trust's vision statement?
8. Trust Board away day   4.30pm
   What issues should be a priority for discussion at the forthcoming away day?
9. Closing round   4.45pm
   What have you most appreciated about our meeting today and what do you most appreciate about the person sitting on your right?
10. Close of meeting   4.55pm

Thinking for a better future

seems to be lacking new ideas. In situations like this, the chair has some options that can help introduce new ideas or free-up people's thinking. What we have found most effective during our meetings in the Trust is to divide into thinking pairs. Here, each person is given 5 minutes to think freely, without interruption, about the issue that is causing difficulty. Alternatively, a more generic question can be posed, such as: 'What might we be assuming here that is limiting our thinking?'. On return to the group, the same question is posed. It was surprising how many new ideas emerged from this process.

Another feature of meetings run in a Thinking Environment is the need to balance appreciation and criticism during meetings. Nancy recommends that participants adopt a five-to-one ratio of appreciation to criticism. As with other features of her approach, this encourages positive and constructive thinking and helps people to feel valued. Although Trust board members recognised the need for this approach and have adopted it in meetings, this raised questions in our minds as to whether it would stifle expression of feelings or insulate the board from bad news that it needed to hear. From his study of group behaviour, Janis (1972) points out that members of a group will often seek approval and appreciation from each other which can sometimes lead them to avoid giving unpleasant or unpopular information. This phenomenon, known as 'groupthink', can lead to poor problem solving and decision making. Our questions on this have been answered, largely through our experience of the cumulative effect of employing the Thinking Environment:

- This approach encourages rather than inhibits individuals from expressing their feelings because they believe that these feelings will be listened to unconditionally.
- People who feel better about themselves have little need to seek approval and will be freer with their thinking.
- The Thinking Environment can create more adaptive group norms which are based around acknowledging different opinions, where they exist, and having the confidence in our ability to resolve any conflict and to develop constructive solutions.

THE IMPACT OF THE THINKING ENVIRONMENT

There are a number of effects that the Thinking Environment has had upon the work of the Trust. Meetings of the Trust board have become more productive and more enjoyable. Colleagues feel as though they have been allowed to have their say and have been listened to, resulting in feelings of being respected and treated as equals. This is not to say, however, that alternative points of view will not be taken. Occasionally, the board lapses into a pre-Thinking Environment stage in which people will interrupt others or not give them maximum attention. This is only natural when learning a different approach. Perhaps the best way to describe the Trust board's meetings is that they are conducted with a sense of ease. We feel that we are carrying out exactly the same amount of business as before but this is being carried out more efficiently and effectively.

Following the Trust board's experience of using the Thinking Environment, plans were put together to extend it to other meetings in the Trust and training was given to those chairing and attending meetings. It is hoped that, eventually, the majority of the meetings in the Trust will adopt this approach.

CONCLUSION

In a broader context, it is difficult to fully evaluate the effect of the Thinking Environment. The objective of the Trust was to improve its capacity to put its values of equality and respect for people with learning disabilities into action. Secondly, it wanted to develop its commitment to staff by releasing their creative potential. The Trust believes that, in the Thinking Environment, it has found a process that is consistent with both these objectives. The principles and practice of the Thinking Environment have led to a greater feeling of ease and confidence amongst many staff that has enabled them to think more freely and creatively in an atmosphere of respect. Its philosophy has also enabled them to feel that the principles which they are trying to employ with people with learning disabilities are mirrored in the way they treat each other. This brings a feeling of connectedness and coherence to their work. The Thinking Environment does not solve all of the problems of an organisation and it does not claim to. It is primarily a way of improving thinking and problem solving; it does not take away frustration at a lack of resources or slowness of change. It does, however, provide staff with the means of approaching their problems more constructively.

References

Abraham C, Stanley E 1992 Social psychology for nurses. Arnold, London

Barnes C 1991 Disabled people in Britain and discrimination: a case for anti-discrimination legislation. Hurst, London

Department of Health 2001 Valuing people: a strategy for people with learning disability in the 21st century. Department of Health, London

Hudson M 1995 Managing without profit: the art of managing third-sector organisations. Penguin, Harmondsworth

Janis IL 1972 Victims of groupthink. Houghton Mifflin, Boston

Kline N 1999 Time to Think. Listening to ignite the human mind. Ward Lock, London

Mullins L 1989 Management and organisational behaviour, 2nd edn. Pitman, London

Nirje B 1980 The normalisation principle. In: Flynn RJ, Nitsch KE (eds) Normalisation, social integration and community services. University Park Press, Baltimore

Oliver M 1990 The politics of disability. Macmillan, Basingstoke

Wolfensberger W 1972 The principle and practice of normalisation. National Institutes of Mental Health, Toronto

Thinking for a better future

Index

Note: Abbreviations used in subheadings are: CHI = Commission for Health Improvement; HEIs = Higher education institutes; IT = information technology; NICE = National Institute for Clinical Excellence; NSF = National Service Frameworks; R&D = research and development; SMINTS = Self-managed integrated nursing teams.

Six Steps to **Effective Management**

Index

Index

Six Steps to **Effective Management**

Index

Index

Six Steps to **Effective Management**

Index